PHYSICIANS OF WESTERN MEDICINE

CULTURE, ILLNESS, AND HEALING

PHYSICIANS
OF
WESTERN MEDICINE

Anthropological Approaches to Theory and Practice

Edited by

ROBERT A. HAHN

Department of Psychiatry and Behavioral Sciences,
School of Medicine, University of Washington, Seattle, WA.

and

ATWOOD D. GAINES

Departments of Anthropology and Psychiatry,
Case Western Reserve University and Medical School, Cleveland, OH.

D. REIDEL PUBLISHING COMPANY

A MEMBER OF THE KLUWER ACADEMIC PUBLISHERS GROUP

DORDRECHT / BOSTON / LANCASTER

Library of Congress Cataloging in Publication Data

Physicians of western medicine.

(Culture, illness, and healing; 6)
lc card. no. 84-26436
ISBN 90-277-1790-7
ISBN 90-277-1881-4 (pbk.)

Published by D. Reidel Publishing Company.
P.O. Box 17, 3300 AA Dordrecht, Holland.

Sold and distributed in the U.S.A. and Canada
by Kluwer Academic Publishers,
101 Philip Drive, Assinippi Park, Norwell, MA 02061, U.S.A.

In all other countries, sold and distributed
by Kluwer Academic Publishers Group,
P.O. Box 322, 3300 AH Dordrecht, Holland.

2-0786-300-ts

TABLE OF CONTENTS

PREFACE

After putting down this weighty (in all senses of the word) collection, the reader, be she or he physician or social scientist, will (or at least should) feel uncomfortable about her or his taken-for-granted commonsense (therefore cultural) understanding of medicine. The editors and their collaborators show the medical leviathan, warts and all, for what it is: changing, pluralistic, problematic, powerful, provocative. What medicine proclaims itself to be — unified, scientific, biological and not social, non-judgmental — is shown not to resemble very much. Those matters about which medicine keeps fairly silent, it turns out, come closer to being central to its clinical practice — managing errors and learning to conduct a shared moral discourse about mistakes, handling issues of competence and competition among biomedical practitioners, practicing in value-laden contexts on problems for which social science is a more relevant knowledge base than biological science, integrating folk and scientific models of illness in clinical communication, are among a large number of highly pertinent ethnographic insights that illuminate medicine in the chapters that follow.

The contributors are to be congratulated for their apt and telling case illustrations, several of which are likely to stay with the reader well after he or she finishes the book. In keeping with the genius of descriptive ethnography, we get to see and experience local contexts of action — a cystic fibrosis clinic in which a fundamental staff conflict discloses the nature of medical interactions in patient care, a busy surgical department attempting to carry out both research and clinical practice while economic, personal and moral issues set the stage for crisis and confusion, a complicated illness trajectory from general practitioner to specialists in which disease and illness become inseparably intertwined, twisting together like a double helix under the pressure of distinctive and conflicting clinical realities. These and other local contexts are interpreted to reveal large themes that link the macro-social world with micro-clinical events: physicians' talk about professional competence, the non-medical determinants of clinical decision-making, the complex, pluralistic practice worlds of everyday medical work, the moral structure of doctoring . . . .

The upshot is a rich, variegated, provocative perspective on medicine that will push readers to begin to rethink conventional wisdom about illness, care and doctoring. In this respect, this large volume does justice to the field of medical anthropology, which, though at an early stage of research on Biomedicine, and following in the footsteps of medical sociology and medical history, but with culture as its subject, demonstrates that Biomedicine is an integral part of local contexts of meanings, norms and power, contexts that provide it with particular and differing styles of action and significance (see Kleinman 1980; Weisberg and Long 1984).

For those hearty souls who can read through it in a single sitting, Hahn's massive report on the worldview, trade, craft and character of an internist will tell them more about internal medicine than anything short of field work. Margaret Lock's masterfully balanced account of medical views on menopause shows the marvelous discrepancies, alternatives, conflicting models, and changing explanatory systems of obstetricians, family doctors and others. Helman's analysis of pseudo-angina is a compelling and exhaustive display of differential constructions of a single illness event and their practical significance for patient and health care system. Rittenberg and Simons disclose the psychiatrists' method is not all that dissimilar (yet different enough to make a difference) from the ethnographer who is working up an indigenous ethnographic category. Pearl Katz must make us all flinch at the social forces driving the surgical knife. There is more besides, including Johnson's masterful depiction of the difficult situation of consultation-liaison psychiatry as a portrait of the ironic confrontation of the "soft" (psychosocial) and the "hard" (biomedical) streams in medicine, which is the best analysis I know of that captures this crucial symbolic contradiction in the odd positioning of a meaning-centered psychiatry in the interstices of a high technology, tertiary care medicine that regularly denies and defeats the human element of care. I should not forget either, Gaines' rich cultural account of the complexities of even this marginal though essential field, psychiatry, that make strict "secular"/"Christian" labels a distortion of a many-sided, negotiated world of practice. The Goods and their collaborators offer us an intricate understanding of countertransference on three interrelated levels — intrapsychic, interpersonal, cultural — that should dispell forever simplistic models of what the therapeutic process entails, and disclose how difficult it is to avoid at least temporary misadventure, even with a combination of sensitive clinical and cultural understanding, when participating in intercultural healing and applying a self-reflexive orientation.

The volume is a case-book filled with stunning illustrations to provoke problem-based learning. Unlike a sociology text or a medical monograph, most of what we read are single-case studies analyzed in depth. Ethnography and interpretation, and to a much lesser degree, cross-cultural comparison, are the chief methods. This is highly appropriate because these are the core methods of anthropology. Here they are deployed by researchers who have had extensive experience working in medical settings. Reading the chapters as an anthropologist-physician, I can almost experience each of the settings and the problems: the accounts are convincingly valid and evocative of major questions in Biomedicine. Clinicians and medical students should find these clinical cameos an appropriate format for learning about the social origins and cultural constructions of illness and clinical praxis. Anthropologists will get a sense from them of the cultural discourses and social realities that constitute Biomedicine as an anthropological subject. General readers will also find the chapters of interest; the latter provide an appropriately concrete grounding for different kinds of social analyses and interpretations, all of which should produce disquiet and concern in the reader about the nature, structure, and significance of various key elements of Western professional medicine.

The chief achievement of this volume is that it is the state of the art in the anthropology of Biomedicine. That state is still more a line of inquiry (and a wavy line at that), very early findings rather than an established body of theory, and heuristic insights, not replicated data or tested hypotheses. But it is remarkable how much ground has been covered in so short a time. After reading the final chapter, I put down the manuscript feeling that I was witnessing an important professional development in medical anthropology: namely, the coming to terms with mundane and ubiquitous Biomedicine in Western society by a field heretofore seemingly obsessed with esoteric culture-bound disorders, foreign folk healers and extra-ordinary healing rituals. This anthropological encounter with our medicine (with the medically commonplace along with the medically unusual) is significant more for what it portends than for what it actually accomplishes. Clearly we are seeing the beginnings of several new anthropologies: the anthropology of the professions and the anthropology of science.

I leave it to the chapters that follow to display what we learn from the anthropology of Biomedicine. Not the least of what I think we learn is the liberating notion that medicine — the whole of it, from sicknesses to therapies and including medical settings, roles and attributions — can be (and should be) rethought in the language of social structure and cultural norms, of interpersonal transactions and differential access to resources, of cultural symbols and social action. And this process of making our medicine into a subject of social enquiry (like other ethno-medicines) is significant also because it creates practically useful knowledge, knowledge perhaps that holds the potential of eventually being applied to liberate physicians as well as patients from narrow, dehumanizing forms of medical praxis that are unhelpful, iatrogenic and that systematically perpetuate dangerous directions in our society's political and moral economy. In this respect too, the anthropology of Biomedicine has the opportunity of intensifying anthropology and its effects.

Departments of Anthropology, Psychiatry,   ARTHUR KLEINMAN, M.D., M.A.
and Social Medicine, Harvard University
and Harvard Medical School

REFERENCES

Kleinman, A.
    1980 Patients and Healers in the Context of Culture. Berkeley: University of California
          Press.
Weisberg, D. and S. O. Long (eds.)
    1984 Biomedicine in Asia. Special Issue. Culture, Medicine and Psychiatry 8 (2).

SECTION I

INTRODUCTIONS

ATWOOD D. GAINES AND ROBERT A. HAHN

AMONG THE PHYSICIANS: ENCOUNTER, EXCHANGE AND TRANSFORMATION

INTRODUCTION

Anthropologists and colleagues have entered a new territory in the heartland of their own society, the Domain of Biomedicine.[1] They have returned with accounts both strange and strangely familiar. Practitioners of Biomedicine assume as essentially and exclusively true their own theory and practice, their "science" which professes the cellular, even biochemical basis of pathology. Anthropologists and medical critics have been struck by this reductionism which excludes alternatives and which asserts a biological universalism and individualism (idiopathic etiologies) which ignore, if not deny, basic anthropological understandings which see cultural and social forces as wellsprings of human behavior, including healing and suffering. Anthropologists have been further challenged by the barriers to communication built into the complex edifice of Biomedicine. At the same time they have also recognized in practitioners of Biomedicine values and premises which they share, parts of a common culture. Anthropologists looking at Biomedicine, thus, have seen versions of themselves as well as alien elaborations of their own culture.

We have gathered here some early anthropological reports from the field. *Physicians of Western Medicine* is a collection of studies of Western Biomedicine. It focuses on a range of biomedical specialists in a number of different contexts which form the domain of the practice of Biomedicine. Some of the physicians who are the objects of our interest are practitioners engaged in private practice while others practice in the context of academic medicine. The physicians in Helman, Hahn, and DelVecchio Good's studies are private practitioners while academically based physicians are the object of research in other chapters such as those by Johnson, Gaines, Rittenberg and Simons, and Katz. Lock's chapter analyzes physicians in both contexts. The selections also contain work on physicians from both within and outside of hospital contexts.

It should also be noted that not all of the practitioners considered in this work are American. Several of the contributions focus on the practice of Biomedicine in other English-speaking countries. For example, Lock's work concerns Canadian physicians as does Katz' study of surgeons. And Helman's chapter, which concludes this volume, is a study of English physicians.

Some of the contributors who have ventured into the field are themselves members of the culture under study, but who have gained a perspective on their own group from the vantage point of anthropology. And, just as our physician-researcher-informants from psychiatry (Herrera and Simons) and general practice (Helman) primarily have utilized interpretive approaches in anthropology to

3

understand biomedical practice and to suggest improvements in it, so too have our colleagues from other social sciences including sociology (DelVecchio Good) and psychology (Cooper).

These anthropological reports illustrate a variety of sociocultural features of biomedical theory and practice. They demonstrate that Biomedicine is a *cultural system* comprised of numerous variations, the "many medicines". Folk theories and traditions are readily incorporated into the actual practice of Biomedicine whether in cardiology (Helman), psychiatry (Gaines) or obstetrics and gynecology (Lock). The studies also show the importance of observation and reporting on actual practices and beliefs, rather than employing negative or positive idealized versions of medical practice, so that it is possible to understand that the healing encounter is a social and cultural event involving communication across cultural or subcultural boundaries. We also find that the practice of medicine is rather unlike its characterization by proponents or opponents. Biomedicine may be seen to be clearly a part of the wider culture, i.e., distinct neither as "science" nor "interest group".

To introduce these studies, we first characterize the "nature" of sociocultural systems and note briefly the antecedents of anthropological studies of Biomedicine, a topic surveyed in more detail in the next chapter by Maretzki. We then turn to examine the relevance of the anthropological study of Biomedicine for anthropology itself and then for Biomedicine and its institutions. Finally, we point out threads tying together the studies collected here.

ANTHROPOLOGY AND MEDICINE

Anthropologists exploring Biomedicine have met resistance both from fellow anthropologists, even from medical anthropologists, and from their biomedical host-subjects. This resistance may have a common source — a blindness to a domain of one's own culture whose powers and prestige make it invisible to member participant observers. Even for many anthropologists Biomedicine is *the* reality through the lens of which the rest of the world's cultural versions are seen, compared, and judged.

Anthropologists have failed to examine their own anthropological culture, including their common reliance on Biomedicine. They have not seen Biomedicine as susceptible to the same sort of cultural analysis to which they readily subject other medical system (Gaines 1979). Until recently (Hahn 1983; Kleinman 1980, 1983), they have given epistemic primacy to *disease*, the understanding of pathology according to Biomedicine, over *illness*, the patients' experience of disorder. They have defined "ethnomedicine" (Hughes 1968) to *exclude* "scientific" medicine (also called "cosmopolitan" [Leslie 1977]); and medical anthropological texts (e.g., Foster and Anderson 1978) have been divided into separate sections on Biomedicine and "ethnomedicines". "Acculturation" has been understood as the conformity of non-Western ethnomedicines to Western; pathological conditions which are labeled in non-Western settings but not in our own, biomedical, nosology are called "culture-bound syndromes". Such definitions and analytic modes are conceptually and historically distorted. They hinder the development of comparative methodology and theory (Hahn and Kleinman 1983).

The resistance of biomedical practitioners to anthropological participant observation has taken two related forms. With notable exceptions, anthropologists and other social scientists have either been denied or given minimal access to medical settings. Petersdorf and Feinstein (1981) report that only 50% of chairpersons of medicine and 40% of pediatrics and family medicine departments claim medical sociology to be a formal part of the medical curriculum. Time allotted to medical sociology is "sporadic" in medicine and pediatrics, and "substantial" only in family medicine. Even when granted access, the status of anthropologists in medical settings has been multiply ambiguous. The uncertain position of the social sciences is suggested by a prepositional plethora distinguishing sociology "in", "of", "for", "from", "at", and "around" medicine (see Eisenberg and Kleinman 1981).

Riska and Vinten-Johansen (1981) have argued that the essential character of the social sciences has been subverted to biomedical ends as social scientists work in medical settings. Discourse on "stress", for example, has deeply penetrated the culture of Biomedicine and beyond, yet has been stripped of anthropological content (Young 1980). The same is true of network theory. Rather than promoting dialogue, the entry of anthropology and fellow disciplines into medical settings has more commonly promoted an enriched biomedical monologue.

In referring to Biomedicine as a "sociocultural system" we do not wish to suggest that Biomedicine is not simultaneously a theory and a practice concerned with representing and affecting some physical and physiological realities. (The editors note here a difference between them which also divides anthropologists more widely; in the determination of human affairs, Hahn gives more weight to an external, "real", "physical" world, while Gaines emphasizes particular cultural constructions of reality as sources and guides of human action.) Rather, we emphasize that Biomedicine is a cultural artifact, a complex human product shaped from human and nonhuman resources, constantly responding to historical circumstances which are in turn human transformations of themselves and their environments. Humans in society constantly recreate structure from structure, in a process which Giddens (1976) characterizes as evidencing a "duality of structure".

A sociocultural phenomenon may be distinguished by three related features:

(1) A domain of knowledge and practice, e.g., medicine, more or less clearly distinguished from other domains. In "Western" societies, the domain of medicine *seems* to participants to be more highly distinguished from other domains than in other societies where it is explicitly associated with religion, politics, economics, and social relations, themselves closely intertwined.

(2) A division of labor and rules of proper action and interaction within the domain, with possibly distinct roles and institutions (Hahn and Kleinman 1983, 1984). Medical "work", e.g., the correction of pathophysiology, is itself prescribed as are relations among different participants in medical settings. The deliberate production of medical knowledge, in the form of research, may also be delimited. The division and rules may replicate the order of the broader society

(Navarro 1976), yet they are also likely to correspond to ideological particularities of the domain itself. The specialty divisions of Biomedicine further correspond to struggles among contenders for prestige and authority within Biomedicine (Stevens 1971). The focal subject of Biomedicine, the human body, thus also bears the scars of conflict and division in the body politic of Biomedicine and the broader society.

(3) A social and cultural means by which the sociocultural system is reproduced and altered. By this process of "socialization" incumbents are explicitly and implicitly taught what it is believed they should know: "premedical and medical education", "internship", and "residency" are formally distinguished elements of the processess of socialization in Biomedicine. But less commonly recognized, informal processes of socialization exist, including the maintenance and alteration of social interaction and its rules. Both precede and continue throughout the medical life cycle in clinical and other settings of medical work.

Such sociocultural elements form a system to the extent that they are interconnected with each other by certain relationships which do not hold, or hold only in attenuated form, among elements outside the system.

That the system of Biomedicine is a sociocultural system implies that Biomedicine is a collective representation of reality. To claim that Biomedicine is a representation is not to deny a reality which is represented, which affects and is affected by what it represents. It is rather to emphasize a cultural distance, a transformation of reality; an ultimate reality cannot be known except by means of cultural symbol systems. Such systems are both models *of* and *for* reality and action (Geertz 1973). Our representations of reality are taken to *be* reality though they are but transformations, refracted images of it.

We emphasize that Biomedicine is one among numerous alternative professional ethnomedicines (see also Lieban 1977; Leslie 1977). All ethnomedicines share a basic epistemological quality: they are *versions* of reality, stocks of knowledge and modes of comprehension and action in reference to, but ontologically distinct from, reality. While newer anthropological studies, such as those presented here, seek to emphasize the equality of ontological status of all ethnomedicines, most members of our society and participants in Biomedicine itself have quite ignored this equality; ethnomedicines may be less equal than anthropologists might like to claim, but they are far more equal than biomedical practitioners have acknowledged. In fact, professional medical systems represent diverse approximations of some biological reality. For example, the biological basis of contemporary and traditional Chinese medicine is reported to be quite distinct from that of Western Biomedicine (Kleinman 1980) though it is yet a biological medicine.

As ideal types, anthropology and Biomedicine seem to differ not only in their epistemology, but also in their fundamental concepts. However, both often lean upon a limited and limiting scientistic empiricism which presents itself in many guises; for Biomedicine, it is pathology as purely a disturbance in biophysiological structure or process (see also Mishler et al. 1981); for anthropology it is explanation in terms of economic, structural or ecological reductionism. Newer approaches in anthropology, however, take a different perspective and focus on meaning and interpretation, thus combining aspects of the work of Weber, Schutz, Geertz, Ricoeur, G. H. Mead and Freud and which are represented in this collection.

While the thrust of Biomedicine is the reduction of pathology to elementary, universal, "natural" biological problems, newer anthropological approaches insist on the interpretation of social processes as an interaction of multiple semantic levels which, while they function together, cannot be reduced to one another. Opposing the trend of Biomedicine, a perspicacious internist, George Engel (1977), has developed a "biopsychosocial model" which is fitting to the medical interests of anthropologists (see also Brody 1973; Hahn and Kleinman 1983).

The tension between the stances of anthropology and Biomedicine engenders significant differences in their practice with regard to the problem of human suffering, a concern which in one sense they share, yet in another they may understand in radically different fashions. We regard the tension between Biomedicine and anthropological theories and practices as a challenge, the acceptance and pursuit of which may be productive for both enterprises. Resolution of this tension may yield convergent enterprises, an anthropological or cultural medicine and a more medical anthropology, both concerned with person-centered problems of suffering, with a theory close to practice, and cognizant of multiple, interrelated sources of causation and relief, including the biological, the psychological and the sociocultural contextual meanings.

THE ANTHROPOLOGICAL STUDY OF BIOMEDICINE

Some of the early interest in the study of Biomedicine derived from the attempt to apply biomedical models of illness, usually psychiatric illness, to non-Western peoples. This interest led to studies of the standard of comparison, Western Biomedicine. George Devereux, a psychiatrically and psychoanalytically sophisticated theoretician, was a pioneer in the examination of Biomedicine (1944, 1949). It was Devereux who first suggested (1980) that core diagnostic entities in psychiatry (e.g., schizophrenia) were probably "culture-bound" disorders, in the sense that they are deeply imbedded in local cultural contexts that shape their form, consequence and significance. More recent work seems to confirm this for the psychiatric "disease" depression (Marsella 1980), as well as schizophrenia (Waxler 1979). It was also Devereux who coined the term "ethnopsychiatry", (1969) later used to subsume Western psychiatry (Gaines 1979, 1982a) just as Western Biomedicine is now subsumed under the rubric of (professional) "ethnomedicine" (Hahn and Kleinman 1983, 1984). Both usages recognize the cultural construction of medical systems, Western and other.

A brilliant but neglected scholar, Jules Henry, considered psychological issues as well as the social organization of medical (mental health) care (1954, 1957). Caudill's noted study (1958) of the social system of psychiatric care followed that of Henry. Such early work, however, seems isolated. It did not lead to the development of an anthropology of Biomedicine or even to a clear recognition of its significance.

As Maretzki notes in the next article of this volume, early studies of Western Biomedicine were primarily conducted by sociologists during the fifties and sixties (e.g., Strauss et al. 1964; Goffman 1961; Jaco 1958; Fox 1959; Freidson 1970; Becker et al. 1961; Merton et al. 1957). The central interests of these studies were the nature of professional roles, role socialization and the powerful influence of institutional ideology and settings. With the exception of work by Fox, little headway was made in understanding the cultural contextualization of Biomedicine. Further, lack of a comparative basis, the stock-in-trade of anthropology, made it difficult for researchers in sociology to recognize the *cultural* principles that organize medical thought and action.

Recent research by anthropologists (and sociologists), most of it unpublished as yet, indicates the growing interest in all facets of medical practice. Following Goffman (1961), organization and underlying ideology of psychiatric practice in a total institution were the foci of Day's research (1978). Robles (1982) analyzed the care functions and their relationship to the wider society of a total institution. The earlier interest in socialization of medical professionals has also reappeared, but there now seems to be increased awareness of broadly cultural issues in training and the relationship of these to medical practice (Light 1980; Borsay 1975; Creson 1976; Gaines and Trego 1978).

There seems to be a new interest developing in the practice of Biomedicine in rural communities. DelVecchio Good's paper in this volume is an example, as are the unpublished works of Midgette (1972), Ripley-Daghlian (1981) and the historical ethnography of Robinson (1975). The practice of medicine in urban areas has also been the focal point for new research (e.g., McMorrow 1978). However, few have attempted to study what Kleinman (1980) calls the 'Health Care System' of a local area, that is, the total system composed of professional, folk, and popular (home-based) sectors and their interactions. This was Kleinman's focus in *Patients and Healers in the Context of Culture* (1980).

Building on an earlier theme in the (sociological) study of Biomedicine are analyses of roles, role strain and other problematics of medical roles (Clausen 1977; Borsay 1975; Schoepf 1975). Other recent research has focused on various aspects of medical discourse including the discourse of psychotherapy (Labov and Fanshel 1977), silence and other aspects of discourse of 'error' in medical practice (Bosk 1979; Paget 1982),[2] the logic of patients' discourse (Young 1981) and difficulties with communicative styles of physicians (Kleinman et al. 1978; Gaines 1982a). Psychiatry has received the bulk of this attention, possibly because it is thought by outsiders to be constituted principally by acts of "talk" (see Johnson, this volume) and thus seems more accessible.

Most recently, an important focus of research has been the understanding of the cultural ideology of Biomedicine through analyses of *physicians* in actual clinical contexts. In such contexts, researchers are able to approach an understanding of the explicit and implicit conceptions and ideas which motivate behavior and which allow physicians to evaluate their own and colleagues' actions and to make sense of their medical experience (see Bosk 1979; Kleinman et al. 1978; Gaines 1979, 1982a, b; Katz 1981; Gaines and Hahn 1982; Hahn and Kleinman 1983, 1984). (Maretzki [this volume] considers in more detail important studies in this area, including earlier work by the sociologist Fox [1959; 1979]).

Though there are many barriers to overcome in research of this type, the research focus on clinical practice seems a most promising one because it provides data not provided elsewhere (e.g., Mishler et al. 1981) to support the claims of both the cultural construction of 'patients'' illness episodes and the praxis of Biomedicine.

ON THE RELEVANCE OF THE ANTHROPOLOGICAL STUDY OF BIOMEDICINE FOR ANTHROPOLOGY

The anthropological study of Biomedicine will illuminate the theory and practice of anthropology in several ways (see Hahn and Kleinman 1983). One, perhaps *the*, central issue distinguishing the range of paradigms and theories in anthropology is the basic nature (i.e., ontology) and the interrelations of the 'material' and the 'ideational' in the determination of human affairs. Ethnomedicines, as deliberate (and collaborative) efforts to affect the valued and dreaded conditions of persons (and or their minds, bodies and relations), are vital arenas in which to explore these fundamental questions. Biomedicine, as a prominent, highly elaborated, materially and technologically oriented ethnomedicine, is a crucial test case.

Beyond questions of matter and idea, the comparative study of ethnomedicines, perhaps especially Biomedicine, addresses a number of other theoretical issues in anthropology. Biomedicine is a core institution of Western society. It affords a subject for the study of power and its manifestations both in 'efficacy' (Young 1976) and in related cultural processes of legitimation and delegitimation (Starr 1982). More generally, it affords evidence for the events through which a society reproduces and alters itself and its constituent institutions (e.g., Navarro 1976; Waitzkin 1979).

The anthropological study of Biomedicine also furthers development of a universal theory of pathogenesis and healing. In contrast to the theory of Biomedicine itself, according to which both pathogenesis and therapy are seen as essentially natural, biological, physiological and ultimately physical events, at least some anthropologists (we among them) insist that human interrelations and the "culture" which they create and recreate are central to both pathogenic and healing events in two fundamental ways. Concepts, explanations, and prescribed reactions to conditions of health and illness are *constructed* in social interactions, both collaborative and conflictual; that is, suffering, welfare, and responses to them are socially defined. These same conditions (and reactions to them) are also socially affected in another way: they are *produced* or caused by human social interactions which distribute the members of society and (other) resources in time and space and by activity. Pathogenic sources and resources for their amelioration are distributed in this same sociocultural process. The pervasive placebo phenomenon and its noxious counterpart, the "nocebo" phenomenon, are significant instances in which constructive and productive processes cooperate; beliefs work to effect what is believed, thus reaffirming belief.

In its contribution to anthropological theory, the anthropological study of Biomedicine will contribute also to the ethnography of U.S. and Western society. The anthropological study of this applied or practical science itself runs against the grain of its subject, for in the prominent biomedical epistemology, medicine (unprefixed by "ethno-") is assumed to lie beyond culture, unlike other "ethno-", "pseudo-", or "proto-medicines" and "superstitions". Medicine is seen as a more or less direct reflection of a unique and unitary reality of nature, namely human physiology and pathophysiology. It is believed to be based in value-free knowledge, and capable of value-free intervention (Mishler et al. 1981). Latour and Wolgar (1979) have shown how the components of biomedical knowledge are systematically stripped of their cultural and historical roots, becoming 'natural', the facts of life; all else-mind, culture, and society, is peripheral. Recent anthropology, in contrast, depicts Biomedicine as "a cultural system" (Gaines 1979, 1982a, b; Hahn and Kleinman, 1984), a more or less coherent and self-consistent set of values and premises, including an ontology, an epistemology and rules of proper action/ interaction embodied and mediated through significant symbols (see Geertz 1973).

The ethnographic study of the culture of Biomedicine will serve not only to document the ins and outs of this hyperbolic professional ethnomedicine, but at the same time to reflect on the observing discipline of anthropology itself. For anthropology and Biomedicine are estranged siblings of a common culture, conceived and born in similar historical circumstances. While there are striking and apparent differences, there also remains a deep kinship. The anthropological analysis of Biomedicine may thus foster a self-examination of anthropology.

Biomedicine provides for anthropology not only fertile grounds for ethnographic study and theoretical investigation, but a fundamental methodological instrument for anthropological and medical anthropological research. When anthropologists observe the conditions of health, illness and care in other socieites (and their own), their common system of reference is that of their own native medicine, Biomedicine, in an often idealized form.

The nosology and even the theory of Biomedicine must be considered among the most systematic, even though partial and misunderstood in fundamental ways (we believe) by its own practitioners. Conditions observed in non-Western settings are labeled, to the best of the ethnographer's ability, according to biomedical notions. Beyond this direct biomedical influence there is reason to suspect an indirect one; where anthropologists cannot discern a biomedical label for some condition, and where indigenous observers seem to profess knowledge of a condition and a label, anthropologists "diagnose" "culture-bound syndrome". This diagnosis may be bound to the lacunae of the nosology of Biomedicine, for by anthropological principles, all conditions are culturally affected, thus none are exclusively so. An anthropological revision of biomedical nosology will make for a more fitting diagnostic nosology, itself culturally unbound.

Finally, the experience of anthropologists in the study of Biomedicine may serve to break down a tenuous distinction between applied and unapplied disciplines and their practice. Participation in the local scene in the course of research is itself action which may or may not in turn "apply" what is learned from that setting. The apparent proximity of anthropology and its biomedical subject may facilitate the participation of "participant/observation". Responsibility and reciprocity with one's hosts/subjects would seem to demand that the observer return information which may aid the host in the attainment of his/her goals. If the observer suspects his own goals to be incongruous with those of his "subjects", it would seem responsible to clarify this as it becomes apparent.

ON THE RELEVANCE OF THE ANTHROPOLOGICAL STUDY OF BIOMEDICINE FOR BIOMEDICINE

The relevance for Biomedicine of anthropological studies is manifold (see Eisenberg and Kleinman 1981). Here, we review some important implications and briefly note several others.

In contrast to studies which take medicine as a homogeneous institution created by social or economic processes, i.e., as a corporate group rather than as a category of people, one of the principal contributions of anthropological studies of Biomedicine is a focus on the diverse beliefs and practices of physicians *at work*. From this work may develop an understanding of the cultural and social organization of medicine which may contribute to more reasonable medical organization and practice. An anthropological understanding of Biomedicine will situate its practices within a cultural context and elucidate the cultural origins, expectations, and values which drive and constrain it. A medicine complacent in its belief that it is uniquely scientific is prone to 'medico-cultural imperialism' in the name of humanitarianism.

Anthropological studies of Biomedicine may contribute to Biomedicine along several interacting avenues mapped out below, i.e., in the provision of a fuller, contextual understanding of clinical practice and clinical processes; by the development of more appropriate clinical care; by fostering greater patient participation in, and thus adherence to, personally and culturally relevant and satisfactory therapeutic regimens; and through the reduction of the cultural imperialist strains of our medicine, especially as it expands into other areas of the world.

Understanding Clinical Practice

Clinicians and researchers within Biomedicine generally believe that their various specialties comprise increasingly sophisticated knowledge and practical systems which are anchored in, and more or less exactly mirror, *a singular* biological reality. While 'exogenous,' extra-clinical factors may be reported in the biomedical literature, such as social status (Brill and Storrow 1960), ethnic affiliation (Katz et al. 1969), and even clinicians' errors (Morrison and Flanagan 1978), such factors are seen as potentially 'avoidable' and ultimately *extraneous* influences on the central enterprise of the clinical encounter. That enterprise is the correction of an empirical reality of histopathological structures or pathophysiological processes.

Contributions to the anthropology of Biomedicine have, on the contrary, demonstrated the hermeneutic or interpretive nature of the clinical encounter and of clinical work (e.g., diagnosis, treatment and management of patients) (Good and Good 1981; Kleinman 1980). Not only are the encounters interpretive, but so too are illness episodes themselves. That is, patient illness episodes must be seen as unavoidably semantic (i.e., meaningful and based upon the patient's cultural interpretations of a problem and the significance of identified problems or conditions) and all clinical transactions between patient and healer must be seen as inevitably hermeneutic (Good and Good 1981; Good 1977; Gaines 1982a; Kleinman et al. 1978). An understanding of the clinical processes and patients' clinical presentations must include all relevant symbolic, i.e., meaningful elements, including the construction of the sickness episode by patient and healer. Such constructions (i.e., Explanatory Models (EMs), after Kleinman [1980]), involve notions of etiology, course, appropriate treatment, processes, and out-come of particular sickness episodes. Clinical outcomes are in large part dependent upon the definition of the clinical situation and presentations embodied in EMs, Semantic Illness Networks (Good 1977) and on cultural conceptions such as that of 'person' which are less easily elucidated (Gaines 1979, 1982b, this volume; Hahn 1982, this volume).

An understanding of the broad, symbolic, semantic and interpretive dimensions of clinical encounters may improve clinical care. Such a perspective recognizes the necessary and integral clinical nature of what are now called 'exogenous' or 'extra-clinical' factors in clinical events. We would suggest that such an approach fosters improved care because it takes account not only of the 'whole person' of the patient, but that of the physician as well. An anthropological understanding of clinical and other medical encounters may foster enhanced therapeutic efficacy for several additional reasons.

Efficacy and Appropriate Clinical Care

As an interpretive enterprise, the medical encounter should be grounded in and responsive to meanings and structures of significance of both patient and healer. We must not forget that patients are rarely pathologists, hence, they do not seek treatment for *diseases*, histopathology or pathophysiology recognized by Biomedicine. Rather, they seek aid for what "ails" them, that is, for their *illnesses*. Illnesses, as has been noted, are personally and culturally constructed and meaningful. A treatment which focuses on *curing*, intervening only in suspected disease processes and which neglects *healing*, the relief of the burden of illness, will produce dissatisfied patients. Such patients frequently will not comply with medical advice because such advice seems inappropriate to the treatment of the illness they recognize. For this reason, adherence to a rigidly biomedical perspective may produce dismal results even in cases where biomedical knowledge is believed to be clear and certain (Twaddle 1981; Knowles 1977). Since the majority of presentations in medical contexts appear without clear signs and symptoms of disease (Kleinman et al. 1978), an exclusively biomedical perspective often may be impotent in the treatment of human suffering. It is because folk healers focus on and treat illnesses in terms of their symbolic meanings that they often seem to be even more efficacious in their healing than are biomedical physicians (Kleinman 1980).

In Biomedicine, lack of clarity of disease signs may lead a patient to be tossed from specialist to specialist, each of whom diagnoses a different entity in line with his or her specialty orientation and distinct from that of other physicians involved in the case (Helman, this volume). And since each practitioner narrowly defines the problem in personally relevant biophysical terms, the patient's understandings about and his or her relevant stresses are ignored, and a central problem, that of the patient's illness, goes unattended.

In addressing 'extra-clinical' issues, an anthropologically informed medicine seeks to provide help for those in need in terms which include culturally varied definitions of illness as well as disease. The thrust of medical care would then be the alleviation of suffering in human, i.e., cultural, terms rather than in terms of *one theory* of the nature of human affliction. It might be suggested here that attention to *illness* is attention to the root source of discomfort and or concern of patients, and as such offers the potential for considerable patient satisfaction. In a litigious social world, this may have significant ramifications for medical practice and related issues such as insurance and, perhaps, the cost of medical care in general (see also Twaddle 1981; Pfifferling 1981; Fox 1977).

A consideration of the cultural worlds of both patient and healer allows for the articulation of concerns of both parties and the negotiation of mutually satisfying therapeutic regimens, regimens which patients will understand and follow (Pfifferling 1981; Kleinman et al. 1978). Such a situation then accommodates both the curing of disease and the healing of illness and obviates the problem of medical practice as the imposition of a single cultural worldview.

Practice and Culture

An anthropologically informed biomedical practice may provide an alternative to the implicit 'cultural imperialism' that is part of much current medical practice. The many efforts to persuade others to accept our definitions of disease and our medicine and widespread disregard for culturally defined illnesses and the socio-cultural contexts of all disease is evidence not only of the imposition of our medical system, but also of our culture's more general worldview including its notions of causation, the nature of persons, intervention strategies, and so forth.

It is important to recognize the cultural basis of both illness and disease conceptions and of the therapeutic forces which are activated to deal with problems which arise. Important also is the recognition that medical conceptions are tied to and interrelated with a host of other cultural conceptions. Because of these ties, the disruption of the medical beliefs and practices of a culture can have far-reaching consequences including the extinction of traditional beliefs (see Onwubalili 1983). Biomedicine can work with other healing systems in order to reduce human suffering without trampling on the cultural systems which provide patients (as well as healers) with social and psychological support.

The cross-cultural comparative evaluation of medical systems is a complex matter which must certainly take into account more than the Western cultural (and hence, biomedical) notions of "saving time" or "trouble" and monetary expense, criteria commonly employed in Biomedicine as if they were medico-scientific bases of action (see Gaines 1982b). Further, notions of "efficacy" always indicate particular constructions of illness and hence vary widely among different ethnomedicines (Harwood 1981; Young 1976; Kiev 1964). Thus, whether or not an ethnomedicine is "efficacious" depends upon the cultural formulation of etiology and cure; a fever, 'caused' by offended ancesters, can be treated "more efficaciously" with antibiotics *only* from the biomedical (and Western) point of view (see Gaines, this volume).

More comprehensive criteria for evaluation must include patients' understandings of success and compliance with their understandings and rules of interaction, and the fostering of patients' social engagement. Our common goal should be a cultural medicine which ministers 'medicoculturally' rather than "medicocentrically" (Pffiferling 1981) and which does not frustrate the administration of appropriate aid to those in need. The pursuit of health requires a cultural medicine, rather than a Biomedicine, which does not implicitly or explicitly impose its own cultural definitions (e.g., "quicker cure") on others.

Almost daily we hear of advances being made in Biomedicine; we hear of new drugs, therapies, improved outcomes and etiological discoveries. But just as medicine seems to be conquering new domains, we see the great expansion of folk and popular therapies, greater recourse to marginal professional healers such as chiropractors, and the greater utilization of naturopathic, 'holistic', homeopathic professionals and their *materia medica*. Simultaneously, we see the development of anti-medical attitudes and actions (see Twaddle 1981) and expanding usage of alternate, folk therapies (Garrison 1977). Scholarly views of Biomedicine thus speak not only of great triumphs, but of "failures" (Kleinman 1978) in medicine and of a limiting "medicocentrism" (Pffiferling 1981). We see prominent physicians attempting to formulate new models of pathology which incorporate nonbiological aspects of human existence (Engel 1977; Kleinman et al. 1978; Mishler et al. 1981).

An improved Biomedicine would seem to be one which is less exclusively bio-medical and more culturally and socially aware. Similarly, an improved medical anthropology may develop out of the study of Biomedicine. Our views of others' conceptions and actions with respect to affliction and healing will doubtless undergo much change as we increase our anthropological understanding of the implicit and explicit assumptions, premises and conceptions underlying Biomedicine. Some of the basic ideological components in both contemporary social and medical sciences have heretofore hindered theory development and practice in both domains.

PHYSICIANS OF WESTERN MEDICINE

The works assembled here focus on different aspects of the ideology and practice of Western Biomedicine. We have arranged the contributions into four sections. The first section is introductory and includes the present paper and one by Maretzki. Maretzki provides for us an analysis of a number of significant works on Biomedicine and biomedical specialists. He also examines the relationship of anthropological and sociological research on Biomedicine and discusses some problems of past work and the prospects for future research on Biomedicine and its specialists.

Section II focuses on internal medicine, the core of Western Biomedicine. The essay by Hahn opens the field studies of our anthology with a portrait of the thought world of a community practitioner of internal medicine. As the central specialty of Biomedicine, internal medicine is often called simply, "medicine". Hahn explores the basic concepts of one practitioner, analyzing one of his central principles, "Treat the patient, not the lab", exploring this practitioner's values and epistemology, and his sources of pleasure and frustration in medical work.

The papers in Section III examine aspects of different medical specialties. Lock reviews biomedical (obstetrical-gynecological) attitudes and practices with regard to menopause. Despite, or perhaps because of, scant knowledge about this process, physicians exhibit a broad range of attitudes and practices. Their approaches are closely tied to their general medical approaches to patients, medication, and the nature of medical practice more broadly. Lock presents case studies of the ethno-medical attitudes and practices of several gynecologists, general practitioners and family physicians to show the influence of cultural or folk models on theory and practice in obstetrics and gynecology.

Rittenberg presents the case of a teenage girl with cystic fibrosis, focusing on one of her admissions to a hospital pediatrics ward. There is conflict among the pediatric practitioners in charge of the girl's care regarding the intensity of treatment to be pursued. Participants of the ward "team" resolve this conflict only when the principal physician's minimal treatment precipitates a decline in the girl's condition. The ominous quality of his failure fosters renegotiation and a collaborative redefinition of the situation and produces a new course of treatment action that leads to improvement in the patient's condition.

Katz analyzes decision-making in surgery. This biomedical specialty is often set apart from other specialties in the folk wisdom of Biomedicine by its member individuals' abilities to "make decisions". Yet in her analysis, Katz is able to show that the bases for surgical decision-making are often non-medical and involve elements of friendship, greed and the avoidance of responsibility. She demonstrates how surgeons obscure the process of decision-making and highlights some of the non-medical factors which organize surgical decision-making.

Focusing more closely, Rittenberg and Simons provide us with an ethno-methodological account of the method and logic of the "gentle interrogation" employed by a psychiatrist as he (Simons) explores the problem which brings a patient to him for the first time. He must elicit a "story" accounting for the patient's presence. He carefully guides the information given, for example, in its degree of detail and its sequence, often reassuring the patient that he is gathering useful information rather than making judgments. The strategy used differs from therapeutic discourse, though it also bears similarities, as well as from everyday conversational encounters.

Good, Herrera, DelVecchio Good, and Cooper examine the case of an Hispanic woman. An interdisciplinary therapeutic team (anthropologist, psychiatrist, sociologist, psychologist, respectively), and three community healers (an *espiritista*, a fundamentalist minister and a *curandera*), exchange and focus upon their different understandings of the patient's condition, symptoms and appropriate therapeutic responses after conflict among them emerges. Therapists' respective cultural backgrounds, including professional training and/or the lack thereof, are seen to shape their visions and comprehension of the patient's problem(s). The issue of countertransference is thus squarely addressed (see also Gaines, this volume). The confrontation serves both to modify reflexively the therapists' individual and collective understandings of the patients, to bring some relief to the patient, and to address pertinent epistemological issues.

In the next paper, Gaines focuses on another dimension of Western psychiatric praxis. In his analysis of Christian psychiatrists, their practices and their relationship to 'secular' psychiatrists, he draws upon previous research on secular' psychiatrists to consider the clinical significance (for patient and healer) of seemingly nonmedical conceptions, such as that of the person. He also examines the nature of the psychiatric profession itself and argues for a recognition of the symbolic nature of this and other healing and or curing 'groups' or 'sectors'.

In Section IV, contributors focus on the often problematic interrelations among the various medical specialties. Authors show that the problems of the medical specialties in interacting with one another have an impact on their respective patients. In the first paper in this section, by DelVecchio Good, we have an analysis of physicians' discourse about physicians. Specifically, she focuses on the verbal evaluations of the "competence" of self, peers and colleagues. She points up the limitations of the traditional sociological approaches to the study of medical professional competition by showing the centrality of cultural/professional *conceptions* of competence in the understanding of professional competition and the social relations thereby engendered or dissolved.

Johnson considers the marginality of consultation-liaison psychiatry among medical specialties. He shows clearly how this ambiguous position in the medical domain results from other medical specialists' perceptions of psychiatry as insufficiently 'medical' (i.e., biological, somatic). We should recognize from this study that a principal dimension of stratification in the domain of medicine is the perception of the degree to which given practitioners are able to intervene on a somatic level in cases of somatic dysfunction or histopathology. Johnson shows the symbolic utilization of medications and somatic manipulations to advance and maintain status in the hierarchy of the biomedical world.

Our last contribution by Helman traces the sickness career of a patient with left-sided chest pain as he moves, and is moved, among various medical specialists in English professional ethnomedicine. Clinical reality, the specialists' diagnoses, changes as the patient moves from practitioner to practitioner. However, the patient's illness is never addressed, and a personally satisfying conclusion is never reached.

SUMMARY

In this volume, contributors cross a new frontier of medical anthropology, the study of the physicians of Western Biomedicine. These healers are the central figures of a key institution in English and European language-speaking communities of the West; they have also had great influence in regions far beyond. In this volume we explore the cultural ideology and practice of Western professional healers in order to better understand our own society, its medicine, generic events of sickness and of healing and our discipline of anthropology.

While biomedical belief and practice are often regarded as unitary or homogeneous, the research presented here demonstrates the heterogeneous views and practices which comprise Western Biomedicine; it demonstrates the existence of many medicines, sometimes in conflict. We note that it is typical for members of a particular culture to disagree; a concept of culture should not suggest an identity of beliefs and practices of its bearers. The works presented here further show that the concepts of Biomedicine form a symbolic complex in terms of which actions are based and judged, and experience interpreted.

Contributors explore the relationship between beliefs and practices found in a variety of medical subcultures and their ties with the wider society and culture of which they are a part. They explore the ways in which key definitions of 'natural', 'work', 'disease', 'self', 'physiological integrity', 'Christian', 'talk', 'chest pain', 'secular', 'syndrome', 'transition' and 'competence' shape the clinical practices and interactions of medical practitioners. We recognize that a truly comparative medical anthropology must be fully cognizant of the formative influence of culture and society on all medical systems whether professional, folk or popular.

In that we focus here on the implicit medical standard whose ethnoclinical categories have been borrowed to classify and evaluate medical phenomena in other cultures, the studies presented here begin to address and lay the foundation for an unbiased formulation of a truly comparative medical anthropology and an anthropological (or cultural) medicine. Explorations of the dynamics of actual medical knowledge and practice in Western society such as those presented here contribute not only to a greater understanding of the cultural context and basis of medical science and practice, but also to methodological and conceptual improvements in the study of human misfortune and the acts and beliefs which surround, sometimes sustain, and alleviate it in our own and other cultures. We therefore hope that the studies assembled here will contribute to the development of improved theory and praxis in both anthropology and medicine.

ACKNOWLEDGEMENTS

The editors thank Mr. Daniel Maltz for his help in locating unpublished sources on the practice of Biomedicine. We would also like to thank Professor Arthur Kleinman for his generous support and encouragement during the preparation of this work, the completion of which is in no small part due to his efforts.

NOTES

1. We use the term, 'Biomedicine' (capitalized) to refer to the preeminent professional ethno-medicine of Western cultures. But we note that it is but one of *several* professional ethno-medicines focally concerned with a version of human biology and pathophysiology. Other professional ethnomedicines so focused include Chinese professional medicine and Ayurvedic (see Leslie 1977).
2. Paget completed a second version of this work which included an improved presentational system for her 'stetch of talk'. Unfortunately, due to space constraints, it could not be published here, but the reader is directed to the original which is otherwise the same (see Paget 1982).

REFERENCES

Becker, Howard, et al.
    1961 The Boys in White. Chicago: University of Chicago Press.
Borsay, Maria
    1975 Subcultural Conflicts in the Cincinnati Free Clinic. Unpublished Ph.D. dissertation. Department of Anthropology, University of Kentucky.
Bosk, Charles
    1979 Forgive and Remember. Chicago: University of Chicago Press.
Brill, N. and H. Storrow
    1966 Social Class and Psychiatric Treatment. Archives of General Psychiatry 3: 340–345.
Brody, Howard
    1973 Placebos and the Philosophy of Medicine. Chicago: University of Chicago Press.
Caudill, William
    1958 The Psychiatric Hospital as a Small Society. Cambridge: Harvard University Press.
Clausen, Joy
    1977 The Natural Experiment: A Method for Studying Conflict Resolution Between Health Professionals and Clients. Unpublished Ph.D. dissertation. Department of Anthropology, University of Colorado.
Creson, Daniel
    1976 The Socialization of Medical Students and Its Bearing on Medical Practice. Unpublished Ph.D. dissertation. Department of Anthropology, Rice University.
Day, Richard
    1978 Organization and Experience in a State Mental Hospital. Unpublished Ph.D. dissertation. Department of Anthropology, University of California at Berkeley.
Devereux, George
    1944 The Social Structure of a Schizophrenic Ward and Its Therapeutic Fitness. J. Clinical Psychotherapy 6: 231–265.
    1949 The Social Structure of the Hospital as a Factor in Total Therapy. American J. Orthopsychiatry 19(3): 492–500.
    1969 Mohave Ethnopsychiatry. Washington, D.C.: Smithsonian Institute Press (orig. 1961).
    1980 Schizophrenia: An Ethnic Psychosis. *In* Basic Problems of Ethnopsychiatry. G. Devereux. Chicago: University of Chicago Press (orig. 1963).
Eisenberg, Leon and Arthur Kleinman (eds.)
    1981 The Relevance of Social Science for Medicine. Dordrecht, Holland: D. Reidel Publishing Co.
Engel, George
    1977 The Need for a New Medical Model. Science 196: 129–136.
Foster, George and Barbara Anderson
    1978 Medical Anthropology. New York: John Wiley.

Fox, Renée C.
1959 Experiment Perilous. Philadelphia: University of Pennsylvania Press.
1977 The Medicalization and Demedicalization of American Society. *In* J. Knowles (ed.), Doing Better and Feeling Worse. New York: W. W. Norton.
1979 Essays in Medical Sociology. New York: John Wiley.
Freidson, Eliot
1970 The Profession of Medicine. New York: Dodd and Mead.
Gaines, Atwood D. and Robert A. Hahn (eds.)
1982 Physicians of Western Medicine: Five Cultural Studies. Special Issue. Culture, Medicine and Psychiatry 6(3).
Gaines, Atwood and Sandra Trego (organizers)
1978 The Anthropology of Psychiatry; Symposium. Southwestern Anthropology Association Meeting. April, San Francisco.
Gaines, Atwood D.
1979 Definitions and Diagnoses. Culture, Medicine and Psychiatry 3(4):381–418.
1982a Knowledge and Practice. *In* Noel Chrisman and Thomas Maretzki (eds.), Clinically Applied Anthropology. Dordrecht, Holland: D. Reidel Publishing Co.
1982b Cultural Definitions, Behavior and the Person in American Psychiatry. *In* Anthony Marsella and Geoffrey White (eds.), Cultural Conceptions of Mental Health and Therapy. Dordrecht, Holland: D. Reidel Publishing Co.
Garrison, Vivian
1977 Doctor, Espiritista or Psychiatrist? Health Seeking Behavior in a Puerto Rican Neighborhood of New York City. Medical Anthropology 1:65–180.
Geertz, Clifford
1973 The Interpretation of Cultures. New York: Basic Books.
Giddens, Anthony
1976 New Rules of Sociological Method. New York: Basic Books.
Goffman, Erving
1961 Asylums. Garden City, New York: Doubleday.
Good, Byron
1977 The Heart of What's the Matter. Culture, Medicine and Psychiatry 1(1):25–58.
Good, Byron and Mary-Jo DelVecchio Good
1981 The Meaning of Symptoms. *In* L. Eisenberg and A. Kleinman (eds.), The Relevance of Social Science for Medicine. Dordrecht, Holland: D. Reidel Publishing Co.
Hahn, Robert A.
1982 "Treat the Patient, Not the Lab". *In* A. Gaines and R. Hahn (eds.), Physicians of Western Medicine: Five Cultural Studies. Special Issue. Culture, Medicine and Psychiatry 6(3).
1983 Rethinking 'Illness' and 'Disease'. *In* E. V. Daniel and J. Pugh (eds.), South Asian Systems of Healing. Special volume. Contributions to Asian Studies XVIII.
Hahn, Robert A. and Atwood D. Gaines
1982 Introduction. *In* A. Gaines and R. Hahn (eds.), Physicians of Western Medicine: Five Cultural Studies. Special Issue. Culture, Medicine and Psychiatry 6(3).
Hahn, Robert A. and Arthur M. Kleinman
1983 Biomedical Practice and Anthropological Theory: Frameworks and Directions. *In* Annual Review of Anthropology. Palo Alto: Annual Review Press.
1984 Biomedicine as a Cultural System. *In* Massimo Piattelli-Palmarini (ed.), Encyclopedia of the Social History of the Biomedical Sciences. Milan: Franco Maria Ricci Publishing Co. (In press.)
Harwood, Alan (ed.)
1981 Ethnicity and Medical Care. Cambridge, Mass.: Harvard University Press.
Henry, Jules
1954 The Formal Structure of a Psychiatric Hospital. Psychiatry 17:139–151.

Henry, Jules
    1957 The Culture of Interpersonal Relations in a Therapeutic Institution for Emotionally
          Disturbed Children. American J. Orthopsychiatry 27(4):725–734.
Hughes, Charles
    1968 Ethnomedicine. *In* International Encyclopedia of the Social Sciences. New York:
          The Free Press.
Jaco, E. G. (ed.)
    1958 Patients, Physicians and Illness. Glencoe, Ill.: The Free Press.
Katz, M., Jonathan Cole and H. Alice Low
    1969 Studies of the Diagnostic Process. American Journal of Psychiatry 125:930–
          947.
Katz, Pearl
    1981 Rituals in the Operating Room. Ethnology 20(4):335–350.
Kiev Ari
    1964 Magic, Faith and Healing. New York: Basic Books.
Kleinman, Arthur
    1978 The Failure of Western Medicine. Human Nature 1(11):63–68.
    1980 Patients and Healers in the Context of Culture. Berkeley: University of California
          Press.
    1981 The Meaning Context of Illness and Care. *In* Everett Mendelsohn and Yehuda Elkana
          (eds.), Science and Cultures. Sociology of the Sciences, Volume V. Dordrecht,
          Holland: D. Reidel Publishing Co.
Kleinman, Arthur, Leon Eisenberg and Byron Good
    1978 Culture, Illness and Care. Annals of Internal Medicine 88:251–258.
Knowles, John, H. (ed.)
    1977 Doing Better and Feeling Worse: Health in the United States. New York: W. W.
          Norton.
Labov, William and David Fanshel
    1977 Therapeutic Discourse. New York: Academic Press.
Latour, B. and S. Wolgar
    1979 Laboratory Life: The Social Construction of Scientific Facts. Beverly Hills, California:
          Sage.
Leslie, Charles
    1977 Introduction. *In* C. Leslie (ed.), Asian Medical Systems. Berkeley: University of
          California Press.
Lieban, Richard
    1977 The Field of Medical Anthropology. *In* D. Landy (ed.), Culture, Disease, and Healing.
          New York: Macmillan.
Light, Donald
    1980 Becoming Psychiatrists. New York: W. W. Norton.
Marsella, Anthony
    1980 Depressive Experience and Disorder Across Cultures. *In* J. Draguns and H. Triandis
          (eds.), Handbook of Cross-Cultural Psychology, Volume 6: Psychopathology. New
          Jersey: Allyn and Bacon.
McMorrow, Leon
    1978 Modern Medicine in Buffalo, New York: An Ethnography of an Urban Institution.
          Unpublished Ph.D. dissertation. Department of Anthropology, State University of
          New York at Buffalo.
Merton, Robert, et al.
    1957 The Student Physician. Cambridge, Mass.: Harvard University Press.
Midgette, Rebecca
    1972 Doctor and Village Medicine in the Central Savannah River Area. Unpublished
          Masters thesis. Department of Anthropology, University of Georgia.

Mishler, Elliot, et al.
 1981 Social Contexts of Health, Illness, and Patient Care. Cambridge: Cambridge University Press.
Morrison, James and Thomas Flanagan
 1978 Diagnostic Errors in Psychiatry. Comprehensive Psychiatry 19:109–117.
Navarro, Vincente
 1976 Medicine Under Capitalism. New York: Prodist.
Onwubalili, James K.
 1983 Sickle-Cell Anaemia: An Explanation for the Ancient Myth of Reincarnation in Nigeria. The Lancet, August 27: 503–505.
Paget, Marianne
 1982 Your Son Is Cured Now; You May Take Him Home. In A. Gaines and R. Hahn (eds.), Physicians of Western Medicine: Five Cultural Studies. Special Issue. Culture, Medicine, and Psychiatry 6(3):237–259.
Petersdorf, R. G. and A. R. Feinstein
 1981 An Informal Appraisal of the Current Status of 'Medical Sociology'. In Leon Eisenberg and Arthur Kleinman (eds.), The Relevance of Social Science for Medicine. Dordrecht, Holland: D. Reidel Publishing Co.
Pfifferling, John-Henry
 1981 A Cultural Prescription for Medicocentrism. In Leon Eisenberg and Arthur Kleinman (eds.), The Relevance of Social Science for Medicine. Dordrecht, Holland: D. Reidel Publishing Co.
Ripley-Daghlin, Barbara
 1981 The Changing Patterns of Health Care in a Rural Vermont Setting. Unpublished Ph.D. dissertation. Department of Anthropology, University of Connecticut.
Riska, E. and P. Vinten Johansen
 1981 The Involvement of the Behavioral Sciences in American Medicine: An Historical Perspective. International Journal of Health Services 11(4):583–596.
Robinson, Janet
 1975 Country Doctor in the Changing World of the Nineteenth Century: An Historical Ethnography of Medical Practice, Chester County, Pennsylvania, 1790–1861. Unpublished Ph.D. dissertation. Department of Anthropology, University of Pennsylvania.
Robles, Nadine
 1982 The Mental Hospital: From Therapeutic to Custodial. Unpublished Ph.D. dissertation. Department of Anthropology, University of California at Berkeley.
Schoepf, Brook
 1975 Human Relations Versus Social Relations in Medical Care. In S. Ingman and A. Thomas (eds.), Topias and Utopias in Health. The Hague: Mouton.
Starr, Paul
 1982 The Social Transformation of American Medicine. New York: Basic Books.
Stevens, Rosemary
 1971 American Medicine and the Public Interest. New Haven: Yale University Press.
Twaddle, Andrew
 1981 Sickness and the Sickness Career: Some Implications. In Leon Eisenberg and Arthur Kleinman (eds.), The Relevance of Social Science for Medicine. Dordrecht, Holland: D. Reidel Publishing Co.
Waitzkin, Howard
 1979 Medicine, Superstructure and Micropolitics. Social Science and Medicine 13A: 601–609.
Young, Allan
 1976 Some Implications of Medical Beliefs and Practices for Social Anthropology. American Anthropologist 78(1):5–24.

Young, Allan
    1980 An Anthropological Perspective on Medical Knowledge. Journal of Medicine and
        Philosophy 5:102–116.
    1981 When Rational Men Fall Sick. Culture, Medicine, and Psychiatry 5:317–335.

THOMAS W. MARETZKI

INCLUDING THE PHYSICIAN IN HEALER-CENTERED RESEARCH: RETROSPECT AND PROSPECT

INTRODUCTION

The study of healers, the healing process and healers' transactions with their clients are central foci in cross-cultural research leading to understanding of the role of medical systems in health maintenance. Healers in traditional, small societies have been studied by anthropologists in considerable detail (e.g., Turner 1967; Lévi-Strauss 1967a). However, it is remarkable that anthropology has heretofore largely ignored the healer of Western Biomedicine, the physician. This paper examines recent studies of Western physicians which compliment those included in this volume. It examines forces external to anthropology which give direction to such studies, the challenges for anthropologists engaged in field research on physicians, and some theoretical perspectives and research foci which have guided research on physicians to date.

Western Biomedicine is a concern of both the social sciences and the humanities. These disciplines have generated interrelated problem foci and strategies for the analysis of data. Anthropology has only recently become *deeply* involved in studying physicians (e.g., Gaines 1979; Gaines and Hahn 1982, and this volume). It is clear that research on the physician of Western medicine is of considerable theoretical importance. To provide a basis for evaluating problems and prospects in the anthropological study of the physician this overview begins with a brief comparative examination of sociology and anthropology, the former being the social science most closely related to anthropology and anthropology's precursor in the study of the physician. The comparison will allow us to elucidate the distinctiveness of anthropological approaches.

ANTHROPOLOGICAL AND SOCIOLOGICAL PERSPECTIVES ON WESTERN HEALERS

Given the breadth of medical sociology and parallel trends rapidly evolving in anthropology, I cannot hope to present an exhaustive review here. Rather I point to some sociological studies which illustrate both overlap with and distinctions from anthropological efforts. Sociology and anthropology have been compared to look-alike relatives from different branches of the same family (Olesen 1974). It is as easy to see parallels between these two disciplines in relation to medicine as it is to characterize their distinctive features (Foster 1974). The parallels with, and duplications of sociological studies of physicians suggest that medical anthropologists might first acquire a familiarity with the sociological literature (Foster and Anderson 1978:175).

R. A. Hahn and A. D. Gaines (eds.), Physicians of Western Medicine, 23–47.
© 1985 *by D. Reidel Publishing Company.*

Viewed from anthropology, the most conspicuous distinction between the two fields is the cross-cultural, comparative orientation of anthropology. Whether ethnographic, focusing on a specific culture, or broader in scope, anthropological studies always assume that phenomena should be seen as part of a wider variety of human social organizational forms and behavioral patterns, or as a combination of biological and social functions embedded in a cultural matrix. The study of physicians by anthropologists is no exception. It assumes an explicitly comparative, *ethnomedical* perspective.

Following Foster, a basic philosophical difference can be detected in the tendency of sociologists to consider biomedical phenomena in terms of professions and medical institutions, whereas anthropologists tend to assume more naturally the perspective of the patient. In so doing, anthropologists reflect an identification and sympathy with the people they study (Foster 1974:3). Where sociologists tend to present the physician as a professional who is ensconced in a high social status requiring adherence to rules, restraints and review, and marked by professional detachment towards the patient's problems, the anthropologist or the anthropologically oriented sociologist allows the professional to emerge as a sympathetic human whose reactions are relevant to the presentation and interpretation of data (Fox 1979b; Gaines 1979), while also reflecting patient concerns and perspectives. Without making too much of a dichotomy based on ideal abstractions, the main point is that there has emerged a distinct medical anthropological focus on institutionalized Biomedicine as a sub-culture of which the physician is a part. While this is also recognized by medical sociologists (see Fox 1979; Freidson 1970a:11), in anthropology the cultural emphasis centrally organizes the overall perspective and sees physicians as part of the wider culture (e.g., Gaines and Hahn 1982).

Anthropologists devote much attention to the individual in the social group. Thus we wonder about the way in which healers assimilate their specialist knowledge with its powerful values and meanings. We concern ourselves with communications with the patient as a lay person who is informed by a diversity of folk values and meanings. We might typically also wonder about the ability of the biomedical healer, given the overwhelming subcultural influences on his or her environment, to maintain effective personal integration with the larger community, with networks of friends, other professionals, and community groups. Our cultural orientation projects our findings against a broader, cultural context, whether in actual analysis or by implication.

Our discipline of medical anthropology has expanded so much in a few years that we have not been able to stand still to assess our research approaches (see Young 1982a). We seem to know intuitively what makes them anthropological, and, therefore, distinct. We know equally well what we see as uniquely "our" is sometimes only relatively so when held against the studies of medical sociologists which have preceded our efforts. It is often stated that the sociological perspective reflects the methodology used, such as the greater reliance on prestructured questionnaires, the superimposition of categories from the outside rather than the use of those generated from within the study population, and the quantification of data. As we discuss some examples of antecedent studies, we should recognize that such statements as the preceding often serve more as demarcations of historical disciplinary boundaries than descriptions of substance.

Yet we can not leave this subject without examining another question: who is to consume all this information and perhaps benefit from studies of the physician? Even if, as individual anthropologists, we are satisfied that good basic research does not need some practical consideration as justification, the question arises in making the arrangements to begin a field study in Biomedicine. The most hospitable environments are those which already have a recognized research orientation, for example, academic medical centers and institutes. Even there very practical considerations and professional status hierarchies may be major determinants of collaboration in, and hospitality toward, social science research (Roberts 1979).

The type of field locations and the opportunities and constraints in the study of physicians are novel for anthropologists. Although there are parallels, both the settings and the state of research differ from the familiar challenge of developing a research project in an unfamiliar culture away from home base. In the professional environment of Biomedicine, the researcher's social membership category is assigned, by sponsors and collaborating subjects, an importance far beyond the participant role with which so many anthropologists approach small non-Western societies. With whom should the anthropologist be identified or compared: health care providers, health care consumers, or a third, non-existing or non-familiar category of "social scientist"? Is there a role for the anthropologist as evaluator or adjunct to the administration of clinical facilities? Or is the closest analogue the role of "volunteer"? The professional self-description "anthropologist" evokes in most persons, including many health professionals, an association with the study of the past, even of primate ancestors of man, or the study of "savages", but certainly not a research role in clinics.

While we will return to this point later, the general implications extend beyond social, ethical, and legal aspects to those of "insider" versus "outsider" roles. They relate to methodological and epistemological facets which have brought forth painstaking self-inspection and the creation of fine, though relevant distinctions, such as the division of medical sociology into sociologies "of", "in", and "for" medicine (Petersdorf and Feinstein 1981). In practical respects, there are potential and real conflicts for the establishment of rapport, trust and confidentiality (Estroff 1981), and the adaptation of the role of social science researcher in the delivery of medical care (Alexander 1979; Chrisman and Maretzki 1982).

FORCES OF CHANGE AS RATIONALE FOR PHYSICIAN STUDIES

The impulse for changing the emphasis of our studies to include the biomedical healer influences a variety of research objectives. These objectives can be distinguished as 'basic', 'disciplinary', and 'applied'. For the first there is an increased sophistication of conceptual and theoretical thinking in the comparative studies of culture which matches the growing complexity of **Biomedicine** itself. We have moved from relatively simple, single theory explications to the synthesis of theories. This force of change is occurring in anthropology, but is not independent of parallel explosions of knowledge in other disciplines and needs to be disseminated to others, including medical practitioners. There remains a general public perception of our discipline as restricted in topical focus to small societies and capable only of capturing simple cultural differences. We need to account to ourselves, and to those among whom we wish to study, for our capacity to understand complex phenomena, including the theory and practice of **Biomedicine**.

Disciplinary changes in the future will positively influence the study of physicians. We need to look to our discipline as a whole, not just to its social and cultural subfields. Medical anthropology has stronger roots in social than in biological anthropology though there are indications that this is changing. We have the unusual disciplinary advantages of generating anthropological research foci along the broad spectrum of fields within the entire discipline, provided individual anthropologists can span the fields. Ecological explorations have demonstrated the falsity of simple reductionism and the importance of a systems approach (Alland 1966; Wellin 1977). Interest in the anthropology of healing as a symbolic process requires an understanding of social, cultural, pharmacological and basic biological topics (Moerman 1979, 1983; Hahn and Kleinman 1983; Brody 1983).

The distinctiveness in the study of physicians by anthropologists becomes blurred by overlapping methodological and theoretical interests. Anthropologists face a very intricate set of problems in their preparation for research, the absorption of relevant facts and their updating, and the dissemination of essential findings. The forces favoring or impeding new directions of anthropological research which include the physician are largely filtered through the institutionalized organization of disciplines which gives shape to disciplinary directions even more than do the capacities of individuals who try to cope with interdisciplinary study.

There are many practical justifications for examining the current directions of the biomedical health care system of which physicians are an integral part (Starr 1982). Some of the most persuasive practical justifications have an economic base, i.e., the cost of health care, Related justifications include professional self-interest. Increased biomedical knowledge generates new specializations and complicates the provision of health care, resulting in increased costs. There is also pressure to intensify and expand professional outlets for practice. A serious student of psychotherapy, Jerome Frank, has claimed that "psychotherapy is the only form of treatment which, at least to some extent, appears to create the illness it treats" (1961:7). Ivan Illich, of course, went far beyond this simple statement in his accusations of blatant medicalization (1975). No matter what data base one chooses, it is evident that there are many interrelated reasons for phenomenal cost increases. Some paradoxical frontiers of present medical practice can be found in heroic interventions, e.g., the application of medical technology to the prolongation of life at all costs. Other arise from inappropriate or cosmetic surgical interventions (Wennberg and Gittelson 1982). All of these forces for change in medical practice rely on social validation. A cost-benefit analysis, including an anthropological perspective, would be appropriate. The cost of health care and its unequal distribution is not outside the purview of cultural analysis as, for example, in the consequences of chronic illness, decidedly a subject for anthropological research (Alexander 1982).

The extraordinary developments in medical sciences and medical technology in the last two decades were paralleled by the rise of a broad public consciousness about their impact on medical care. We can distinguish in the reactions of consumers of Biomedicine several overall reactions: those related to a search for holistic medicine, the special concerns of women with appropriate health care, and the search for ethnically relevant health care (Harwood 1981; Press 1982). These powerful orientations increasingly have an impact outside the health care delivery institutions. They also influence individuals within, including growing numbers of physicians who state their views about desirable health care (e.g., Ingelfinger 1976; Jellinek 1976; Thomas 1971; Weed 1981).

To translate holism into social science concepts which can serve systematic studies of the physician is, indeed, a task in which medical anthropology has a role. The biopsychosocial model and its implications for medical education and practice is one possible point of articulation for anthropology (Engel 1977, 1982). It can be related to different medical specialties, particularly to family medicine and primary care in internal medicine, but also to other biomedical primary care specialties.

Because a feminist approach to cultural phenomena has become a significant focus in anthropology, and one which draws on appropriate social science concepts to document the cultural assignment of gender roles, this interest in relation to physician education and activities is a most important topic for anthropological studies. Recent investigations of male dominance in obstetrics/gynecology, based on participant observation and informal interviews, could be one stimulus (Scully 1980; Lock 1982, and this volume). These studies of the culture of Biomedicine are more than basic contributions to the social sciences. They imply the need for change of current practices. There has been a long delay in recognition within the social sciences of a male-centered bias in many so-called 'human' concerns, including medicine (Lorber 1975).

Our entry into studies of the physician is based on the notion of healing as an overarching cross-cultural concern of medical anthropology. The Western physician is the most widely recognized, powerful and legitimized healer in our society. With our research in smaller societies and traditional healing activities as a contrast, we recognize the effect of health care institutions; they have generated in our research framework a medicocentrism with the result that culturally shaped illness experiences are fitted into rigid biomedical frames imbued with Western beliefs and values (Pfifferling 1981). For medical anthropology a focus on the physician as healer is not limited to our own Western societies, but is relevant for studies of medical systems in all human societies. The physician role is spreading into all corners of the world, along with the rise of national health care systems and private medical practice.

Traditional healers and biomedical practitioners are joined in total health care systems through the help-seeking and illness behaviors of clients (Kleinman 1980; Salan and Maretzki 1983). Parallel behaviors in seeking help for medical problems from alternative (to physicians) healers is equally evident in our own society (e.g., Garrison 1977, 1978; Snyder 1983). This fact, commonly ignored or discouraged by physicians, has various implications for the doctor-patient relationship in terms of compliance and clinical outcome (Kleinman 1980).

The 'Man-over-Nature' thrust (Kluckhohn and Strodtbeck 1961) is central to the ethos of Biomedicine in the United States. Scientific speculation and pseudo-science leak in at the edges where objective knowledge is insufficient or does not exist (see Katz, this volume; Maretzki and Seidler 1983). These edges are constantly shifting (Duffy 1979). They change the nature of institutionalized biomedical health care as in the case of osteopathic medicine which is marginally "in", and chiropractice which is not (Riley 1980; Skipper 1978; Wardwell 1980; see also Wallis and Morley 1977). Ideas differ for individual practitioners. Patients, even if they accept enthusiastically or with reserve the powerful results of science and medical technology, do not share with physicians either the biomedical knowledge base or the physicians' rules of action. Patients and healers, as Gaines and Hahn demonstrate (1982, and this volume), rely on folk models of illness and idiosyncratic interpretations which vary greatly and may or may not include biomedical information.

Patients' knowledge is influenced by the popular presentation of biomedical facts and the information ('health education') received in clinical practice. The biomedical healer and the patient are locked into clinical situations wherein problems are differentially conceived and distinct styles of communication impede communication across cultural boundaries (Kleinman et al. 1978). The similarity with contact situations in other anthropological investigations is apparent, as is the contrast with the practice and style of non-Western folk and Western professional healers. Healers in traditional cultures more often share a worldview with their patients. Their healing techniques are usually public and utilize familiar strategies and metaphors (Turner 1967; Lévi-Strauss 1967b).

CHALLENGES OF FIELD RESEARCH ON PHYSICIANS

In assessing the challenges of doing anthropological research on physicians, there is probably no baseline of "ordinary" challenges to use for comparison. Whether in remote communities, in regions of extreme climate, in urban centers, or in hospitals or clinics, each situation may make unique demands. Individual anthropologists differ in background and the qualities they bring to field situations. For these reasons it is hard to generalize and to give manual-style suggestions. In general, health care settings as field sites for anthropology present great challenges and hence one's approach should not be left to chance (Chrisman and Maretzki 1982).

The study of physicians must draw upon special skills in interpersonal relations as well as on an ability to handle oneself in very complex, rule-oriented institutions. The contrast with other anthropological field sites is that these settings are much less forgiving than, for example, most traditional tribal or village communities (e.g., Gaines 1982b). In clinics and hospitals even small errors in personal style of interaction and non-adherence to rules may have serious repercussions for the researcher. It follows that such research is best approached with extremely thorough preparation and complete professionally responsible immersion during the study period. As an example, the anthropologist in the clinic will soon discover how important it is to give clinic staff a schedule of presence in the clinic, and to adhere to stated times, or adequately inform the staff of changes. This is one important detail in recognizing essential conventions. But it may also constrain the anthropologist.

Knowledge of health systems is a prerequisite for physician studies. These systems in their varieties and complexities have been well described and analyzed by social scientists (e.g., Caudill 1958; Mechanic 1976, 1979; Starr 1982). Humanists involved in the study of ethical and legal aspects of medical care have recently added further insights and experiences. A period of prior experience by the fieldworker in a clinical setting is advantageous, if not mandatory. An arrangement for initial "supervision" with an experienced clinician, tolerant of social science approaches, is helpful. This provides reactions and information relating to the experiences of the fieldworker. The supervision model is common in clinical training (Light 1980). It is thus very appropriate to transfer it to research preparation.

Health care settings generate intricate interprofessional and interpersonal relationships with direct implications for social scientists who are not a part of the regular staff. Many of these are reflected in the experiences of anthropologists who have assumed the roles of teachers and/or researchers in various clinical settings. In the Introduction to *Clinically Applied Anthropology* (1982), Chrisman and I abstracted very specific points which have emerged from our own experiences and those of the other contributors (1982:1−24). Unless the anthropologist manages to develop close and trusted working relationships, and focuses on a problem area which the physicians can acknowledge as useful, essential *rapport* is not likely to develop. The well-known, though not readily documented defensiveness of the medical profession, which tends to curtain off professional activities from public view, presents formidable obstacles to such studies. That such obstacles can be overcome to the mutual satisfaction of the researcher and research subjects has been ably demonstrated in studies in this volume and in others I will mention briefly below. Each study must be appreciated in terms of the overall challenges and the creative efforts undertaken to overcome those challenges. Some were carried out in the more benign and open climate of a few selected medical schools where social scientists apparently have been more welcome and assimilated into medical context than elsewhere.

An example of a "classical" study of physicians is Renée Fox's early research with physicians and patients at the frontiers of medical knowledge and practice of that time (1959). The uniqueness of her work lies in the formulation of an investigator's role which allowed her access to the physician-patient dyad. As a result she shared in the information normally considered the private domain of this relationship, and available only in the service of curative intervention. More than just ordinary research skills, it look special interpersonal talents to be so effectively included. These qualities cannot necessarily be imparted through social scientific training.

Considering that few social scientists have the appropriate background, Fox's study is also a testimony to the researcher's need to absorb rapidly, and without interference, the enormous amount of medical information and communicative styles of the physicians' culture. Fox's own explanation is that physicians are confronted with two types of uncertainty: that arising from the imperfect state of medical knowledge, and the physician's own incomplete or imperfect mastery. In this situation the researcher functioned as a sympathetic listener and as a non-threatening human support. Fox's study, like those of others, also suggests a greater receptivity to social science by young physicians, especially residents who are still in formal medical training and more involved with the process of their own professional development.

The non-threatening, emphathetic role which Fox as a social scientist chose in her field research illustrates the importance of interactional style. It also opens another important topic, the role of bias, impartiality, or objectivity in relation to the role and identity of "insider" and "outsider" mentioned before. Minimally, the awareness of one's biases is necessary to function as a researcher. If the bias is very unfavorable towards the physician, or in relation to the biomedical health care system in general, the anthropologist is handicapped, as would be the case in any field situation approached with a negative orientation. The reverse, an overcommitment, or too strong an identification with the clinical professional, has similar risks for the researcher and the research product. These risks have engendered a series of different positions on the nature of involvements of anthropologists as researchers in clinics, differences with continue to be discussed in lively debates (Medical Anthropology Newsletter 1980; Bennett 1982; Russell 1982).

Discussions of relationships, identity, and identification, bias and active involvement bring us face to face with problems of an ethical and legal nature. In the study of the physician these occur at two interrelated levels. At a basic level, the researcher, through the study of the physician, shares information which concerns patients, and therefore involves the researcher in ethical and legal obligations requiring close attention and responsible handling. Examples appear in several medical sociology studies of physicians, most notably in Bosk's work (1979) on the handling of technical and moral errors by surgeons. The second level concerns the nature of reporting which we will briefly review in relation to Joan Cassell's discussion (1980) of Bosk's research.

As a researcher, Bosk had to remain neutral to the consequences of errors which were discussed in his presence by physicians who trusted him. Seen from another angle, he participated in covering up details and identities sufficiently to protect those who committed errors. How this can lead to serious conflict for a researcher is part of the general nature of paradoxical situations where the participant research role involves exposure to conflicting loyalties. Comparable ethical dilemmas have been faced by urban researchers who study activities which are legally defined as criminal (Weppner 1973). It is a credit to Bosk that an extremely sensitive area of professional activities could be studied in the operating theater and in morbidity and mortality conferences. The study is, as well, a credit to the faculty and residents who agreed to participate as subjects.

Joan Cassell ties Bosk's findings, and the analysis he offers on the handling of technical and moral errors, to the ethics of anthropological fieldwork in general. In so doing, she offers us a view which appropriately closes a circle. She links the insights gained from a study of physicians to the potential errors in our own professional handling of the research task in fieldwork. Bias, unfavorable or favorable, she asserts, leads to technical error in anthropology if, as in her example for the study of physicians, a personal negative bias results in a falsified hypothesis which, through further failure to examine significant variables, results in a crusade or even in crucifixion rather than an objective research product. Such technical errors, Cassell suggests, easily lead to the moral error of blaming those who are considered by anthropologists to be outside their "moral communities" (Cassell 1981:166–167). Traditionally, anthropologists have favored the powerless, and here is where we may expect to err. But over-identification with the powerful can have the same effects in the opposite direction. The study of physicians, in that sense, offers unfamiliar challenges which go to the core of the anthropological research roles and their products.

PROBLEM FOCUS IN PHYSICIAN STUDIES

The study of physicians by anthropologists evolves at a time when the American public view of health care and the role of the physician reflects a broad range of sentiments (Capra 1979; Cousins 1973; Illich 1975; Knowles 1977). By listening to conversations and surveying the public media and literature, it is easy to gather expressions on both extreme and intermediate positions. The physician emerges as a savior of lives, as provider of relief for the chronically sick, as a curer of the sporadically ill, as authority in providing judgments of broad social significance based on professional knowledge, as a model for those deciding on an occupation role, as a general representative of a desirable social position, of wealth, and probably still — in the majority of interpretations — with male, rather than female, characteristics.

On the opposite side, villainous roles and motivations are projected on to the physician: those of dominance and excessive control, male chauvinism, excessive greed for extraordinary financial compensation, excessive power exceeding a more narrowly defined place of medicine in the social fabric, and others. These public expressions are bolstered by reports challenging physicians' activities as professionals and as individuals which arise from legal cases, from malpractice proceedings, from criminal acts in which physicians may be involved, and which, no matter how personally explained, are publicly linked to the physician's status in society and the sanctity of the professional role. As a public hero, the physician may be expected to be above moral reproach, even by strict standards. There are comparisons made with the priest in discussing the importance of confidentiality and other spheres of conduct. Public perceptions, when translated into a systematic research approach, are a relevant focus for social science research.

Understanding the Western physician can not be separated from the total context of American medicine (Fox 1979a). Anthropologists naturally reduce the abundance of contextual issues to those most amenable to cultural analysis. We suggest three separate, but related problem foci: the social context of medical practice, the nature of 'problems' as they are diagnosed by the physician, and psychosocial and cultural factors in illness. The two general topics organizing this brief overview of physician studies are (1) the physician as part of a professional organization and the institutions created by and for the practice of professional skills, and (2) the physician as a clinician in the interaction with patients. In the latter topic, there are potential comparisons with other healers. The elaboration of professional status, definition, and specializations in the medical profession are, though present (Unschuld 1979), not matched in other cultures, except as borrowed from the Western model.

A third possible topic is that of the physician as a human being, thrust into a role demanding unusual adaptation. This important perspective on the physician will be least examined here because there is, as yet, little in the social science literature that stands out. The issue of the physician as social being has not only led to the physician's self-examination, especially by psychiatrists, but it is an essential factor in understanding the physician's call to the profession, and the molding by each physician of the core element of practice, the doctor-patient relationship. Where this relationship is threatened by a 'difficult-to-manage-patient', there is a danger of negative, unproductive reactions by physicians (McCue 1982). Beyond individual episodes of physician frustration, there is the more general syndrome of physician burn-out and the "impaired physician" (Vaillant et al. 1970).

SOCIALIZATION OF THE PHYSICIAN AS A MEMBER OF A PROFESSION

Sociology and anthropology logically turn to investigate how individuals function in social aggregates by studying their socialization. The existing studies of professional socialization in medicine which interest us most are those utilizing participant observation and informal interviewing. No social scientist with an opportunity to closely observe medical education can escape being impressed by the overwhelming forces acting on the physician-in-training.

In the classical sociological studies of medical socialization, there is no agreement as to the specific nature of professional role learning. The core of the argument centers on the learning of specific values and attitudes to become effectively integrated into the professional ethos of Biomedicine. Howard Becker and his collaborators began their classical study (Becker et al. 1961) with the basic problem orientation: what happens to these young people who enter medical school to learn the technical skills of a physician? How do they learn to internalize the expected role, and what psychological coping mechanisms emerge during their course of studies (see also Mumford 1970)? The question of how it is possible to survive this overwhelming, transformative experience, from entering layman student to, four years later, a diploma-carrying professional, had earlier attracted other social scientists (Merton et al. 1957), more traditional in the use of sociological methodology.

Becker et al. argue against those who see a professional self-image emerging during the four years of medical study (e.g., Huntington 1957), nor do they accept other views of students' gradual development of coping skills, such as negotiating within a hierarchy of professionals, emotional detachment, and time allocation (Fox 1957; Fox and Lief 1963). Instead, Becker et al. (1961:420) argue, on the basis of their participant study in the University of Kansas Medical School, that students are never given sufficient responsibilities in patient care to provide clues which could lead them to confuse their student status with that of a doctor.

In the course of my own observations of medical students in Hawaii, I have seen them learn History Taking and Physical Examinations (HPE) during their first year, and graduate progressively to more clinical tasks, always supervised by residents and attending physicians. By the fourth year of training the essential elements of the professional role have been learned. At that time the "we" feeling of a medical student in the presence of physicians excludes not only the patient as outsider to the professional identity, but in most cases also the social scientist, even one who holds a faculty status in medicine. I have observed that by the time of graduation the essential values and attitudes of the physician have been formed and are well established. Relevant here seems to be the acceptance of direct responsibility for problem-solving and care of the patient as the student internalizes that sense of responsibility.

Renée Fox, who for so long has been a keen observer of physicians from the time of their training through many stages of professional career development, captures the almost elusive human qualities involved. Her short, sensitive presentation portrays the basic aspects of the 'human condition' which need to be faced in learning the professional role effectively (1979b). Here we encounter an empathetic and humanistic approach to the understanding of the physician's task through a view of professional socialization. This approach is markedly different from the more distanced statements in other sociological studies. Since Becker et al. mention the foment in medical education at the time of their writing (1961:430), it is also possible that there has been a shift which requires less of the defensive, cynical attitude found in their student subjects. Instead, a more positive professionally oriented commitment may accompany the gradual increase in challenges of medical education.

Psychiatry offers the most puzzling perspective on the physician as a healer, one who needs to reconcile conflicting professional role challenges. Role related stresses and identity problems are well-known to psychiatrists who treat physician colleagues (see Johnson, this volume).

The social perspective on the role of the psychiatrist is a topic of constant interest in psychiatry as well as in the social sciences and humanities. Central to this topic always is the issue of when a diagnosed mental illness is the pathology of an individual, and when it is more broadly understood as deviance from some group's social values and expectations. Thus an individual's lack of social integration may not be a condition of maladaptation due to a disease process, but one of maladaptation to one's social environment deriving from values or ideology from another environment. Trained as physicians in Biomedicine, there is a challenge to this group of physicians which is unique. That is, they require more knowledge of psychological and sociocultural principles than is systematically taught in medical school or psychiatry residency training.

Light's balanced, yet incisive ethnography (1980) of psychiatric residency training describes this phase of professional socialization. A sharp picture emerges of the cultural context in which psychiatry is practiced and taught (e.g., socialization rather than patient care was the main concern in the training program Light observed [1980: 212; see also Roberts 1977]). Light describes the power position from which these physicians bestow labels on their patients, in contrast, for example, to psychologists. In entering this powerful and relatively closed system of patient care, Light recognizes the unusual degree of pressure on residents. His book reveals the process of training and residents' coping mechanisms developed to maintain their own identity and sanity, given the pressure of glaring contradictions inherent in their specialty.

Light's methodology is the key to this insightful study, a receptive research environment the prerequisite for carrying it out. First-hand observations for an extended time period through participation in all phases of the residency program provided the insights he offers. The ethnography unfolds with almost drama-like qualities as residents face one challenge after another.

As social scientists, we can appreciate Light's book. Whether or not psychiatry will, is another matter. A layman remains an outsider to the profession. Though a sociologist, Light functioned like an anthropologist in a remote community. But the fascination of many psychiatrists with the analyses offered by an anthropological approach applied to Western professionals with complex identity problems could quickly fade if sensitivities are hurt.

It is only one step further to take the position that the study of American psychiatry can and should be approached as any other ethnopsychiatric investigation (Gaines 1979: 381). Gaines sees the psychiatric profession as a culturally shaped institution whose members have been part of particular cultural traditions long before entering professional training. Within psychiatry there are a number of ideological positions which imply quite diverse conceptions of mental illness. Gaines points out the folk conceptual bases of these in contrast to psychiatric discussions of variation which see psychiatry grounded in different scientific schools of thought (e.g., Lazare 1973). These are brought to bear on individual patients from different ethnic backgrounds who present with conditions which have their origin and meaning in distinct cultural traditions.

Lacking a unified theory of etiology, the fact that diagnoses are made in cultural contexts and of conditions presenting in a cultural package of the patient's history and symptomatology, combined with the variety of possible therapeutic strategies, all suggest how residents in the same training program emerge with quite diverse models of mental illness. Gaines recognizes that professional training of psychiatrists illustrates the organization of diversity, and that at a higher level of abstration the psychiatrist as a professional shares a great deal in style and action with any of his/her colleagues. An even greater range of psychiatric beliefs and behaviors has been demonstrated in subsequent studies (Gaines 1982a, c, this volume).

ETHICAL AND MORAL DILEMMAS FOR PHYSICIANS

Psychiatry is not the only specialty with internal inconsistencies. All of medicine has internal conflicts though it often appears to outsiders as smooth and uniform. Many conflicts are of an ethical and moral nature. Learning to cope with the management of errors in a surgical practice is the subject of Bosk's study, mentioned earlier. Bosk's work is a penetrating social science exploration of social control through responses to the errors of surgical residents in training. In a searching and fair manner Bosk analyzes a set of practices which are stark and potentially demoralizing to practitioners in traning.

The implicit and relevant contextual background for Bosk's study is the ever-present effort of physicians to maintain professional control, and in so doing to avoid the imposition of standards from the outside. Technical errors can be forgiven since correction through skill review and further learning offers a remedial solution. Confession, an essential response to technical error, is proof of adherence to group standards and results in forgiveness (1979:179). Severe and repeated moral errors lead to expulsion of those in training. Moral errors are more serious than technical errors, more threatening to the continued functioning of the professional without serious outside interference.

Bosk (1979: 189) disputes Freidson (1970a) and others who allege a reluctance in the profession to enforce standards of practice along with efforts to sweep errors under the rug (also see DelVecchio Good, this volume). Bosk appeals to the corporate sense of the medical profession and illustrates the severity of socialization to ethical professional standards. There are few topics about physicians more hidden to outside examination than those elicited by this research. For this reason, Bosk's discussion of his field experiences as an adjunct member to surgical teams of residents and attending physicians provides an important example for others who plan research (1979:183—213).

THE PHYSICIAN FROM NON-WESTERN, DEVELOPING COUNTRIES

Medical anthropologists who study in non-Western communities often view the role of Western Biomedicine introduced into traditional societies as tangential to their research interests, though the situation may be changing as 'cosmopolitan' medical systems begin to impinge everywhere on traditional systems of medicine (Dunn 1976). What happens when individuals from one of these traditional societies, still close to their own cultural roots, even though mission-educated, are trained in Western countries as physicians? This question led De Craemer and Fox into research in the Belgian Congo (now Zaïre), resulting in a report, *The Emerging Physician* (1968).

An important anthropological issue is how these physicians, many of whom had previously been prepared to serve as medical assistants in their own country, assimilate their own cultural ideology to that of the sub-culture of professional medicine. Unlike their Western-raised colleagues, these physicians had to make a number of adjustments to their particular African culture and the new Western patterns in which they were subsequently trained. Several of these physicians were descendants of traditional healers. Through their long-standing contacts with Europeans an ability developed among them to integrate traditional and modern medical approaches. The results of this study need to be interpreted in the light of Janzen's work in Zaïre (1978) and subsequent discussions (Janzen and Prins 1981) which allow the cosmopolitan medical system quite a limited role in the overall health care system of the country.

We can expect that anthropologists will find the dimensions I have mentioned regarding physician studies in the West considerably complicated in studies on physicians from developing countries. Such physicians are expected to link personal, traditional cultural knowledge with scientific knowledge in their practice of medicine including psychiatry. A point of some relevance here, too, is the community and public health orientation of new African physicians. This orientation is appropriate to the challenges of their role in their developing countries, but it is likely to generate a set of conflicts not limited to this one geographic region. Conflicting motivations, including the wish for higher remuneration, the desire for political involvement, and other motivations which arise from newly gained status are all widespread. We can expect such concerns to be of increasing interest to anthropologists who seek to portray traditional cultures against the background of their rising national health care interests and goals (Maretzki 1984; Salan and Maretzki 1983).

When the non-Western physician is fully included into anthropological studies of healing, new challenges will arise for comparative studies. George DeVos has given us some food for thought. Commenting on Reynold's (1980) discussion of Japanese therapies, DeVos (1980) suggests that it will not be easy to find appropriate espistemological bases for comparison. Different meanings attach to divergent situations. We may find that the Western physician will have difficulties in breaking through culturally shaped modes of thinking about illness, but that non-Western physicians may be able to bridge different cognitive models on the basis of personal cultural experiences. Our 'etic' and 'emic' distinctions are too simplistic to help us over such epistemological barriers. The challenge will be to remain firmly grounded in disciplinary efforts while exploring these horizons.

THE CLINICAL PRACTICE OF PHYSICIANS

For research purposes a distinction should be made between diagnostic and curative aspects of clinical practice. Both foci may be considered in the same study. Other topics, for instance the internal communication of clinical findings and patient progress during treatment, could be a third area of research. Anthropological investigations of this nature have barely begun. There are few precursors in medical sociology. I should again mention Fox's classic study emphasizing the physician-patient relationship under conditions of unusual stress (1959).

Szasz and Hollender in psychiatry (1956), and numerous other psychiatrists and other physicians since, have closely examined conceptually and clinically the nature of this core aspect of medical practice, the doctor-patient relationship (Balint 1957; Morgan and Engel 1969; Bowden and Burstein 1974; E. Cassell 1979). It is essential to appreciate this central theme in biomedical practice to see its importance in any research on the physician. Its principal elements are the physician's responsibility for the patient and the reciprocal trust of the patient. The full impact of this core theme can only be understood through participant observation.

In many biomedical situations, successful diagnosis and treatment require a close physician-patient relationship. But even where essential, this ideal is not often obtained in clinical practice. In primary medical care this relationship is considered basic, and therefore a goal of good practice. This can be contrasted with the episodic care of Emergency Room or some walk-in clinics. The crucial distinction between what physicians sometimes describe cynically and derogatorily as "veterinary care", as opposed to good medical care, hinges on a mutually satisfying relationship. Because many physicians are concerned about this central aspect of medical practice, medical anthropologists will find here opportunities for research. As anthropologists we were reminded long ago that there are more than verbal dimensions to effective communication; "*any* disturbance of the information processing systems should automatically be classified as a mental health problem" (Hall 1973). A microanalysis of doctor-patient interaction, following ethnosemantic approaches, illustrates the progressive structuring of interaction, the way in which each speaker in the doctor-patient dyad acknowledges or fails to acknowledge the other, and in so doing develops an effective or less effective communication (Robillard et al. 1982).

In the training of physicians until the present, more is left to modeling after experienced physicians than to systematic training of effective interaction styles. Perhaps, we would not even have moved, as we have, towards an increased understanding of the nature of miscommunication between physician and patient if it were not for the awakening of ethnic consciousness in the United States (Harwood 1981; Weidman 1978).

Recent waves of culturally distinct immigrants and sojourners from various parts of the world present with cultural problems in the clinical which call for appropriate responses (Pfifferling 1981; Weaver 1981). Problems with such patients have created an awareness, mostly outside Biomedicine, that *all* physician-patient encounters have a cultural dimension, even when the patient's general cultural background overlaps with that of the physician (Helman 1978; Blumhagen 1980).

In the diagnostic process, the patient's ability and willingness to share information by providing as accurate and valid a medical history as possible is not just a function of memory or education, or of English fluency. Gaines has pointed out that conceptions of self and person vary cross-culturally and greatly affect medical histories (1982a). Hahn (1982, and this volume) also discusses the role of the concept of the person in the practice of one physician, a general internist. Basic to the potential of a satisfactory relationship are opportunities for effective verbal communications (Weaver 1981).

With communications as the basic process for a data base, the nature and creation of medical knowledge is a topic of broad significance (Young 1981, 1982b). Young presents the perspective of the patient's communication of his/her state of health and sickness and raises questions about common anthropological interpretations; the applications in medical information exchange are quite obvious and directly implied. The essence of Young's presentation is that what he calls "actors" present their health and sickness status on the basis of ideology and knowledge and that, "he (the actor) continually evaluates it (his knowledge) against his intentions, expectations, and perceptions of events . . ." (1981:379). He points out further that scientific knowledge and ideological knowledge are not necessarily contradictory forms of belief (Young 1981:385). The key to Young's complex discussion is the physician's inclusion or non-inclusion in clinical work of social determinants of knowledge.

DIAGNOSTIC, RECORDING AND TREATMENT DECISIONS

The patient's socially and culturally informed presentation subsequently is processed by the physician into diagnostic and treatment decisions which also have social concomitants. Bosk (1980) has analyzed rituals which both validate the process of the decision-making and help to bridge uncertainty, thereby strengthening the physician's respect for the authority of those further up in the hierarchy. This analysis, of course, raises interesting questions about the diagnostic process in private practice where these mechanisms of social exchange and social control are less accessible, or totally inaccessible, so that the decision-making burden can not be shared, except during informal exchange in group practice or in social conversations. Gaines (1982b) explores a number of clinical cases where existing psychiatric definitions (diagnoses) were altered by the communication of relevant anthropological knowledge, theory and/or methodology. The work highlights the interpretive basis of diagnosis (see also Good and Good 1981).

Record keeping and health care team communications are other areas of physician centered activities which reflect basic cultural conceptualizations as part of the diagnostic process. The medical chart serves as a central information and storage system. The challenge for this record is that it should be relevant, accurate, comprehensive and parsimonious. The Problem Oriented Medical Record (POMR) is a physician initiated modification of recording patient problems which has spread widely through the medical system within a few years, but not without a substantial amount of criticism and resistance (Pfifferling 1977).

The purpose of the POMR is to list all problems presented by a patient; it therefore goes beyond the narrow organ pathology centered focus and includes psychosocial and cultural dimensions. "Objective" data and "subjective" data are listed separately, and an analysis helps in suggesting strategies for intervention.

Pfifferling, who followed and documented the reception of this innovation in two medical centers, claims that the physician can decide medical strategies appropriate to the patient's problems on an individual basis consonant with the overall objectives of medical treatment (1977). He expects that the POMR will result in a greater awareness, allowing physicians objectively to view their own rituals and magical thinking in medicine. The evaluation of effects of the POMR awaits further study, though Pfifferling warns of the obstacles to engaging in such research.

Treatment is probably most central to an ethnomedical focus on physicians. It is the goal of health-seeking behavior and, therefore, the essence of the physician's practice from the layman's point of view. Understanding efficacy in treatment is possible with a variety of approaches, including epidemiological research at one extreme and specific outcome studies of individual sickness episodes at the other. Jerome Frank's research (1961) on psychotherapy effects is widely known among psychiatrists as well as psychologically oriented medical anthropologists because it draws on comparative ethnographic materials. How psychiatrists have gone about evaluating their treatment through therapy outcome studies, and with what results, is reviewed in an article by Luborsky et al. (1975). Fuller Torrey, another psychiatrist, used his anthropological training and interests to observe treatment by healers in several cultures. He also surveyed the anthropological literature for other examples in order to present a popularly oriented study which equates psychiatric treatment approaches with those of different healers (e.g., shamans) throughout the world (Torrey 1972). These are some of the bridges that have been established between anthropology and psychiatry. More scholarly and original are the contributions to *Magic, Faith, and Healing* (Kiev 1964) — all this indicates the predominant role of psychiatry in comparative research on treatment.

Studies of some relevance to an understanding of treatment in a comparative perspective, including Western forms, seem preliminary when held against the work of Arthur Kleinman, and that of others who played an important role collateral to him. Many of them, social scientists and physicians, have published in the journal *Cultural, Medicine and Psychiatry* edited by Kleinman. The core work, however, is Kleinman's book, *Patients and Healers in the Context of Culture* (1980). In it he presents very detailed research data on treatment forms and outcome in a

Chinese culture (Taiwan). In so doing, he provides the broad conceptual framework
needed for such comparative studies, integrating anthropological and clinical
orientations, and the appropriate understanding of the physician's tasks and limitations. Key concepts such as clinical reality, curing, healing, explanatory models,
all are explored on the basis of findings and related back to the broad perspective
which Kleinman has developed in conjunction with Leon Eisenberg (see also
Eisenberg and Kleinman 1981).

Kleinman's orientation is grounded in the distinction of disease, as the mal-
functioning of biological and psychological processes as these are diagnosed in
biomedical practice, and illness, the subjective psychosocial and cultural experience
and meaning of a perceived state of sickness (1980:72). This implies that curing
and healing as processes can only be understood in terms of the broad psychosocial
and sociocultural context of illness construction (see Good 1977). It follows
that in modern biomedical care physicians may cure, but cannot heal (Kleinman
1980: 363–364). The evaluation of effectiveness of treatment has to be made on
the basis of patient perception, not just physician's judgment. Coming to terms
with differential interpretations of "clinical reality" is a core task of physicians
(Kleinman 1980:375).

Kleinman's work is recent, but its impact on new directions in medical anthropology and medicine are already evident. In fact, the present volume, and the series
of which it is a part, owe much to the insights of Kleinman. Since Kleinman also
perceives a role for medical anthropologists as clinical consultants (not therapists)
in the diagnostic and treatment strategy planning of physicians (1982), the importance of his work may not be judged only on the basis of understanding derived
from research, but by more critical and sensitive criteria of professional roles in
clinical practice.

Earlier I pointed to the broad range of anthropological activities, and the fact
that there is a biological sub-specialization in anthropology. We assume that as
further research develops, and more bridges are built between Biomedicine and
medical anthropology, research on the effectiveness of treatment will turn to
links between biological processes in the human organism and cultural processes,
and that this will permit new study targets for anthropologists investigating the
physician as healer.

CONCLUSIONS

It is fair to say that a new direction in medical anthropology is emerging in which
studies of the biomedical physician will assume an important place. I have outlined
some antecedents for such studies and the expansion of the field. The chapters
in this book add new and original research results and theoretical innovations.

Seen from the wider perspectives of anthropology, the social sciences, or from
that of Biomedicine, these efforts may be judged as modest in scope. But subjects
explored in this volume, such as semantic illness networks, folk theories in Biomedicine, the relation of biomedical science to culture and others, are much more

important than those engaged in health care planning and services seem able to acknowledge.

It is prudent to adopt a scale for assessing the impact of new ideas which retains a sense of realism. The American health care system is exploding in many directions simultaneously. The expansion of scientific knowledge leads to new containment of diseases, faster we hope than diseases develop and take hold; chronicity is an increasing difficult problem for a 'curative' medicine (Alexander 1982). Techno-logical refinements in treatment are not only costly, they multiply the system's complexities. The wish for a more holistic approach to health clashes with these developments, yet it is a growing and revolutionary force. Costs of health care are immense, but these are not the only determinants, as policy makers seem to think, of the problems besetting the health care system. The anthropological approach to understanding culture and organism provides for different views of the development of obstacles in health care and effective responses to them. Central to the anthropological orientation is the often crucial influence of the cultural basis of biomedical intervention and healing.

If all of this manifold cultural context of practice were communicated to the individual physician in Biomedicine, perhaps more physicians would see the value of cooperating with medical anthropological studies of the many-sided role of physician as healer. We, in turn, would be able to offer research approaches that are geared to the great and complex diversity of cultural forces impinging on this key professional health role.

We can take the position that all the research we wish to generate about the physician in Biomedicine is part of the academic process of the search for knowl-edge and its exchange among disciplines, a function which most of the works cited here have had. But we cannot sidestep the question of how far beyond this we wish to go, or may be driven, as medical anthropologists; for our field of inquiry has very practical human importance. Are we following Kleinman's recommenda-tion to enter clinical and public health settings and become engaged as consultants, thus drawing upon the research we generate for practical applications? Should we, as medical anthropologists, expect to put our shoulders to the wheel in some practical role in health care systems or their development? There can be no doubt that the study of the physician of Biomedicine brings the medical anthropologist in contact with different uses of knowledge and opens up professional roles different from those we once knew as students of small scale societies. The study of the physician, his/her ideology and praxis, promises to be a difficult enterprise. The problems and the prospects are clearly indicated by this volume and other examples of our first, halting efforts to illuminate our subject, the physicians of Western medicine.

REFERENCES

Alland, Alexander, Jr.
  1966 Medical Anthropology and the Study of Biological and Cultural Adapatation. American Anthropologist 68:40–51.

Alexander, Linda
    1979 Clinical Anthropology: Morals and Methods. Medical Anthropology 3(11):61–107.
    1982 Illness Maintenance and the New American Sick Role. In Chrisman, Noel and T.
           Maretzki (eds.), Clinically Applied Anthropology. Dordrecht, Holland: D. Reidel
           Publishing Co.
Balint, Michael
    1957 The Doctor, His Patient and the Illness. New York: International Universities Press.
Becker, Howards S., B. Geer, E. C. Highes, A. Strauss
    1961 Boys in White: Student Culture in Medical School. Chicago: The University of
           Chicago Press.
Bennett, Linda (ed.)
    1982 Reconsidering Appropriate Roles for Medical Anthropologists in Clinical Settings:
           Case Studies. Medical Anthropology Newsletter 14(1):18–26.
Bosk, Charles
    1979 Forgive and Remember: Managing Medical Failure. Chicago: The University of
           Chicago Press.
    1980 Occupational Rituals in Patient Management. New England Journal of Medicine
           303(2):71–76.
Bowden, Charles L. and Alvin G. Burstein
    1974 Psychosocial Basis of Medical Practice: An Introduction to Human Behavior.
           Baltimore: The Williams and Wilkings Co.
Blumhagen, Dan
    1980 Hypertension: A Folk Illness with a Medical Name. Culture, Medicine and Psychiatry
           4(3):197–277.
Brody, Howard
    1983 Does Disease Have a Natural History? Medical Anthropology Quarterly 14(4):3ff.
Capra, Fritjof
    1982 The Turning Point. New York: Simon and Schuster.
Cassell, Eric
    1979 The Healer's Art. Baltimore: Penguin Books.
Cassell, Joan
    1981 Technical Error and Moral Error in Medicine and Fieldwork. Human Organization
           40(2):160–168.
Caudill, William A.
    1958 The Hospital as a Small Society. Cambridge, Mass.: Harvard University Press.
Chrisman, Noel T. and Thomas W. Maretzki (eds.)
    1982 Clinically Applied Anthropology. Dordrecht, Holland: D. Reidel Publishing Company.
Cousins, Norman
    1979 Anatomy of an Illness as Perceived by the Patient: Reflecting on Healing and Re-
           generation. New York: W. W. Norton.
De Craemer, Willy and Renée C. Fox
    1968 The Emerging Physician. A Sociological Approach to the Development of a Congolese
           Medical Profession. Stanford: The Hoover Institution, Stanford University.
Duffy, John
    1979 The Healer: A History of American Medicine. Champaign, Ill.: University of Illinois
           Press.
Dunn, Fredrick L.
    1976 Traditional Asian Medicine and Cosmopolitan Medicine as Adaptive Systems. In
           Leslie (ed.), Asian Medical Systems. Berkeley: University of California Press.
De Vos, George
    1980 Afterword. In David K. Reynolds, The Quiet Therapies. Honolulu: The University
           Press of Hawaii.
Eisenberg, Leon and Arthur Kleinman (eds.)
    1981 The Relevance of Social Science for Medicine. Dordrecht, Holland: D. Reidel Publ. Co.

Engel George L.
   1977 The Need for a New Medical Model: A Challenge for Bio-Medicine. Science 196:
         129–136.
   1982 The Biopsychosocial Model and Mental Education. The New England Journal of
         Medicine 306(13):802–805.
Estroff, Sue E.
   1981 Making It Crazy: An Ethnography of Psychiatric Clients in a Community. Berkeley:
         The University of California Press.
Foster, George M.
   1974 Medical Anthropology: Some Contrasts with Medical Sociology. Medical Anthro-
         pology Newsletter 6(1):1–5.
Foster, George M. and Barbara G. Anderson
   1978 Medical Anthropology. New York: John Wiley & Sons.
Fox, Renée C.
   1959 Experiment Perilous. Philadelphia: University of Pennsylvania Press.
   1975 Training for Uncertainty. In R. Merton, G. Reader, and P. L. Kendall (eds.), The
         Student Physician. Cambridge, Mass.: Harvard University Press.
   1979a Essays in Medical Sociology: Journey Into the Field. New York: John Wiley &
         Sons.
   1979b The Human Condition of Health Professionals. University of New Hampshire Dis-
         tinguished Lecture Series.
Fox, Renée C. and H. I. Lief
   1963 Training for Detached Concern in Medical Students. In H. I. Lief et al., (eds.), The
         Psychological Basis of Medical Practice. Berkeley: University of California Press.
Freidson, Eliot
   1970a Professional Dominance: The Social Structure of Medical Care. New York: Atherton
         Press.
   1970b Profession of Medicine: A Study of the Sociology of Applied Knowledge. New York:
         Dodd Mead.
Frank, Jerome D.
   1961 Persuasion and Healing: A Comparative Study of Psychothreapy. Baltimore: The
         Johns Hopkins University Press.
Gaines, Atwood D.
   1979 Definitions and Diagnoses: Cultural Implications of Psychiatric Help-Seeking and
         Psychiatrists' Definitions of the Situation in Psychiatric Emergencies. Culture,
         Medicine and Psychiatry 3(4):381–418.
   1982a Cultural Definitions, Behavior and the Person in American Psychiatry. In A. Marsella
         and G. White (eds.), Cultural Conceptions of Mental Health and Therapy. Dordrecht,
         Holland: D. Reidel Publishing Co.
   1982b Knowledge and Practice. In: N. Chrisman and T. Maretzki (eds.), Clinically Applied
         Anthropology. Dordrecht, Holland: D. Reidel Publishing Co.
   1982c The Twice-Born: 'Christian Psychiatry' and Christian Psychiatrists. In A. Gaines and
         R. Hahn (eds.), Physicians of Western Medicine: Five Cultural Studies. Special Issue.
         Medicine and Psychiatry 6(3):305–324.
Gaines, Atwood D. and Robert A. Hahn (eds.)
   1982 Physicians of Western Medicine: Five Cultural Studies. Special Issue. Culture, Medi-
         cine and Psychiatry 6(3).
Garrison, Vivian
   1977 Doctor, Espiritista or Psychiatrist? Health Seeking Behavior in a Puerto Rican Neigh-
         borhood of New York City. Medical Anthropology 1:65–180.
Good, Byron
   1977 The Heart of What's the Matter. Culture, Medicine and Psychiatry 1(1):25–58.
Good, Byron and Mary-Jo DelVecchio Good
   1981 The Meaning of Symptoms: A Cultural Hermeneutic Model for Clinical Practice.

In L. Eisenberg and A. Kleinman (eds.), The Relevance of Social Science for Medicine. Dordrecht, Holland: D. Reidel Publishing Co.

Hahn, Robert A.
1982 "Treat the Patient, Not the Lab": Internal Medicine and the Concept of the 'Person'. *In* A. Gaines and R. Hahn (eds.), Physicians of Western Medicine: Five Cultural Studies. Special Issue. Culture, Medicine and Psychiatry 6(3):219–236.

Hahn, Robert A. and Arthur Kleinman
1983 Belief as Pathogen, Belief as Medicine: "Vodoo Death" and the "Placebo Phenomenon" in Anthropological Perspective. Medical Anthropology Quarterly 14(4):3ff.

Hall, Edward T.
1973 Mental Health Research and Out-of-Awareness Cultural Systems. *In* L. Nader and T. Maretzki (eds.), Cultural Illness and Health. Washington, D.C.: American Anthropological Association.

Harwood, Alan (ed.)
1981 Ethnicity and Medical Care. Cambridge, Mass.: Harvard University Press.

Helman, Cecil G.
1978 'Feed a Cold, Starve a Fever' – Folk Models of Infection in an English Suburban Community and Their Relation to Medical Treatment. Culture, Medicine and Psychiatry 2(2):107–137.

Huntington, Mary Jean
1957 The Development of a Professional Self-Image. *In* R. Merton, R. G. Reader and P. L. Kendall (eds.), The Student Physician. Cambridge, Mass.: Harvard University Press.

Illich, Ivan
1975 Medical Nemesis: The Expropriation of Health. London: Clader and Boyars.

Ingelfinger, John M.
1976 Listen: The Patient – Once Again. New England Journal of Medicine 295(26): 1478–1479.

Janzen, John M.
1978 The Quest for Therapy in Lower Zaïre. Berkeley: University of California Press.

Janzen, John M. and G. Prins (eds.)
1981 Causality and Classification in African Medicine and Health. Social Science and Medicine 15B (3).

Jellinek, Michael
1976 Erosion of Patient Trust in Large Medical Centers. The Hastings Center Report 6(3):16–19.

Kiev, Ari (ed.)
1964 Magic, Faith and Healing: Studies in Primitive Psychiatry Today. Glencoe: The Free Press.

Kleinman, Arthur
1980 Patients and Healers in the Context of Culture. Berkeley: The University of California Press.
1982 Clinically Applied Anthropology in a Psychiatric Consultation-Liaison Service. *In* N. Chrisman and T. Maretzki (eds.), Clinically Applied Anthropology. Dordrecht, Holland: D. Reidel Publishing Co.

Kleinman, Arthur, L. Eisenberg, and B. Good
1978 Culture, Illness and Healing. The Annals of Internal Medicine 88:251–258.

Kluckhohn, Florence R. and F. L. Strodtbeck
1961 Variations in Value Orientations. New York: Row, Peterson and Co.

Knowles, John (ed.)
1977 Doing Better and Feeling Worse: Health in the United States. New York: W. Norton.

Lazare, Aaron
  1973 Hidden Conceptual Models in Clinical Psychiatry. New England Journal of Medicine
      288:345–351.
Lévi-Strauss, Claude
  1967a The Sorcerer and His Magic. In C. Lévi Strauss, Structural Anthropology. Doubleday
      and Co.
  1967b The Effectiveness of Symbols. In C. Lévi Strauss, Structural Anthropology. Doubleday
      and Co.
Light, Donald
  1980 Becoming Psychiatrists: The Professional Transformation of the Self. New York:
      W. W. Norton.
Lock, Margaret
  1982 Models and Practice in Medicine: Menopause as Syndrome or Life Transition? In
      A. Gaines and R. Hahn (eds.), Physicians of Western Medicine: Five Cultural Studies.
      Special Issue. Culture, Medicine and Psychiatry 6(3):261–290.
Lorber, Judith
  1975 Women and Medical Sociology: Invisible Professionals and Ubiquitous Patients. In
      M. Millman and R. M. Kauter (eds.), Sciences. New York: Anchor Press.
Luborsky, L. et al.
  1975 Comparative Study of Psychotherapy: Is It True That, "Everyone Has Won and All
      Must Have Prizes"? Archives of General Psychiatry 32:995–1008.
McCue, Jack D.
  1981 The Effects of Stress on Physicians and Their Medical Practice. New England Journal
      of Medicine 306(8):458–463.
Maretzki, Thomas W. and E. Seidler
  1984 Realities of Mental Health Service Development: A Case Study. In P. Pederson and
      A. Marsella (eds.), Cross-Cultural Mental Health Services. Beverly Hills: Sage Publica-
      tions.
Maretzki, Thomas W. and E. Seideler
  1983 Biomedicine and Naturopathic Healing: A Historical View of a Stormy Relationship
      in Germany. Unpublished manuscript.
Mechanic, David
  1976 The Growth of Bureaucratic Medicine. New York: John Wiley & Sons.
Mechanic, David
  1979 Future Issues in Health Care: Social Policy and the Rationing of Medical Services.
      New York: Free Press.
Medical Anthropology Newsletter
  1980 Open Forum: Clinical Anthropology 12(1):14–25.
Merton, Robert, G. Reader, P. L. Kendall (eds.)
  1957 The Student Physician: Introductory Studies in the Sociology of Medical Education.
      Cambridge, Mass.: Harvard University Press.
Moerman, Daniel E.
  1979 Anthropology of Symbolic Healing. Current Anthropology 20:59.
  1983 General Medical Effectiveness and Human Biology: Placebo Effects in the Treatment
      of Ulcer Disease. Medical Anthropology Quarterly 14(4):3ff.
Morgan, W. L. and G. L. Engel
  1969 The Clinical Approach to the Patient. Philadelphia: W. B. Saunders Co.
Mumford, Emily
  1970 Interns: From Students to Physicians. Cambridge, Mass.: Harvard University Press.
Olesen, Virginia
  1974 Convergences and Divergences: Anthropology and Sociology in Health Care. Medical
      Anthropology Newsletter 6(1):6–10.

Petersdorf, Robert G. and A. R. Feinstein
    1981 An Informal Appraisal of the Current Status of 'Medical Sociology'. *In* L. Eisenberg
          and A. Kleinman (eds.), The Relevance of Social Science for Medicine. Dordrecht,
          Holland: D. Reidel Publishing Co.
Pfifferling, John Henry
    1977 Records and Revitalization: The Problem Oriented Medical Records System in a
          Clinical Setting. Ann Arbor, Mass.: University Microfilms International.
    1981 A Cultural Prescription for Medicocentrism. *In* L. Eisenberg and A. Kleinman (eds.),
          The Relevance of Social Science for Medicine. Dordrecht, Holland: D. Reidel Publ.
          Co.
Press, Irwin
    1982 Witch Doctor's Legacy: Some Anthropological Implications for the Practice of
          Clinical Medicine. *In* N. Chrisman and T. Maretzki (eds.). Clinically Applied An-
          thropology. Dordrecht, Holland: D. Reidel Publ. Co.
Reynolds, David
    1980 The quiet therapies. Honolulu: The University Press of Hawaii.
Riley, James N.
    1980 The Quiet Therapies. Honolulu: The University Press of Hawaii.
          Social Science and Medicine 14B:111–120.
Roberts, Cecilia M.
    1977 Doctor and Patient in the Teaching Hospital. Lexington, Mass.: D. Heath Co.
Robillard, A. B., G. White, and T. Maretzki
    1982 Between Doctor and Patient: Informed Consent in Conversational Interaction. *In*
          S. Fisher and A. Todd (eds.), The Social Organization of Doctor-Patient Interaction.
          Washington, D.C.: Space Center for Applied Linguistics.
Russel, John C.
    1982 Responsibilities of Anthropological Researchers in Clinical Settings. Human Organiza-
          tion 42(1):63–69.
Salan, Rudy, and T. Maretzki
    1983 Mental Health Services and Traditional Healing in Indonesia: Are the Roles Com-
          patible? Culture, Medicine and Psychiatry 7(4):1–40.
Scully, Diana
    1980 Men Who Control Women's Health: The Miseducation of Obstetrician-Gynecologists.
          Boston: Houghton Mifflin Co.
Skipper, James K. Jr. (ed.)
    1978 Medical Sociology and Chiropractice. Sociological Symposium 22.
Snyder, Patricia
    1983 The Use of Nonprescribed Treatments by Hemodialysis Patients. Culture, Medicine
          and Psychiatry 7(1):13–32.
Starr, Paul
    1982 The Social Transformation for American Medicine. Cambridge, Mass.: Harvard
          University Press.
Szasz, Thomas S. and M. H. Hollender
    1956 A Contribution of the Philosophy of Medicine – The Basic Models of the Doctor-
          Patient Relationship. Archives of Internal Medicine 97:585.
Thomas, Lewis
    1971 The Technology of Medicine. The New England Journal of Medicine 285(24):1366–
          1368.
Torrey, E. Fuller
    1972 The Mind Game: Witchdoctors and Psychiatrists. New York: Emerson Hall Publishers.
Turner, Victor
    1967 Forest of Symbols. Ithaca, N. Y.: Space Cornell University Press.

Unschuld, Paul
    1979 Medical Ethics in Imperial China: A Study in Historical Anthropology. Berkeley:
        University of California Press.
Vaillant, George, J. R. Brighton, C. McArthur
    1970 Physician Use of Mood-Altering Drugs: A 20-Year Follow-Up Report. New England
        Journal of Medicine 282(7):365–370.
Wallis, Roy and P. Morley (eds.)
    1977 Marginal Medicine. New York: Free Press.
Wardwell, Walter I.
    1980 The Future of Chiropractice. New England Journal of Medicine 302(12):668–690.
Weaver, Charlotte A.
    1981 Role Evolution of Language Translators in a Major Medical Center. Unpublished
        Ph.D. dissertation. The University of California, San Francisco.
Weed, Lawrence, L.
    1981 Physician of the Future. New England Journal of Medicine 304(15):903–907.
Weideman, Hazel et al.
    1978 Miami Health Ecology Project Report, Volume 1. University of Miami (offprint).
Wellin, Edward
    1977 Theoretical Orientation in Medical Authropology: Continuity and Change over the
        Past Half-Century. In: D. Landy (ed.), Culture, Disease, and Healing. New York:
        Macmillan Publishing Co.
Wennberg, John and A. Gittelson
    1982 Variations in Medical Care Among Small Areas. Scientific American 246(4):120–
        135.
Weppner, Robert S.
    1973 An Anthropological View of the Street Addict's World. Human Organization 32(2):
        111–121.
Young, Allan
    1981 The Creation of Medical Knowledge: Some Problems of Interpretation. Social Science
        and Medicine 15B(3):379–386.
    1982a The Anthropology of Illness and Sickness. In B. Siegel, A. Beals, S. Tyler (eds.),
        Annual Review of Anthropology 11. Palo Alto, California: Annual Reviews. Inc.
    1982b When Rational Men Fall Sick: An Inquiry Into Some Assumptions Made by Medical
        Anthropologists. Culture, Medicine and Psychiatry 5(4):317–335.

SECTION II

CORE MEDICINE

ROBERT A. HAHN

A WORLD OF INTERNAL MEDICINE: PORTRAIT OF AN INTERNIST

> Nothing is black or white. I'm beginning to
> think there's no such things as black or white.
> When they're dead, they're white.
> – Barry Siegler, M.D., Cartown, U.S.A., 1979.

CONTENTS

A. A STUDY OF THE WORLD VIEW OF A PRACTICING INTERNIST: INTRODUCTION

The following portrait attempts to penetrate and represent the thought-world of a single practitioner of general internal medicine, to depict the premises, attitudes, and values which guide, express, and rationalize this practitioner's experience of medical work. I seek to formulate the coherence and incoherence of his thought, its dominant metaphors, and the troubles and the pleasures of his work. I explore the ways in which the work of general internal medicine, "physiological integrity", corresponds to the consciousness, action, and environment of one practitioner. I refer to this man as "Barry Siegler", though this is not his name.

Internal medicine is the mind, if not the heart, of 'Western' medicine — Biomedicine. It is called simply "medicine". It is medicine's medicine, the generic and central specialty to which other specialties refer for the last word on our underlying ills, our "diseases". Internal medicine is perhaps the most rational of Biomedical specialties, advocating action by systematic calculation of the patient's

51

internal pathophysiology, in preference to more direct, surgical penetration for unobstructed vision and intervention.

While their techniques are often lethally and vitally powerful, internists are inclined to favor reason over force, and integral strategy over topical action. Medicine is thus known among fellow specialties as "conservative": To "go medically" is purportedly to intervene more cautiously, to act mainly from outside the body's boundaries, "non-invasively"; perhaps it is to respect more fully the body's constitutional and physiological processes. Yet even non-invasive medicine may be more or less "aggressive", actively intervening or forbearing entirely — "doing nothing", to allow a so-called "natural" course.

The present portrait is the first of four. From these four I will attempt a composite exemplifying the core of medical practice, general internal medicine. I will then compare this U.S. medicine with what anthropologists have reported of "non-Western" healers, for example indigenous Amazonian curers, Chinese shamans, and African diviners. A first object of this comparison is an understanding of the nature of medical thought and practice, and of pathology and healing, by an exploration of their varied sociocultural settings.

It has been pointed out to me that four subjects (in comparison to a population of 350 000 U.S. physicians, 71 000 internists, and a fraction of general internists) is a very small number, one from which generalization is not possible. I have been concerned to plumb the depths of the conscious worlds of a few practitioners rather then to survey a larger sample. I have followed these individuals where they led me rather than asking only predetermined questions and accepting only predetermined answers. The contrast in approaches parallels that between some versions of anthropology and of sociology.

The four internists I have studied were not selected in a random fashion. Yet these four physicians are exemplary in two senses: they are representative of their profession, its values, premises and practice, representative also of cultural features of the broader society. In addition, they are exemplary in fulfilling professional and societal expectations in a highly competent fashion. Though my own medical ignorance by no means allows rigorous evaluation, I have an intuitive sense (perhaps akin to the sense which patients have) that these practitioners are fully capable in what they do. My intuition may derive in part from the clear respect these men are given in the medical community, in part from the thought-out knowledge they express in encounters with colleagues.

In the present study I am not so much testing theoretical hypotheses as exploring a phenomenon, taking a theoretical position as background. In my comparative study of four internists in cross-cultural perspective, I will more systematically explore the fit (and misfit) of healers' beliefs in the dynamics of society.

The theoretical focus underlying the present study is *work*. I am only peripherally concerned here with work as paid labor. I focus on work as the directed expenditure of effort; I thus include "housework", "recreation", and "contemplation", even "sleep" (e.g., "dream work") and other forms of "rest". Work is the effort and concomitant product of action (and inaction).

I am concerned with two faces of work, the personal and the social. In their exertions, persons at once express themselves and reciprocally absorb those parts of the world touched by their expressions; expression (a pushing out) and internalization (a taking in) are consequences of work. A basic human project is the "work of self", a work by and of self, for, and perhaps against self. The construction, maintenance, and continuing adaptation of self is an ongoing collaboration of persons and their environments.

By these same exertions and their by-products, human work creates and recreates society — the structure and unfolding process of interacting humanity. Giddens (1976), following de Saussure, has used the phrase, "duality of structure", to refer to the human response to a given social order in the production, even the reproduction, of further, consequent social orders. I am recommending work, the human expenditure of effort, as the event mediating both societal and personal creation, growth, and reproduction. I thus propose a union of the works of George Herbert Mead on the *social construction of self* and Karl Marx on the *production of society*. Both of these phrases are deliberately ambiguous. At once, persons and the societies in which they live create themselves and each other, and are thus created by themselves and each other.

Mediated by social relations of work, individuals are connected to others by two complementary processes of communication: internalization and expression. Through internalization, society — its understandings, values and rules — is literally incorporated within persons. Persons are made to be social, to take within themselves the culture of their society; they are socialized. By expression, what is within, internalized, comes out, intended or not. Expression may accomplish many things, including the representation of an individual's version of his/her society, its culture, and the world. In this study of physicians, I examine expressed belief to explore individuals' versions of the culture of Biomedicine. I interpret what these physicians say in different settings to abstract a system which lies within, a system which may be thought of as generating situationally appropriate expressions of belief.

While I examine individuals as the possessors and expressors of belief, I do not think that the individual is either the beginning or the end of the matter of belief, but rather, the medium. An individual's beliefs are his/her version, a turn or twist, of what is believed by consociates. Moreover, the expression of belief is constrained by the rules of social behavior; it is guided by the believer's motives and by his/her understanding of the social situation which he/she addresses. Expressions of belief then continue to socialize others, by an internal response to what is expressed. I examine the beliefs of individuals as vital signs of this social dynamic.

In medicine and its specialities work is defined in a certain way. Some tasks fall within its scope, others do not; these sorts of information, technique, and response are appropriate, others are not. The bounds of work, and work within those bounds, entail a theory — a theory that the bounded phenomena are sufficiently isolated or discrete that they may be separately identified, predicted, and treated — separately, that is, from what lies beyond those bounds. Devoted work assumes also that such efforts are of sufficient value to call for their isolated pursuit.

In general internal medicine, the work was succinctly defined by one of my informants as "physiological integrity". In this case study of Barry Siegler I explore some implications of the division implied by this definition. It is a division which corresponds to distinctions deeply embedded within our culture (see Fox 1979; DeTocqueville 1969) — mind-body dualism, pragmatism, empiricism, individualism, and a tension between realism and nominalism. The manifestations of these are explored in my analysis. Taussig (1980) and Young (1980) have argued that some of these principles constitute a part of what might be called "the capitalist metaphysic". The division corresponds also to some of Barry's personal characteristics — to his own personal troubles with the personal troubles of others. At work within these boundaries of physiological wholeness, Barry finds much satisfaction as well as some frustration; at the beyond these boundaries, frustration and anxiety loom large.

My comparative study is 'based on' and refers to a body of information produced by the method which is the hallmark of anthropology — participant observation. It is the standard method of the field; yet it is hardly standardized, and it is not clear just what its standards are, and in what ways, if any, it is a method. Essentially, in participant observation the researcher is present and thus participates in some fashion in the scene which he/she also observes and analyzes. The observer's presence may, but need not, lend a close familiarity with the subject observed; the observer may even come to share in the experience of those he/she observes. His or her presence may also affect the scene and phenomena observed, and should thus be taken into account in knowing what is "there" without this presence.

That such a study as this is 'based on' the 'data' 'collected' in the field is a partial illusion which survives an empiricist and inductivist theory of knowledge. By this theory, knowledge appears in discrete bits of 'data', kindly given in or by our environment. Scientists (and other knowers) go out into the field with collecting 'instruments' to gather these data into larger and larger bundles which may then be 'written up'. According to this theory, knowledge is built simply on empirical foundations; it reflects the (one and only) reality.

While such a theory is perpetuated by the language if not the thought of much anthropological writing, it is contradicted by the principal tenet of this same discipline — that human thought and (other) action is ordered by 'cultures' which vary extensively among societies and their divisions. While there is some sort of objecting, objective 'reality' beyond our culturally ordered perceptions, this reality is stingy. It gives little, as the etymology of 'datum' misleads us to believe. Rather, it is human thought which gives form to reality; I thus use "information" rather than "datum". Humans apprehend or take what they know at least as much as it is given to them. This cultural ordering interacts in a complex dialectical fashion with the seemingly harder orders of the objective world.

My representation of physicians' work and worlds is thus a response to my own cultural situation. It is cast in my idiom, formulated by my principles, directed toward the solution of my problematics. My representation of Barry Siegler is mine as well as his, an interactive product, from its most empirical, objective, factual 'evidence' to its more inferential and speculative conclusions. The ethnographer's presence in his ethnography is not invisible, as phenomenology and ethnoscience might have us believe; the ethnographer's presence is manifest.

Yet, while recognizing my presence in my representation of others, I also maintain that I have produced a document which both enters the thought system of of the physician and shapes the very formulation of this system in ways which make sense in its own terms. Thus, in writing of Barry Siegler, I order and title divisions of my analysis with key idioms from Barry's speech. I move to understand his metaphysics, his morality, his theory of knowledge, and his values; and in doing so, I use his own understandings of these matters — "God's mechanisms", "Judgment", "Pictures", "Patients", "Pandoras", "Surprising as Hell", and so on.

Of all people, anthropologists should not deny the quality of their own work as social, cultural, and personal event. Yet the author's personal engagement in such work is commonly ignored in anthropological research (as it is in medical practice). While such work may perhaps be undertaken without engagement or reflective awareness, lack of reflection may also signal the author's suffering and self-denial, and hinder intimate knowledge of the informant as subject. Failure to recognize engagement (i.e., in 'countertransference') yields a misunderstanding of the resulting work itself on the parts of author as well as reader (Devereux 1967). Rosengarten (1981) reflects on the importance of love in his relations with the subject of his 'autobiography' of Nate Shaw. I would add that other passions may intrude as well — anger, resentment, hatred; no one of these excludes others.

I met Barry Siegler through a colleague, and asked him if I might follow him in his medical work, to learn what he did and what he thought. (Barry himself later referred me to the next physician with whom I worked.) Though he did not seem especially concerned, I promised confidentiality and anonymity to both him and all of his patients and colleagues whom we would see.

Over the course of five months in 1978, I accompanied Barry Siegler on daily hospital rounds, consultations at a hypertension clinic, occasional office visits, and night and weekend call. Barry most often introduced me as "Dr. Hahn", as if I were a member of the medical team. Indeed I suspect that even when he introduced me as "an anthropologist", some patients understood me to be a medical specialist like a cardiologist or a nephrologist. Barry would occasionally introduce me as a researcher studying the practice of medicine in the U.S.

My participation in the scene I observed was minimal. I attempted not to interrupt the press of medical work, the work of doctors and patients. As we moved between medical events Barry would often share with me his reaction to events and persons he encountered, perhaps to get them off his chest, perhaps to inform me, perhaps for both of these or for some other reason. In rounds I would occasionally ask questions; or I might be offered unsolicited explanations. In a minimal reciprocity, I took phone messages, reminded Barry that he had been paged on the loud speaker system, and recalled phone numbers. Barry would sometimes refer to me as a witness to others in the rounds team that he had said or done something. I was with him for a longer period than were the residents who worked with different physicians, and who may have been beginners. I would occasionally watch them make what I knew was, by Barry's standards, a mistake.

My ignorance of medicine proved both a handicap and an advantage. Though I learned some medicine on the job, I was never sufficiently well versed in its principles and logic to be able to evaluate properly decisions made, to assess the alternatives or understand the subtleties of their purposes and consequences. My ignorance also gave me the pleasure of encountering a new language, the dialect of medical talk, rich in its own forms of discourse and in a vocabulary which overlapped with common usage, but which was in many ways distinctive. Medical talk maintains a separation from patients, and a distance also from the immediacy of their suffering. Referring to cancer as "CA" and to an amputation as "BK" — below the knee, may afford this double defense. I attempted both to see the profusion of color in this language and to understand its medicalized interpretations — elevated, cut and cleaned — antiseptic. Barry speaks this dialect with fluency and grace, and from this vantage point, was a pleasure to hear. He too seemed pleasurably aware of its etymology and even of its poetry.

The majority of my information is verbal, consisting of selected portions from hundreds of hours of Barry's talk with patients, residents, nurses, colleagues and me. The talk I have recorded is principally meta-medical: it is *about* as well as being a *part* of medical work. I have worked in the interstices of Barry's medicine, in the cracks or interludes between the calculations of how much of what medicine is required for this or that condition, between the gathering and giving of narrowly medical information, between visits with different patients. I have not been concerned with the details of medical logic, but with the framework in which it is set, and with reactions to it — its uncertainties, its purposes.

I have attempted to discern the multiple connections between language genres in Barry's usuage in order to construct a system which might account for his verbal and other expressions and actions. Barry is highly articulate in his work, capable of effecting desired results. I have tried to represent his facility. His expression reveals a pathos inherent in medical work, one not well confronted by our medicine.

I have paid close attention to idioms and epithets and to concepts which illuminate Barry's understanding of this work, its fundamental elements, its sources, its objects and his. Barry repeats variations of several epithets in many settings, and I have accordingly given great weight to these, carefully exploring their sense. I analyze the life of his metaphors to discover how close a literal interpretation accompanies metaphorical allusion. When literal usage is nearby in time, the idiom is more than empty or dead metaphor. Thus, for example, in Barry's talk I believe references to God, sex and excrement are more than simply metaphoric idioms. Literal reference is close by in the background.

My own feelings about Barry will be apparent in the portrait. I was and remain highly ambivalent, greatly admiring this man for his medical competence and his social and political agility, wishing to be closer to him, yet at the same time greatly resenting his medicalized vision which ignored what I take to be the core of persons, resenting also his vulgarized physical expressions and his abusive remarks about patients and others, especially about women and about those he held in moral contempt. Perhaps I have been insufficiently compassionate with the plight of his work, myself overwhelmed by his harsh expressions of suffering.

Little of this dark side did I suspect as I began my work. I knew of Barry only as a physician repeatedly paged on the hospital loudspeaker system, when I was engaged in other work (as social scientist on Pediatric 'rounds'). I knew that he was highly sought after and highly respected. He was the first physician I approached for my study, and I was delighted that he accepted my request without hesitation. I have not sought, as one of my colleagues (an internist) has criticized me, to ideologically represent medicine and its practices in some prejudged fashion, a caricature. The other doctors I will describe are each very different in attitude; my more personal reactions to them differ as well.

Despite what I believe is my penetration of his cosmological framework, I do not feel that I have shared Barry's more intimate feelings in his medical work. This itself is telling, and I believe he avoided and hid these intimacies from himself almost as much as he hid them from me. Barry is articulate and expressive, but also guarded, defensive, and not highly introspective.

I believe that, as with the other internists I observed, Barry derived some personal satisfaction in being thought of as sufficiently interesting to be observed closely over a few months' time by a serious anthropologist. But, thoroughly pragmatic, Barry was ambivalent about academics, as I describe below. I believe he was as often irked as stimulated by my probing, and by some of the 'liberal' values which may have been hidden or explicit in my questions, my beard, and my comfortable, nonconformist dress (though still within the mode of jacket and tie).

Though I did not ask him, I believe that Barry also has mixed feelings about me. He warmly accepted my request to accompany him in his work, though he was cautious about my joining him in office visits because, he said, it would slow him down too much, and he already "ran behind". In the hospital and clinic, his more public work, Barry was exceptionally open to me. I believe that my presence affected his performance little, though people who had worked with him told me that in my company, Barry was gentler in his relations. While at some level highly self-aware, he did not seem constrained. Only once or twice did he ask me not to repeat something he had said — his legitimate right, my obligation.

I do not think that he understood my quest for his cosmic framework and metaphysics, notions which he might deny having or considering clear or worthy. I believe he accepted my company as another of his contributions to the circum-medical world. Highly competent in his work, he had nothing to hide. He would serve as a model in the community, as he already does in his teaching, but now also through my work.

I doubt that Barry would like my portrait of him. I was unable to arrange time in his schedule to talk with him about my findings. Yet, perhaps perversely,

I take this conjectured attitude of avoidance and denial as further evidence for the validity of my representation. I believe that (just as I seek it out) Barry avoids the personal, the obscure corners, the psychiatric facets of others and himself. He is visibly anxious and threatened by the deeper troubles of others. Medicine is an approach which translates passion into patho-physiology, allowing him a more distant contact. I do not think that internal medicine is always approached in this way. I am claiming that it provides such a path, and that Barry attempts escape by means of it. I also believe he does not succeed. His language is fully passionate, however indirect.

B. BARRY SIEGLER: PERSON AND WORK

Barry Siegler practices general internal medicine in "Cartown", an American city of 200 000 people. He has worked here continuously since he began to practice more than twenty years ago.

"Call me Barry, Barry is fine," he said when I asked how I should address him. Now 53, Barry was born, raised, and educated in Chicago. He is married and has a close family with several grown children. One of his children is starting, another finishing medical school; one is a pharmacist, another a school teacher. When home from medical school, Barry's daughter joins him in his hospital rounds. His influence on his children is strong; he remarks ironically, "They did not learn." Barry's wife is not employed. He says of her jokingly, "She was the only smart one; she married me."

Barry is of average height and medium build. Sometime before I met him, he had begun jogging and had lost 20 pounds — so he told one of his patients. He runs regularly at night or on weekends, sometimes for more than an hour. Occasionlly he runs outside, but says he finds this boring, and he prefers to run in his basement while listening to cassette tape recordings of talks on current medical knowledge.

Barry dresses neatly, without flamboyance. As often as not he wears a sports jacket and tie, occasionally a suit. He very rarely wears a white coat on hospital rounds, but he commonly wears one in his office. He always carries his stethoscope, hung or draped around his neck; he uses it frequently.

Barry was raised as an Orthodox Jew, and while he rejected Orthodox practices when beginning college, he still maintains a strong Jewish identity. He is troubled eating ham, and he is acutely aware of who among his patients and his co-workers is Jewish, and who Middle Eastern or German, and thus possibly anti-Semitic. On one occasion he was especially concerned that a Jewish patient be quickly treated so that she could be home for religious holidays.

Following a college premedical education, Barry served in the Army as a medical aide and technician. He once remarked to me of this experience, "When I was a lab technician in the Army, I could deal with anything but snot . . . ." Bodily effluents are powerful and complex symbols in Barry's corporeal world, in ways I analyze below.

Barry completed his medical school training in Chicago, moved away for his internship and residency in internal medicine, and settled in Cartown. While many of the specifics of medical practice — knowledge of pathophysiology and therapeutic techniques — have changed since the time of Barry's medical training, several general principles from that period remain firmly rooted in his thought. His insistence on the diagnostic "listening to the patient", his use of direct, firsthand observation rather than technologically mediated means of knowledge, his emphasis on the consideration of multiple rather than single patient characteristics and on rational in preference to inductive exploration — all derive from the period of his medical education, and all are now prominent in his own teaching. Such principles are the grounds on which he criticizes contemporary medical education and practice.

Barry recalls also principles he was taught which did not make sense at the time, but which he came to understand through practice.

This is what they used to describe in medical school all the time as "sixth sense" .... Never knew what the hell that was. And it finally dawned on me after being in practice that there is nothing like a sixth sense; it's just your experience, what you've seen. You can draw upon what you've heard other people describe, what you've seen yourself, what you've read, and your different approaches to putting things together.

Barry is the senior partner in a three-man group of general internists. The membership of the group has changed over the years. Recently, a fourth partner was asked to leave. I questioned Barry on what had happened, whether there had been a difference of policy. He reluctantly said only, "No, there was a difference of habit"; characteristically, he did not want to express the troublesome differences any further.

With his current partners, relations seem amicable. Barry says he is pleased by their cooperation; beyond their set division of work, they voluntarily help each other. The three share an office suite and nursing and administrative staff. In order to use the office effectively, they divide the hours they spend there so that usually only one of them, or at most two are there at a time. They overlap briefly in the afternoon when they meet to assure a daily review of hospitalized patients, administrative matters, and other news.

I asked Barry about the similarities and differences between his partners' medical practices and his own.

I think they're pretty close; by and large they are. We differ in some areas. They are more aggressive, freer with meds, faster to discharge, too fast labelling people as "crocks", taking a stance and not backing off. I think that's just — I was like that exactly, and maybe I still am at times.

Since the three partners alternate in visiting the same patients in hospital rounds, they are continuously aware of each other's assessments and responses. Most often there seems to be agreement. Occasionally, Barry will note that a partner has failed to treat as he, Barry, believes necessary. For example, when a resident informs him that a partner has recommended surgery on an older patient with circulatory problems, he replies, "I go medically on them regardless . . . ." On another occasion, when a resident tells him that a partner has not "put a patient on" coumadin, an anticoagulant, Barry is troubled and irritated, and exclaims "Ah, shit!" I believe he is annoyed here both by the partner's failure to treat in this instance, and by a more persistent difference of practice. Barry is highly sensitive to the unobstructed flow of blood in his patients, and he believes that anticoagulants are too often insufficiently used, with fatal results. "I run scared of pulmonary emboli," he says (of blood clots which lodge in vessels of the lung, obstructing oxygen uptake and damaging lung tissue).

In the group practice, each partner has his own patients, patients with whom he is most familiar and to whom he is primarily responsible. Barry has had some of his patients and their families since he began his practice. He notes that his patients grow older as he does. Each of the partners does rounds on the others' hospitalized patients, takes night and weekend call for the others, and sees the others' patients when their primary physician is away. Patients are thus given both the long term continuing care of one physician, and the "coverage" by this physician's partners during his absence.

Barry's patients and those of his partners may be divided into three kinds: there are his own and, less often, his partners' (or even his community colleagues') patients whom he sees in the office; there are the group's patients whom they have admitted to the hospital either because of the severity of a problem, or for a more routine procedure requiring brief hospital stay; and there are hospital patients on whom Barry or another of the partners is asked to consult. Processes of consultation indicate a community in which knowledge is divided and exchanged.

While the final and most public goal of Barry's work is the physiological well-being of his patients, actions toward this goal are surrounded by a much broader field of acts, relations, and institutions. This 'circummedical' field (the term is mine, not Barry's) includes the institutions within which medicine is practiced, their physical apparatus, their personnel, and the still larger societal institutions of which medicine is a part. Each of these has its properties and rules of interaction; each constrains and/or facilitates Barry's more strictly medical work. Barry notes that work in the circum-medical field is "a part of medicine that people don't appreciate". A large part of his thought and energy are directed toward circum-medical arrangements, and Barry is agile here as he is within the field of medicine itself.

Barry sometimes refers to this work in the same idiom by which he refers to medical work with patients — an idiom of "treatment". Beyond his talk of treating his patients and his insistence on not treating numbers or 'labs' (that is, the results of laboratory analyses), Barry speaks, for example, of treating older patients by "treating their physicians". He must know how these physicians themselves 'operate' in order to treat them, so that they in turn will treat patients as Barry himself believes proper; he administers to patients by administering to the psyches of their primary physicians. Barry similarly complains of physicians who "treat lawyers" — that is, who treat patients in a manner to avoid lawsuits rather than for appropriate medical indications. Treatment in the circum-medical arena thus entails psychological sociological, political, and economic knowledge of the structures and rules which shape each realm.

Barry participates extensively in the administrative and political activities of the medical community in which he works. He has recently been President of the County Medical Society. He founded and now directs the local PSRO (Professional Standards Review Organization), which surveys the hospital stays of all federally funded patients in order to assure proper, but not excessive expense. Barry believes that physicians can best control the inevitable encroachment of government into medicine by participating early and actively in the process. Participation, he knows, runs against the grain of many of his colleagues — his own too, as he says, "Physicians like to be their own *macher* (Yiddish — boss, agent)".

Barry has served as Chief of Medicine at one of the hospitals, and during my stay with him, he was asked to serve as Chief at another hospital. He declined, he told me, because of personality conflicts. He has participated also and continues to participate on Cartown University and community committees concerned with medical matters — the selection of faculty in the University Department of Medicine, the opening of a local HMO (Health Maintenance Organization), and the purchase of an expensive CAT (Computerized Axial Tomography) Scanner by a second Cartown hospital.

Barry did not support the purchase of a second CAT Scanner for the community. While he believed this machine is "a tremendous instrument, and the information is really, really, really excellent", he felt that, given its great expense, one machine in the community was sufficient. The members of the County Medical Society did not agree, and their delegate voted for purchase in the State Regional Council. The machine was purchased, and is widely used, by Barry as well.

While he served on a committee to consider and plan the development of an HMO for Cartown, Barry has doubts about this form of medical practice. He would not want to practice in one. He feels the salary system undermines motivation and would undermine his own:

I think I'd be much less efficient, because . . . I would probably, if I were human, over a period of time begin to slacken off and do, ah, and work at the same pace as the slowest person in that group, because I've seen that happen . . . . Why the hell don't I just do what he does, get the same thing.

He adds that in HMOs patients don't always return to see the same doctor, "And the satisfaction, a lot of personal satisfaction in contact, diminishes."

Barry's life is scheduled far in advance. He knows when he will take his vacation next year, which weekends and nights he is "on call", which mornings he will make rounds in which hospital, and the hourly contours of each day. These plans are generally changed only for emergencies — those of patients, colleagues, and his family. Patient emergencies are the business of being on call, but these and other emergencies may also interrupt the remainder of the schedule as well.

Barry's time is structured by degrees of medical engagement — of access by patients, and of his reciprocal obligation to respond. Each partner has intense time "on", but certain time "off" as well. Each is "covered" by his partners when he is "off". These states significantly define the physician's role. Barry once referred to periods spent in the hospital as "clump time" and to periods at home waiting to be called as "scattered time". While in the hospital, medical work is continuous; call at home leaves him continuously susceptible to medical interruption. Emergency call reaches the office as well. When I first went to meet Barry in his office, to explain my study and to ask to accompany him, he had left the office without warning to go to the hospital where his patient was admitted with an "MI" (myocardial infarction, or heart attack). I left to return another time; scheduled patients were delayed.

Barry's schedule marks out his location and the general scope of his work there at different times, but not which patients he will see or what specific problems he will have to treat. The schedule provides slots for work whose size is limited in several dimensions. Certain problems can be dealt with in the hospital, but not in the office, or in the afternoon hospital working visits, but not in hospital rounds, or in the intensive care unit, but not "on the floor", and so on. Barry tries to fit the work into his schedule. If parts do not fit, they are abandoned or postponed, or the schedule expands, extending Barry's day, deferring and reordering other appointments. He "runs behind".

Barry is oppressed by two sorts of temporal constraints: Too much to do in the allotted time, and the urgency of action imposed by what are too often literal "deadlines". Time is differently shaped accordingly: excess draws it out, imminence intensifies each moment.

Barry's day beings with rounds, sometimes at one, sometimes at the other of two (out of four) Cartown hospitals to which he and his partners admit patients. He is accompanied by the residents and sometimes by medical students on his service. The rounds run from 7:30 to 9:00 am or shortly after 9:00 am, when Barry goes to the group office, several miles away. He has breakfast in the hospital, often with the residents and students (and during the period of this study, an anthropologist), and in one of the hospitals with an obstetrician friend or another physician. Talk at breakfast is often about recent recreational activity, sports events, or food. Sometimes, Barry will be in the hospital before breakfast, to read his patients' electrocardiograms and other laboratory reports.

During rounds, Barry walks with his followers through the busy hospital floors on which his patients are staying. The rounds "team", from three to eight people, may include not only the ever-present residents, but also pharmacists and pharmacy students, nurses, and social workers. Barry often has patients on medical and surgical wards, sometimes on obstetric and rarely on psychiatric wards, and in both the ICU (Intensive Care Unit) and the CCU (Cardiac Care Unit). On each ward, the team stops at the nursing station to collect the "charts" of Barry's patients from a central rack. Before each patient is visited, the resident responsible for this patient presents or updates "the case", referring especially to recent clinical observations and the latest information from laboratory studies. The resident also reviews or modifies his or her diagnosis and therapeutic recommendations, or notes problems in their formulation.

Most of Barry's hospital medicine, including diagnosis and therapy, is conducted with residents in rounds and follow-up visits. It is often on hospital rounds that appropriate information is elicited and evaluated, that false or irrelevant information is sought out and discarded, and that decisions regarding therapy and its termination are made. Much of Barry's medicine is thought rather than action.

In the hospital the medical residents and students are perhaps the most important persons among his circummedical relations. While they are only on his "service" (and on their clerkship in medicine) for periods of several weeks, perhaps months, it is they who spend most medical time with hospital patients. (Nurses spend much more time with Barry's patients than he does; beyond their nursing care, however, they are acting on medical decisions made by Barry, his partners, and the residents. In this capacity, their role is at most assistant and advisory.)

The residents pass their week and weekend days, often nights, in the hospital gathering information from patients, analyzing, and initiating or altering therapies. While Barry and his partners are the attending physicians for these patients, the residents carry out much of the diagnosis and therapy. (A physician who attends, "the attending", is the one who is responsible for the medical care of a patient or group of patients, e.g., a ward.)

Barry claims that ninety percent of medical practice is learned after medical school. In accordance with his extensive pragmatism, he also believes in learning by doing and by being held responsible. He tells the residents that the patients are not his, but theirs: "You are the attending on all these. I'm just a bystander".

In part this authorization is rhetorical, for Barry maintains a close watch over these subordinate apprentices. He questions them, socratically, but he also corrects them definitively, and he is visibly disturbed when he thinks they have made a false diagnosis or initiated a harmful 'therapy'. During the course of my study, one resident irked him especially, a man from the Middle East. I was not sure whether Barry's irritation was simply with the resident's medical errors, or whether his medical errors were judged by his foreign origins, more specifically, his Moslem background. Of this resident he commented, "The first rule of medicine is 'Do no harm'. His rule is 'Do something'." Barry is suspicious of foreign practitioners as well as of affirmative action minority medical students and residents from within the country.

In the teaching rounds Barry does not hesitate either to support a resident's plausible or correct assertion. Nor does he hesitate to express his own uncertainty or ignorance on any matter. Uncertainty is a central, though dreadful part of the work. He uses it to teach; he urges backing off when uncertain, and he recommends holding alternative hypotheses.

Barry's teaching is carried by two verbal genres: *within-medicine* citations of knowledge about physiology and pathology, and *about-medicine* principles —

general principles of medicine, its reasoning and its values. Within-medicine talk, the majority of his discourse, includes specific talk about the characteristics of patients, for example, blood chemistry, temperature, radiological findings, and general reports from population studies, about the course of pathophysiology, the efficacy of certain drugs under specified conditions, and so on. About-medicine, or meta-medical, talk includes a great variety of remarks about how medicine is done, and mostly about how it should be done. Much of this talk consists of epithets, formulae repeated frequently with variant versions, in many circumstances. The epithetical status of this talk is attested by Barry's quotation of it, for example, "That's why we say, '. . .'," by its frequent repetition, and by its sonorous composition. Barry's epithets are not idiosyncratic; they may be current in medical circles elsewhere. In both 'within' and 'about' genres Barry shows considerable verbal agility, using strong language, yet attuned to subtleties, undertones, and shades of meaning. He cuts and he smoothes, questioning and affirming, and with these instruments he assures the expedition of his work.

Following the resident's presentation and Barry's response, the rounds team enters the patient's room. One of the team may draw a curtain to separate visually and symbolically this patient's space within a room of several patients. Barry or the resident will greet the patient, and may introduce others in the team to the patient, either as "other doctors who work with us," or as "Dr. So and So", "Dr. . . .", and so on.

Barry often greets familiar patients by first name, regardless of age; a few of these reciprocate, calling him "Barry". Most address him as "Doctor" or "Doctor Siegler". He will call female patients, "Hun" (Honey) or "Sweetie", and encourage them, "That a gal". Male patients he often calls "Guy". He will address new or "consult" patients by their family names, but may still comment, "That a gal", "That a guy". In their absence, for example, in corridor talks with the residents (most often beyond the patient's ear shot), he may refer to them in the same way.

In Barry's work with patients, touch is multiply important. He often shakes hands with new or old patients. During the rounds visit, he may put his hand on the patient's shoulder, or hold a hand, particularly with a female patient, and especially if the patient seems emotionally upset. Almost always, as he leaves a patient, he will again shake hands, touch the patient's shoulder, or gently squeeze the patient's foot. Sometimes he simply holds up his open hand, palm toward the patient, and says, "Take care". These are touches and gestures of greeting and reassurance. I did not ask, but I believe Barry would interpret them as such. I believe also that these gestures of contact are symbolic for him the same way as they are for patients, further reassuring him of a connection, a licence to touch, and a power to affect.

There is another kind of touching, a medical one. In knowing about patients and their conditions, Barry insists and relies heavily upon his senses, principally sight, touch and hearing. He resists the distortion and distance fostered by technological medicine. Touch is an essential sense. He applies his stethoscope to the patient's body to listen to the patient's blood flow and heart sounds, bowel sounds, and respiration. He percusses also to evaluate pulmonary and bowel function, and liver and heart location and size. He palpates bowel, liver, neck, arm pits, and many pulses. He "does" 'pelvics' and 'rectals', and with a tongue depressor, examines throat and mouth. He feels the skin, and flexes joints to assess mobility and neurological condition. He may also "dress" and "undress" wounds, and remove dead tissue. Less often his contact penetrates; he may withdraw blood or other fluids by syringe, or he may inject medicines.

The boundaries between salutatory and medical (salutary) touchings are unlcear, intersecting with overlapping distinctions between diagnosis, therapy, and even pathogenesis. In the greetings of entry and departure, Barry may discern diagnostic signs in the patient's response; he believes he comforts as well. Medical touchings may also reassure, but they may disturb, expose, and penetrate. Diagnosis may be therapeutic; it may also be pathogenic, iatrogenically, as Barry is well aware. And therapy may be diagnostic, suggesting if not confirming a diagnosis by its effectiveness or its failure.

By the patient's bedside (the prototypical 'clinical' setting), the contrast between talk directed to the patient and talk among the medical team is striking and significant.

If the patient is comatose, little or nothing may be said to him. If stuporous or somnolent with drugs, little more than greetings pass. If asleep, the patient is often awakened. Barry most often asks patients who are awake and alert how they feel, and he may probe them on particular symptoms. In turn he may tell them in a simplified, concise, but straightforward fashion his current diagnosis, prognosis, and/or prescriptions. In doing so he uses little medical terminology, and explains it simply when he does. He gears his talk to what he takes to be the alertness, the intelligence, and current knowledge, understanding and interests of the patient. Most often he does not present sufficient information to allow the patient to evaluate the alternatives and to consent well informed.

He has doubts about the capacities of some patients. When I say to him that a patient we have just seen did not seem very intelligent, he replies:

Well, that's what you say when you're talking to patients, you know. How do you know? (*laughs*). How do they understand what you're saying? It's so hard. God!

On another occasion he remarks:

You've got to instruct people in really simple things. If you give a woman a vaginal suppository, you've got to tell her to take the foil off first.

Barry believes that patients should be informed of their conditions only to the extent they wish to know. To a contemporary insistence on full disclosure to patients, he objects,

That's inhumane. A lot of people don't want to know. A lot of people go to their graves hoping they're going to make it.

In contrast to talk to patients, talking among the medical team is more quiet, sometimes whispered; the number of syllables per word increases, and the rate of speech accelerates. It is a different dialect, spoken to exclude. Within the dialect, Barry may ask the nurse for the patient's height by saying, "What's the height," in a manner which is impersonal, anonymous, and exclusionary. He may say of a somnolent patient, "Look at the sensorium." Less often, Barry may ask a medical colleague for a characteristic of the patient, using the patient's name and everyday language, "Mr. Jones' blood pressure", when the patient is familiar and alert. In the following interaction, most of Barry's talk is directed to the assisting nurse:

— What's the height?
(*Nurse:*) 59 inches, 213.
Barry: (*to patient, a Native American*) You ought to grow an inch or so more.
— This (*gestures upwards*) way, not this (*gestures sideways*).
(*to nurse*) Femoral pulses are of good quality. Testes are normal. There is a small cyst at the inferior pole to the left, of the right . . . of the right testis, about a half centimeter.
(*to patient*) Cough please . . . Cough again. Cough again . . . Looks good. Looks good, sir (*much louder*). A little too much beer, but otherwise OK . . . Take care now.

The patient's talk is not only or primarily taken at face value, as an expression of his or her thoughts and feelings; rather, it is most often taken as an index of his/her bodily functions, that is, diagnostically. Thus talk with patients is translated into the language of medical talk, and there it is examined for its formal properties, coherence, affectional tone, correspondence to reality, and alteration from normal. An interest in the patient's world is suspended if not lost in an exploration of physiological disturbance as it is manifested in the patient's self-presentation.

In the halls, Barry will often greet other physicians, nurses, and hospital staff. At one hospital he warmly chats with an older Jewish cleaning woman, "Bessie", who, he tells me, fled from Germany during the War. With nurses, Barry will sometimes request information about patients, or additional pieces of equipment for some procedure; or he may ask or tell them to make certain observations about a patient, or to change the patient's diet. Also with nurses, he often makes sexual or flirtatious remarks; while such remarks are made with an undertone of jest, the remarks themselves suggest that there is a weightier issue to be made light of.

Barry's relations with physician colleagues in the hospitals and the Cartown medical community are complex and highly indicative. In these relations are reflected his conception of himself, the integrity and limits of his specialty and his capacity within it, his attitudes toward other specialties and those who practice them, and the rules of behavior which operate within the medical community and its segments.

The principal collegial relations are those of referral and consulation. When a physician consults with a colleague, he retains responsibility for the patient's treatment, and he may or may not follow the consultant's advice; when a physician refers a patient to a colleague, treatment responsibility shifts, at least temporarily, to the second physician. (A study of a medical community in terms of the exchange cycles of patients and their problems among medical and other practitioners, by consultation and referral, would be fascinating and rewarding; while "doctor shopping" by patients is notorious, the parallel patient and problem trading by physicians is little considered.) Barry both makes and receives both patient referrals and consults. He may refer a patient for limited medical procedures, for example, surgery, with the expectation that the patient will return to him from long term care. Or, he may refer a patient to another physician's long term care. A permanent referral may occur when either he or a patient finds incompatible each other's interests or practices. Some patients remain despite the trouble they may make for him. Half jokingly, Barry comments on one patient and the physician who referred her:

He referred her to me twenty years ago, and I've never gotten even with him.

Barry is attempting to limit new patients in his practice, and so is reluctant to accept new, long term referrals. From my observation, he accepts many of the frequent consults made to him. In these exchange relations, he is sometimes disturbed, as when the patient's attending physician requests the consultation too late or immediately before a planned discharge of the patient; here the referring physician may be more concerned with legally protecting him/herself than with helping the patient. Barry is irritated also when the attending physician has made mistakes, or continues to do so by not following Barry's recommendations. He complains, for example, of an old community physician who, he says, "treats symptoms". He asks himself sarcastically, "Why doesn't he retire?" He complains also of surgeons in the community, for whom he frequently consults, that they do not use anticoagulants sufficiently, leading, he thinks, to later problems of clotting (e.g., pulmonary emboli or stokes). He complains of obstetricians who fail to consider systemic problems. "You can't treat a woman like a pregnant uterus".

Difficulties arise not only with the attending physician, but also with the patient's problem which may be difficult to diagnose or treat. Physicians generally consult when they feel incompetent, and the matters on which they consult are likely to be complex, beyond the scope of general medical practice. The intensity of consultation work became sharply clear to me one morning when Barry remarked to the rounds team, with tempered equanimity, "We were asked to see him when his heart stopped".

Barry also consults about his own patients with other physicians — with surgeons, neurologists, psychiatrists, anaesthetists, obstetricians, pathologists, radiologists, and others. He himself is unsure in these areas, and is glad not to work there.

I think this guy (*the patient*) if he's not psychotic, is severely neurotic. I'm the poorest psychiatrist. I am as poor a psychiatrist as I am a dermatologist.

(*Of oncology*) It's a horrible specialty. I can't imagine doing that. But thank God some people are willing to do that . . . . Cancer is a big ball game. You've got to treat it with big guns on day one.

Barry relies on these experts. Yet he is often troubled by two aspects of relations with them: their violations of the etiquette of the medical community, and the medical content of some of their advice. Delays in the responses frustrate him, particularly with emergent crises.

That's communication again with surgeons. We just don't get it. I get very irritated by that – not knowing what's going on with patients.

Just call him up and ask him for numbers to treat with. I don't know why it takes three weeks to get a report from a hematologist.

It's interesting to me: When a surgeon can't make a diagnosis he disappears, leaves the case.

In the same vein, when they do communicate, consulted physicians may not do so properly or in sufficient detail. They may fail to justify their recommendations and orders. Barry may then override their recommendations.

Screw him. Fuck the anaesthesiologist. He can call us! That frosts me . . . . He didn't call. He just wrote the order. That's not the way it's done . . . . I had a run in once with an anaesthesiologist.

Cancel it. I have absolutely no compunctions about cancelling an order. And if he objects, I say, "Well, I won't send you any more patients."

Violation of these social norms in the circum-medical arena multiplies the problems which haunt Barry's more medical work.

Barry is sometimes disturbed also by the contents of consultants' proposals. He is wary of further testing for what he believes is already known, especially where further testing may delay available therapies. He rejects treatments whose side-effects seem to him to outweigh their benefits.

We're going to get oncology, and if they say "5-flourosol", we're going to negate that . . . . Chemotherapy isn't worth shit. All those rotten side effects, but it didn't stop that damned tumor.

Occasionally Barry's disturbance with a consultant's response is a mix of medical judgment, community etiquette, and broader constraints. He believes, for example, that radiologists sometimes fail to commit themselves on a "reading" because they do not wish to be held (legally) responsible.

They hedge. It's very difficult for them to say it's black or white. They say it's grey.

Here the failure to communicate a clear diagnosis is constrained by a circum-medical, legal worry; yet the failure is justified in terms of the nature of the work itself, that is, unclear pictures. Barry is annoyed by the recent legal preoccupation of physicians: "If you have to treat the lawyer, then get out of medicine."

Barry's field of collegial relations is by no means one of battle. He is most often friendly with colleagues, patting them on the back, smiling, and joking with them, as well as exchanging news and information about patients. Barry's position of respect and prominence in the medical community is evidence of his social as well as his medical skills.

To patients, colleagues, and subordinate medical personnel, Barry most often presents a gentle manner, speaking softly and smiling frequently. This manner may give way to a controlled, sharp tongued anger, for example, when a resident begins an ineffective and harmful 'therapy' with only a vague rationale. Sometimes a deeper anger and rage seem to lie beneath his common gentleness, as when he makes an angry remark following a seemingly calm phone conversation, or as when, on rounds, he is very friendly and reassuring to a patient in the patient's room, and complains angrily about the patient afterwards in the hall. I present evidence below to show that behind a gentle, surface ease, there lies a deeper frustration and anger. I believe the anger is partially rooted in the tension between the power and the impotence of the medicine he practices. He is aware of the anger, and not quite clear about its object.

I'm a terror sometimes. I get very angry sometimes. I like to think my anger is directed at shitty nurses and shitty doctors.

At the same time Barry has a persistent sense of humor which manifests itself not only in the instructive remarks and asides he makes to residents, nurses, and fellow doctors, but also in the stories he repeats, for example:

Did you hear the joke about the reporter who goes up to Nome, Alaska? In the winter, in February. Did you hear this story? You know, and there's 18 feet of snow and the winds are blowing 90 miles an hour, and it's 60 below zero, and you can't find anybody except in a bar. And he goes in the bar, and he sees some guys and he says, "Hey guys, what do you do here for entertainment in the winter? And they say, "We, we, we, we hunt and we screw." And he says, "What can you possibly hunt this time of year?" And they say, "Someone to screw". (all laugh)

Tell you the story about how doctors never change their minds once they've made a decision: Did I tell you this?
(RAH) No.
And, they tell a story in one of the southern medical schools about a kid who saw a patient in the hospital, ill and ah, and the guy said, "Well, I know what your problem is, sir. You've got locked bowels." And the guy said, "But I got diarrhea all the time." He said, "That's right. They're locked in the open position", (laughs)

Sexuality and excretory functions are common idioms of his humor and of his anger. These idioms are current in Barry's circum-medical relations, tying these manifold relations to his practice of medicine and to his capacity to confront the pathologies of patients.

Barry always tries to leave the hospital for the office around 9 am, so that he does not make office patients wait. He rushes to leave, impatient; he often postpones until the afternoon what he planned or hoped to do in the morning. Still, he notes, patients sometimes wait as long as two hours to see him. Most patients are scheduled far in advance; others, "squeeze ins", call with problems felt to be urgent, and are seen if the partners and/or staff concur on the urgency. I suspect that except in the most extraordinary of circumstances, perhaps a serious plea from a valued community colleague, only Barry's or his partners' own patients

would have this immediate access to his attention. Barry says that he himself
waits about five minutes every five years, when patients do not show up.

Barry's patients are scheduled between 9 am and the early afternoon. One day
when I accompained him, he saw 28 patients between 9 am and 2:45 pm, approximately 12.3 minutes per patient. Some of this time was spent other than in the
patients' physical presence; yet not all treatment takes place during the patient
encounter. Outside of patient visits, Barry completes and signs 'forms', talks with
his other staff and partners, goes to the bathroom, and makes phone calls. Barry
works without break; he eats no lunch.

Usually I can reasonably see six, five or six an hour. Sometimes with squeeze-ins, with the
schedule as it is, with the fullness of the schedule, there might be as many as eight, sometimes
nine in an hour. And I can't see that many, obviously. So I fall way behind. Then I keep running to catch up. So, the other day, oh there was lots . . . the other day I was running two
and a half to three hours late all day, for most of the day.

Barry's office visits with patients differ from his hospital rounds. In the office,
most patients are familiar, most of their problems routine. Many patients have
come to him for years as have the families of some. Visits most often concern
more established issues on which responses are standard, uncomplicated, and
with regular outcome, – mild acute diseases or chronic ones nor requiring hospitalization. "These are the 'simples'," he says, "routine chronic disease and things
like that." "That's all we do in the office, take the stitches out that someone
else put in." In office visits, Barry may check to see that the patient is taking a
medicine as prescribed, and that there are no new side-effects; he will inquire also
about the patient's more personal life. Barry seems to enjoy these visits, as do
this patients.

The office provides Barry relief from the too-regular "tragedies" of hospital
work. On several occasions of great frustration in hospital rounds, moments at
which he is unable to relieve a "disaster", Barry half humorously expresses a
wish for more "juicy pneumonias", that is, for (patients with) diseases which
are potent, yet easily and reliably treatable. Here he balances the high tension,
excitement, potency and impotence of hospital work with more certain and comfortable, but less "interesting" success of office work.

In the office, too, the staff is familiar with the routines of Barry and his partners.
Procedures are followed smoothly, with minimal need for communication or
explanation. When doing pelvic exams, Barry will most often have one of his
nursing staff "chaperone", telling the patient, "Let's have a gal give us a hand".
Nurses also show the patients to the small examination rooms, take their "vital
signs", and later may give the injections which Barry prescribes. They and the
other office staff will also prepare most of the "paper work" and some of the
records which are kept. Before Barry goes in to examination rooms to see each
patient, the nurse may inform him of particular problems the patient has mentioned, or of some other feature of the patient she thinks pertinent to the visit.

Barry is visibily affected by his patients' characteristics and by their conditions.

He challenges me to guess the age (96) of a patient in remarkably good health. He is greatly troubled by others, exclaiming to me later, "God, a lot of these people look great, but Jeez, they've got their problems." He winces when a patient tells him he is short of breath thus indicating circulatory problems. He gets angry when a patient with "essential hypertension", now short of breath, admits not restricting the salt in his diet:

Why don't you knock it off. You got to make some judgment whether you want the difficulty breathing, or whether you want the salt.

He expresses to me his anger also at another patient's husband who left her for another woman, upon which the patient's disease worsened, and the patient entered the hospital.

Her husband — I could wring his balls off, if I could get a hold of him.

After office hours, Barry returns to the hospital to visit patients, work with residents, study laboratory reports, and write or dictate notes and orders. One afternoon a week he is physician at the local hypertension center. In addition, he has meetings to attend. He often returns home only at 9 or 10 pm, and then may still be called, requiring that he return to the hospital if he cannot "handle the problem" over the phone. At home, in the evening, he will often jog in order to relax.

Barry rotates night and weekend call with his two partners, so that he is on every third night and every third weekend. Call is more frequent when one of the partners is on vacation. On weekend call, Barry makes Saturday and Sunday morning rounds in both hospitals, on all of the group's private and all of their "consult" patients. He will most often spend the whole morning in the hospitals, and he may be called back later if some problem arises which he, the resident, or a nurse feels requires his direct attention. The office is closed on weekends, but the partner on call will be available to patients by phone, through an answering service, and patients will be admitted to the hospital if necessary.

Barry looks forward to time off. "Any time I'm off is good". he said when I asked if he had enjoyed a free weekend. He sometimes expresses a need for time off when none is scheduled. He notes the difficulty of getting back into the work after he has been away; the momentum has been lost. On his longer vacations he drives with family members to a cottage up north, where he hunts and jogs. He says he enjoys both for the peace and relaxation they bring.

C. GOD'S NATURE, GOD'S MECHANISM, AND MORAL CERTAINTY

Barry's universe is at once natural, given — God given, and largely unknown. Barry is a religious man, not in the sense of dogmatic conviction or extensive ritual practice, but with deep personal identity and commitment. When I asked him at breakfast one morning what remained from his Orthodox upbringing of an attitude toward God, he replied,

Intellectually it doesn't make any sense to me; emotionally it does. I don't believe in the image of God, I believe in something — Nature. If you let things alone, don't screw around, Nature takes care of them.

This response accurately represents Barry's understanding; it accords not only with his more explicit statements, but also with the world suggested by his expressions of occasional satisfaction and frequent frustration, expressions in which religion, both invocative and blasphemous, is buried at little depth beneath the surface of explicit idiomatic meaning. Detailed religious doctrine and belief, beyond Jewish identity, is by no means apparent in his consciousness, as it is expressed. Barry's religious stance lies, rather, in a distant but firm and overarching order.

The interpretation of Barry's religious (and blasphemous) remarks is not straightforward. An idiom of heaven and hell, blessing and damnation, and God, or the Good Lord, permeates Barry's speech in a manner which seems to hover between metaphorical and literal reference. Rhetorical genres coalesce and split apart. His description of his sense of religion (above) is a literal one, and there are others like it. More often, however, his religious allusions are partially metaphorical expressions of anger and/or frustration at his inability to achieve some end, perhaps because someone else is uncooperative. Barry also makes religious allusions in talk with patients, for example, "The Good Lord doesn't want you yet". In making these remarks, Barry may laugh or smile, or raise his hands skyward, suggesting the commonly reported native informant who says, "Other people here believe such things; me, I don't". Here I explore the breadth of Barry's religious references, taking them literally, but allowing that he may use them metaphorically as well. For someone raised in orthodoxy who professes some religious belief, religious allusions are likely to be more than casually idiomatic.

The Nature to which Barry refers is distinct from the 'nature' of science, one which may be unknown, though perhaps knowable, but which is devoid of spirit — disenchanted. Barry says he believes in Nature; he professes faith beyond (partial) knowledge. Moreover, this Nature is essentially purposeful. It takes care of things, if only too-mortal humans do not interfere. I refer to Barry's world as a "deified Nature". What is the world of God's Nature, its powers, provisions, and constraints on human activity, which emerge from Barry's religious allusions?

In God's domain lies the ultimate fund of knowledge, and the control of human access to this fund. While probably not intended literally, the number and the intensity of 'religious' idioms which Barry uses at least hint at an underlying religious framework.

One of the most common causes of pancreatitis is the auto-immune thing — so-called "idiopathic", or God knows what case.

I haven't seen everything, God knows. I see something new everyday.

Human access to knowledge is severely limited, to Barry's deep frustration.

We're really so damned limited. There ought to be a lot more we can do for these old people besides give them a place to sleep and eat.

Barry's God is distant, inaccessible. He expresses his anger toward an oncologist who delays in responding to his requests for information about the treatment of his patients; he compares the oncologist to an otiose God — withdrawn, unreachable: I said, "Shit, trying to call you is like trying to call God".

While removed, God is yet provident. At least metaphorically, the Good Lord is said to provide not only life itself, but also healing "mechanisms" and relief from suffering, even through death. My field notes on Barry begin with his remark, "Williams expired through the night. That's a blessing!" He also made statements such as these:

The Good Lord provides for some good mechanisms to heal, if you just don't screw around too much. (*His daughter asks why the healing of a punctured lung takes place.*) Who the hell knows why. If you just let him (*holds up his hands*) do his work, and don't try to prevent him . . . (*laughs*).

He had about a hundred things wrong with him. And by the grace of God, he got better.

God seems also to provide these troublesome oncologists to do their difficult work.

But thank God, some people are willing to do that . . . . Cancer is a big ball game. You're got to treat it with big guns on day one.

Barry curses his ignorance, his inability to diagnose, to know what to do once a diagnosis has been reached, and to predict with certainty what will happen.

How the hell do you know what medications do?

The Goddamn medications and their side effects.

Mr. P did it. He wiped out his heart . . . . You know, there's no Goddamn way on the face of the earth that you can predict these things. He's on coumadin (*an anticoagulant*), bed rest, and what the hell can you do? It's so Goddamn frustrating.

Even when a patient does unexpectedly well, Barry's inability to know or predict remains a sign of his impotence. Of a cancer patient who has no pain, he comments, "Some of these people run courses that are just surprising as hell". While the turn of events is favorable for the patient, Barry's inability makes it "surprising as hell". The patient's course and condition are a measure of success. Barry's potency in positively affecting this course is itself a vital measure.

Disease itself is a curse, some deaths — those of seemingly healthy and young people, a "goddamn waste".

Some days there are people with cancers all over hell.

What a goddamn waste. Only 34 years old. He had a hyperthermic reaction in surgery . . . . (*Barry is informed of the patient's family refusal to donate the patient's organs.*) That's a waste. That makes it a bigger waste.

God's work does not seem to be consistently good, according to Barry's moral remarks. Too often God does not seem to provide directly the relief which patients and their conditions call for — relief, perhaps found only in death.

(I ask how long a patient with "terminal cancer" will live.) If she's got that the Good Lord would be kind to her, if it's very soon.

He's so sick, that poor guy. Why the hell doesn't the Good Lord take him?

There is tension here between Barry's conception of "The Good Lord" and this God's seeming inaction, his allowance of suffering and death. Barry suggests that The Good Lord may not be so good. "Why the hell doesn't the Good Lord . . .?", he asks. He asks not because he expects or even wants an answer, but to vent his anger.

In justifying his belief in Nature emotionally rather than intellectually (see (a) in Figure 1), regarding this Nature as primarily responsible for healing (see (b)), Barry sets up a number of what seem to be tensions among his own beliefs. Justification within his scheme involves a basic paradox. As I explain in detail below, Barry's thought associates (c) emotion and judgment (or philosophy) as non-rational human processes. He seems to avoid both. He contrasts them (d) to science, the ultimate basis (e) for his medical practice. Yet, in the explanation of Nature and the healing which Nature provides, he is satisfied with emotion as a justification. Science and emotion, explanatory grounds which he most often holds to be exclusive if not contradictory, here justify the same phenomenon.

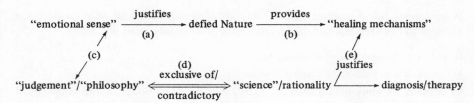

Fig. 1.

Barry is by no means a theologian; nor, I am sure, would he want to be one. Theology lies in the domain of judgment, and Barry mocks what he calls philosophical issues, citing (his own version of) the Medieval question, "How many angels are there on the head of a pin?" as an example of irrelevance and irresolution. Though the tension between science and judgment/emotion clearly runs through his thought and his work, not only as he justifies belief in Nature, but also in his deeper attitudes toward self and patient, he does not raise or confront it as an intellectual issue.

I cite further paradoxes both to suggest Barry's lack of interest in such questions, and also to suggest another principle which makes fuller sense of his beliefs. If Nature provides healing, and if this is the goal of Nature, why, then, is there disease and suffering? And, if disease and suffering are Natural phenomena, are they not somehow good, to be left alone? If not to be left alone, when is interference proper; and when does interference become "screwing around", a cosmic promiscuity hindering rather than fostering Natural healing? And, if human healing powers are limited in a Natural fashion, why should Barry be so frustrated?

Barry would probably regard such questions as little more than the question of angels on a pin head. Yet I would suggest that these paradoxes indicate the incompleteness of his religious explanation for an understanding of much of his thought and action. The religious view stands, sometimes opposed, by another implicit explanation: Moral Certainity. By moral certainty, some events and acts are clearly right, others clearly wrong: Disease and suffering (medically defined) are certain evils; efforts to remedy and relieve them certain obligations, and failures to act certain offenses, wrongs. This principle is implicit in Barry's thought and action; Barry does not himself voice it, and might even deny it, for reasons I clarify below. I have given it a name. I argue that Moral Certainty is a principle which justifies much of his medical and circum-medical action. It resolves by fiat some of the paradox implicit in his religious thought. He is compelled by this principle; it is a foundation of his commitment to his work.

Moral certainty accounts for the morlaism which Barry shows — his ambivalence toward the treatment of an alcoholic, his reluctance to support the treatment of a "promiscuous", poor, single mother, and his doubts about the quality of physicians who have been given special access because of their minority status. (These attitudes may accord with a common American principle of individualism that people are and should be responsible for their own situations. They correspond also with Barry's own insistence on being his own *macher*, or boss.)

Moral certainty, opposed to moral relativity, accounts for a significant facet of Barry's relations with his patients, that is his presumption of their interests, his apparent knowledge of what is best for them. Most often he need not ask the patient because he knows. And he may inform the patient in a manner he believes will most likely elicit consent to what he, Barry, thinks best.

Finally, moral certainty makes sense of disease and other evils in a Nature which is the essential source of healing mechanisms. It explains Barry's puzzlement at Natural tragedies. Moral certainty provides the firm grounds for questioning Natural events. It accounts also for the "hell" of surprises that events have turned out well despite his predictions and his interventions. It goes so far as to justify intervention itself, for there seems to be little other reason to intervene in a world in which Nature provides the essential source of healing.

I am suggesting that Barry's universe is anchored in two powerful structures: his Jewish upbringing which persists in a defied Nature, and a deep moral sense by which he knows what is right, what evil. The two structures are often mutually supportive in Barry's work, but they are not consistently so. On some issues, moral certainty contends directly with the defied Nature. The "Good Lord" does not always act in a manner which Barry knows to be good. At such times he comes to doubt the wisdom and powers of God's Nature itself. Here his moral sense prevails. He knows the proper course of action; he is impelled to act for an end which he knows implicitly to be worthy.

D. SCIENCE, JUDGMENT, AND THE INDIVIDUAL

A focal objective of Barry's work is the correction of systemic physiological disturbance in his patients, and the relief of concomitant suffering. Often he succeeds.
It is his knowledge — general knowledge of the principles of physiology and pathophysiology, and particular knowledge of individual patients, which allows him to
predict and to affect the courses of patients' conditions. It is the faults in his
knowledge which lead him to fail where he fails, and the gaps and limits of his
knowledge which often lead him not to act at all. These limits are of profound
and perpetual significance to Barry. They foreshadow health and disease, life
and death in his patients; they demarcate his powers and his effects. Within, and
especially near the severe, but uncertain limits of his knowledge, Barry derives the
pleasures of his medicine; beyond these limits lie prominent sources not only of
his patients' suffering, but of his own suffering as well.

In this section I follow the distinctions which Barry makes among the domains
of knowledge — principally a distinction between "science" and "judgment". I
then follow the course of science in Barry's composition and use of "pictures"
— conceptions of the conditions of patients. Barry conceives of these pictures in
strikingly different ways — in a realism which reifies conditions in fixed, Platonic
forms, and in a nominalism which regards pictures as at best useful illusions, a
conception which predominates in Barry's view. These extremes are moderated
by a pragmatism which has ramifications throughout Barry's unphilosophical,
even antiphilosophical philosophy. I distinguish the various sources of general
knowledge and knowledge of particular patients, and I discern some relations
among these sources. I discuss the troublesome failures of pictures to accurately
correspond to the realities of patients' diseases. When pictures fail, and Barry
after them, his distinction between science and judgment collapses, and all is
painfully a matter of arbitrary belief.

Science and Judgment

A distinction between "science" and "judgment" or "philosophy" runs through
Barry's thought and expressions. It defines what he takes to be the epistemological
bases of his work, and sets off a domain in which he works comfortably from
another which he avoids, sometimes fearfully.

Then we come to the philosophy of this thing, not the science. What are we doing? (*Medical
findings on a patient do not clearly indicate a course of treatment*.)

She's fit to have the surgery, but she and the surgeon should be aware that she's an added risk.
It's still a judgmental thing on their part. You can't say it's contraindicated, but you can say
it's an added risk. She's a nice gal. That's a nice consult.

Barry uses the term, "judgment", in two different senses — a generic ("unmarked")
one which includes all cognitive processes, and a specific ("marked") one which
includes processes based on value, excluding those based on science. (The term is
thus semantically like the category, "animal", which, in a broad (unmarked)

sense, includes the category, "human", and in a narrower (marked) sense contrasts with "human".) The examples above illustrate the narrower, specific usage. In the broader usage, Barry says, for example,

Judge them (*i.e., signs and symptoms*) by the company they keep.

This is the sequence of films. They're all different techniques. It's pretty hard to judge them. They don't look strikingly different to me.

These "judgments" are not distinct from his science, but are a part of it. In the analysis which follows, in order to explore the dynamics of the essential contrast between different forms of a knowledge, I consider only the narrower sense of "judgment", that which is opposed to "science".

Science provides the ultimate grounds of Barry's medical knowledge. Yet Barry clearly asserts that while medicine is in principle a science, it is not yet so in fact. Medical knowledge is vastly deficient, and it is this deficiency which makes a part of his work so excruciating. Yet what knowledge there is in medicine is finally based on the facts and principles of a science, however weak.

There's a lot of unpredictability, where, where you know, we're not that scientific really, in terms of what we can do with the numbers and figures that we have.
(*RAH*) Is that, you think that's a matter of principle, or ah?
No, it's a fa . . . , it's a matter of fact.
(*RAH*) You think of it, it's a matter that we don't, we don't know . . . .
That's right. Oh sure. We think we're knowledgeable now, but we're very, very dumb and very ignorant, and the knowledge, yet the knowledge that we have now is much greater than it was ten, fifteen years ago . . . .

Science is the realm of fact and logic, and stands in contrast to the realm of belief and emotion. I am by no means fully aware of the details and complex links in the chains of reasoning in Barry's medicine. From his working explanations, however, I draw several inferences about the structure of Barry's medical reasoning and its elements. Many of his comments attest to explanatory principles and more systematic, 'theoretical' knowledge. When a resident does not understand a diagnosis or a therapy, Barry may elaborate an explanation connecting a variety of 'findings' about the patient with general principles of pathophysiology. He thus gives evidence of a larger theoretical scheme which makes sense of his observations and which justifies his actions.

In contrast, much of Barry's knowledge consists of patterns of correlation and sequence. This and that occur together such-and-such percent of the time; this follows that at such-and-such a rate. The events connected by these relations include not only the course of the patient's condition, but the effects of intervention as well. For much of what Barry knows he has no explanation, or only a partial one. Or, he may once have had an explanation, now forgotten.

Some breast cancers may cause on elevated acid phosphatase, and I don't know why.

I honestly can't remember the physiology of that . . . I'm wrong as often as I'm right.

I don't know. I don't know how they work. I don't think anyone knows how they work. (*Resident asks how expectorants work.*)

The knowledge of science is not valued for itself, but because it is useful. Barry is most often a pragmatist: worth and truth are both defined by efficacy, that is, by what works in the achievement of his objectives. The objectives themselves are natural, taken for granted. The details of a theory are worthy of recall when they facilitate the solution of medical problems.

Barry uses the term "academic" to connote knowledge which is useless and wasteful.

At this point, it's really very academic. (*Which came first, the patient's kidney problem or his hypertension.*)

You can argue the academics of it, too. But, from a practical point of view, she's gotten worse.

Academic medicine is exceedingly expensive. No one is in a hurry to do anything.

I'd like to work in some academic institution so I could disappear four or six hours at a time.

They're (*American College of Physicians*) really very academic, and I don't care much for them.

In a similar "Ivory Tower" idiom, Barry refers to the university committee which assured that my research would protect my 'human subjects' as "Knights of the Round Table", suggesting mythological unreality and illusory, misguided power. Likewise, Barry thinks little of a course on the philosophy of medicine which his son is taking. Barry's attitude toward "academics", both persons and their studies, is strong and ambivalent. He resents and envies the leisure of academia, its freedom from commitments to tight schedules and to the press of clinical call. Yet he often relies on academic consultants and on the scientific knowledge which is produced in academia. About these sources, too, he is ambivalent.

Barry's reaction to research medicine and to annual research meetings betrays an anger beyond rejection. I asked one morning if he thought of conducting research, and he responded, "I have absolutely no desire to do so". And of the annual meetings, "The annual meetings are absolutely horrible. They're just atrocious. They're really rotten". I suggest that these strong sentiments are allied with his frustrations with uncertainty — his need, yet his inability to predict, to know what will happen and what should be done. It is the same resentment he shows for academics who produce imperfect though vital knowledge, but are often not then directly responsible for its pressing application or its failure.

As a body of efficacious fact, science most often dictates action, to Barry's way of thinking. When one knows the relevant facts and principles, one knows how to act. Logical necessity has totally subsumed moral necessity; morality has become invisible.

So you've got to go the route with that ... You've got to go to full heparinization (*anticoagulation*). You've got no choice. This could be lethal.

The notion of "having no choice" is significant. The constitution of pathology and the impulse to treat pathology are so strong, so deeply ingrained in his thought and conduct, that they are no longer thought of as choice. The social basis of judgment and action are transformed into an immutable, natural logic.

Only where the facts of science indicate a close and precarious balance of

risks and benefits is the mandate for action no longer clear. Science has not yet
provided a unique option, "no choice". Action then becomes of matter of choice,
"a judgmental thing".

That's a judgmental thing, and I don't have any better idea what to do than you. You have
to balance . . . . What the hell do you do? I would treat her with heparin, but at a reduced
amount.

You can take either side on that. Both sides are right and both sides are wrong. (*On the merits
of kidney transplanation*.)

Here science provides basic information, non-judgmentally. Yet, since both action
and inaction have balanced benefits and risks, the choice between them is unclear.
Judgment takes over, non-scientifically.

Judgment, also called "philosophy", is the domain of value, ethics, "what you
like". Barry's talk suggests that there are other sorts of judgments as well, but I
have not heard him name these. He mentions only economic judgments, concerned
with cost in dollars; these are important in Barry's thinking. Barry believes judgments to be matters of individual choice, all (or many) choices being equally
justifiable. On matters of judgment, "I don't think there are any right answers".
He says he does not object to any decisions made on philosophical questions,
because all choices are equally good (or bad). He hints also that such questions
and their answers are often irrelevant, extraneous, picayune, comparing them to
his paradigmatic, worthless puzzle, "How many angels are there on the head of a
pin?"

Pictures

Barry refers to his conception of the patient's problem, most often a physiological
one, as "a picture", "a story", "a thing", and less frequently with the more common
medical term, "an entity". He refers to the processes through which characteristics
of the patient come (or fail) to compose a picture as "making sense" (or "not
making sense"). The characteristics themselves are said to "make sense", and
Barry also says of himself that he "makes sense of" or "gets a handle on" these
facts (or fails to do so). It is the "picture" or "thing", an explanatory hypothesis
which "makes sense" or by which Barry "makes sense" of systemic physiological
observations, that allows the intervention and prognosis which may be possible.

Wow, I don't believe it. It doesn't make any sense. Just because a piece of lab data comes
back from a computer doesn't make it accurate.

How can it be normal? It's got to be either hypoplastic or hyperplastic . . . .

It just doesn't make any sense, I don't believe it. I don't care what they say.

I don't know if there is such an entity. I don't know if anyone thinks there is such a thing.
(*Resident asks about "chronic appendicitis"*.)

It makes sense with what he has.

I can't put it into any one thing yet. A lot of things come to mind . . . . to try to
put this all together into one sort of thing — I've been unable to do this.

You know, the whole picture would fit so well with the carcinoma. I can't get out of my thought the fact that that would explain everything so logically.

That's a story for labyrinthitis . . . . You can look for neoplasms. You're spinning your wheels.

I haven't seen everything, God knows. I see something new every day.

The contrast between the characteristics themselves make sense and Barry's making sense of them is important, since the former ignores and the latter recalls the subjective or constructive nature of knowledge. If purported facts fail to make sense, the anomaly must inhere in the facts; but, if Barry is unable to make sense of the facts, it may at least be possible that the difficulty lies in Barry's sense-making activity rather than in the purported events to be made sense of. These are respectively metaphors of realism and nominalism, of naturalism and constructionism.

In Barry's thought, pictures and things are both moving and fixed. They are moving, setting a dynamic "course" through time, in that they depict sequences of events of bodily parts and physical systems. They are thus processual, and here the "story" metaphor seems more apt. Pictures are also fixed in that they are more or less static generalizations, presumably based on populations of patients in whom identical or nearly identical sequences have been observed. The problem of a particular patient either does or does not conform to the picture, in a binary fashion. Pictures may be known in great detail or sketchily, and better for some conditions and courses than for others. Yet, to whatever degree known, the essence of a picture is its fixed course. It is this property which allows (tautologically) prediction of the events occurring to patients of whom a given picture is true.

To extend Barry's own metaphor, pictures form a gallery of many halls. Barry speaks of "sorts of thing", the ways that pictures, which themselves order facts about a patient, are ordered into larger arrays. The guide to Barry's gallery is not clearly discernible, yet it would seem to be based on those same signs of which pictures are composed. Observation that a patient presents certain signs would send Barry looking in one section of the gallery.

Alongside Barry's heightened awareness and concern for the ambiguities of fact and artifact (e.g., the way in which what is taken as fact is a human product, an artifact), he is aware also of the relativity of picture and picture-element, that is, the pictorial nature of the parts of pictures themselves, as well as, conversely, the part of pictures in larger pictures or in galleries of pictures. As I discuss in more detail below, Barry recognizes the importance of eliminating what is reported as fact, which is invalidly biased by the means of observation. Such purported "evidence" distorts the larger picture. I suggest, then, that since he sees elementary "data" as themselves highly informed and created artifacts, he might regard these seeming elements as themselves smaller pictures. Thus, what he calls "pictures" would be composed of pictures, themselves parts of larger pictures.

Barry is acutely aware of another relativity as well, the historical changing of the pictures in his own gallery and the galleries of the profession more widely. He is wary of currents in medical thinking, and he is often opposed to these, for his own reasons.

I don't get excited about serum ammonias like everyone else does.

That's what a lot of people think. They think ammonia is everything, but really it means zip [that is, nothing].

Brompton's isn't worth a damn. Brompton's is a fad.

It's (*use of a feeding tube with upper gastric bleed*) one of the many things, the many, many, many things I don't think make sense.

Pictures and those more elementary observations (signs and symptoms) which compose them, work in a dialectical fashion in the diagnostic process. At early encounters with a patient, when either the patient him or herself or his/her particular problem will most likely be unknown to him, Barry begins by collecting observations from increasingly detailed reports by the patient, and from grosser to finer observations of his own of the patient's physical condition and "presentation". At this point, Barry may have vague hypothetical "pictures", sketches perhaps, awaiting in his preconscious or even in unconscious thought. As his observations accumulate, perhaps guided by pre- or unconscious pictures, a sketch may be undermined and discarded, or it may be given support and be brought to consciousness for further exploration. Barry often stresses to residents the importance of maintaining several, alternative pictures. At this stage, he might tell one of them, "I can't put it into any one thing yet. A lot of things come to mind".

At some point in diagnosis, there is a significant perceptual event. The picture emerges to predominate in Barry's diagnostic search, and more elementary observations are then gathered for use in evaluating the patient's characteristics as elements of the picture. Barry might now says of a sign or symptom, "It makes sense with what he has". The picture is tenuously pinned to the patient as hypothesis. Subjectivity and construction − the idea that pictures are constructed artifacts − are dropped from Barry's expression, and further reports proposed as fact are now evaluated in terms of what has been established, though tentatively, as fact or picture.

Barry is well aware of the powers of pictures in diagnosis. Though he does not talk about them in an abstract way, he commonly makes reference both to the rational guidance for which pictures are essential in diagnosis, and to the perceptual bias to "see" what is not there and not to "see" what is there, following the picture one expects.

Diagnoses may be made or reported not only to decide a course of treatment, but also to effect the treatment. Barry may present a diagnosis to a patient in a manner intended to convince the patient to comply with his recommended action, an action which he or she might not take, given a different diagnosis or given the same diagnosis in another rhetorical manner. For example, Barry regrets telling one patient in his office that she was doing well, because (he thinks) she then failed to follow his recommendation and ended up in the hospital. On one occasion, Barry suggested to a nurse that a patient who read the "PDR" (*Physician's Desk Reference*, explaining effects and side effects of medicines) be told that he had tachycardia (accelerated heart rate) so that he would then conform to the recommended treatment; the patient would be frightened into compliance. Perhaps Barry was not serious in this suggestion, for he told me that he did not believe that scaring patients was effective in inducing compliance. He believes that people are most difficult to convince or change, even for their own good; and while he occasionally remarks that decisions about the course to follow should be left entirely to the patients, he uses diagnostics rhetorically, in order to persuade.

While diagnoses are most commonly made in order then to treat, on some occasions, when diagnoses are uncertain and when the proposed treatment is benign, without significant risk, the treatment may be given partly in order to make or confirm a diagnosis, retrospectively. Resolution of the given disease problem is some evidence that the problem was one generally cured by this treatment; conversely, complete failure to resolve is evidence that the problem is another, not one commonly relieved by this means.

Knowing Pictures, Knowing Patients

Barry's science comprehends knowledge both of general principles and of particular patients. That is, it includes statistical and theoretical knowledge of populations, based on studies by other researchers, and particular, experiential knowledge of individual patients by Barry himself and by his colleagues. Between these two elements of his science, populations and individuals, general and particular, there is both mutual support — when individuals provide further evidence for generalizations, and when generalizations guide the response to individuals — and a tense opposition, when Barry's own experience runs against the currents of medical thought, and when statistics fail to predict the course of given patients.

Barry's gallery of pictures has several sources: his early medical training which provided a firm basis, the distant public information in "the literature", the closer, more personal information from colleagues, and his own experience. Barry is highly selective of the information which he accepts to confirm and especially to revise his pictures. His gallery of pictures is stable, itself exerting a strong conservative influence on new acquisitions. Barry is extremely skeptical about findings in "the literature". He says, "The stuff you read in the literature, 90% is bullshit, maybe 95%, maybe even 98% .... You can quote me".

He seems to reject the statistical reports of population studies when they are contradictory or extraneous to his own principles. Of an epidemiological study relating low bulk fiber diets and intestinal cancer, he remarked to me, "I really don't know what the heck you can make out of studies like that". But when the conclusions of a study support his own beliefs, he accepts them. He cites a large population study in support of his dominant belief in the importance of anticoagulation in certain circumstances:

That's an important study, because thousands of patients were followed. Some people don't like it, and say it wasn't well done. Well, if you don't like something, you can always find something wrong. But I firmly believe this is an important study.

I've seen too many die at 21 days, "uncomplicated" .... The only problem is what crystal ball do you have to have to know the course of an uncomplicated MI (*myocardial infarction*)?

.... Not someone's chief, but statistics: two years of coumadin (an anticoagulant), 10 000 people, 10 000 MIs .... They don't talk about the original study. They talk about what the chief of service says.

Barry suggests at once that this is an important study, thus indicating a real, effective result, and that knowledge, even in science, is a matter of faith, of "firmly" believing. As with laboratory results, Barry uses statistical studies selectively to confirm what he already believes. The standing knowledge by which he works significantly shapes new knowledge he may come by.

Barry gives much credence to his own experience. Especially on some questions he has strong convictions, and his experience is confirmatory. For example, regarding anticoagulation, he says,

I feel very strongly about bleeding. I'm chicken 'cause I've seen bad things happen.

And regarding a therapy recommended by a resident, he says ironically:

I have no problem with you doing that, but I've never seen it work; in my limited experience.

Barry also speaks with ambivalence of the significance of personal experience. Personal experience contrasts with systematic, large population "fact". Personal experience, along with "emotion" mislead to the overestimation of one's own observations.

I wish I could be very scientific and say, "Hey one and one is two, or two and two is three, but ah, or two and two is four, excuse me. But, ah, I think everything you do in medicine is, ah, is, is hopefully based on fact, but clouded by experience and emotion". You know, that's true of everything.

The personal experience which he greatly favors is direct and mediated by few devices or institutions of assessment. As described earlier, Barry makes extensive use of direct experiences of the patient's condition, by percussion, palpation, pulsing, and visual observation of the patient's body, and by the patient's "presentation".

(RAH) What is important, then, the symptoms, the signs and symptoms? Very much, and, and, ah, the presentation of the patient, how they present. Not only what they say, but in things they don't say or how they say it, as well as what you find. If you can listen, you can get a diagnosis most of the time. This was taught to us as students, and it's true. It's very, very true.

Of the less direct means of evaluating patients, laboratory studies, Barry says they are "supportive". The laboratory "supports and confirms what you're doing". Where the laboratory reports contradict his prior beliefs, the reports are all but ignored, "thrown out". He recounts to me telling a medical student about the diagnosis of "a coronary":

He says, "What were his laboratory studies yesterday?" — the first thing he said to me when we got to the floor. And I said, "Why?" He said, "Well, we want to know if he had a coronary." I said, "Is that the only way you can tell if he's had a coronary?" And he kind of looked at me startled, and ah, ah, I said, "We, you know, we have to, you have to start thinking about what you get from the patient, and what you think of what the patient tells you, and what you find as you look at the patient as to what he has. And if the laboratory doesn't agree with what he has, you throw the laboratory out."

Barry takes "what he (*the patient*) has", that is, the hypothesized picture, to be the known standard which the lab may support but not weaken.

Barry reasons carefully in his scrutiny of lab reports. He is acutely aware of their mechanical and social sources. He is, pragmatically, an "operationist", in the philosophical sense, maintaining that what one measures is the act of measurement. A measurement may, but often does not, correspond to some phenomenon of interest in the patient. Too often it corresponds more with its mechanical source, for example the cuff used to measure blood pressure, or with its social source, for example some person or institution who/which habitually measures in a distorted fashion.

You might cure his high blood pressure by measuring with a big cuff. (*Ironic, that is, the patient did not have high blood pressure, but was thought to have it because of inaccurate measurement.*)

Could she have had an infarct, or did the technician place the electrode differently?

You have to understand there's some problem in that. Dr. Jones thinks everyone is in cardiac insufficiency.

He sees microprolapses in everyone. I think the incidence is 20%. He sees 90%.

(*I ask, "The radiologist read the film wrong?"*) No, he read the wrong film. That's happened several times.

If it comes from B-Laboratory, I'll tell you what it says.

Barry is likewise aware of himself as instrument in his more direct observation of patients:

I can't feel it (*a certain pulse in a patient*). I think I'm influenced by the fact that he shouldn't have it.

In knowing patients and in looking for the proper picture, Barry insists upon intuition as well as rationality. The two may be relevant at different stages in diagnosis: intuition as a source of hypotheses, reason in their evaluation.

The initial impression is often the right one. Very often it is.

There's no question in my mind what he's got, but I can't prove it to you (*the resident*).

He looks better, but I can't measure it.

Reason also is vital, the ultimate scientific justification for action (and/or inaction). Barry also refers to reason as "thinking", and "making sense", and to its absence as "without rhyme or reason".

Just because it's done doesn't make it the right thing to do. Think about what you're doing.

I don't want you to do these things merely because I want you to do them. You can argue with me and be off 180 degrees. (*Joking?*)

It's bullshit. It's really bullshit, the way we do things without rhyme or reason . . . . It developed for 11 months after an X-ray. (*He inveighs against preventive medicine, because a patient's cancer developed following a screening.*)

The powers of reason, however, are limited. One may reason to conclusions or alternative conclusions, but the truth of the matter is validated in what works.

When you get nausea in a hospital patient without explanation, look at medications. You just can't sit and say, "It might happen, it might not". But medications are an important source of nausea, unfortunately. The only way you can tell if she's vomiting from it is to stop it.

When you add it all up, and you say this can do that, and this can do that, all you can do is measure the effect in the person.

He recommends two strategies for finding the right picture. One is the maintenance and exploration of alternative pictures.

Don't put all your eggs in one basket. I just made that up. If things aren't working the way you think they should, don't be rigid in your thinking.

In medicine, this strategy approximates what is more formally referred to as "differential diagnosis". It explores all of the diagnoses suggested by the initial information, then eliminating each alternative by further evidence, until a correct diagnosis is achieved. The order of elimination may follow the probability that each diagnosis is the correct one, or the urgency of each diagnosis, given that it has been correctly made, or perhaps the ease by which each alternative can be eliminated. (That is, one is likely to look at the most plausible hypotheses first, or those whose presence would be most dangerous, or those easiest to eliminate as false.)

A second strategy is "standing back" or letting a condition alone to see if it or one's conception of it then resolves. Standing back is a posture of delay; it engages intuition and gestalt, a physiological holism.

Stand back and look at the whole thing . . . . Rely on first impressions.

Oftentimes, if your're not sure what it is, sit on it, and look at it again in a week. It may be back to normal.

In a deliberate suspension of the diagnostic search, the apparent problem may resolve itself either by disappearing, becoming no longer problematic, or by becoming recognized and understood. The parts would then come to be seen to compose this or that picture.

Surprises and Shades of Doubt

Failure to discover the patient's picture, failure of the picture to predict the patient's course, and failure to know how to affect that course when known; failure haunts Barry in his work. In failure, his metaphor shifts from one of "pictures" and "stories" to another of "horror stories", "tragedies", "catastrophies", and "disasters". He recognizes that his powers are partial and threatened. He is deeply frustrated. Hell and damnation crowd in.

That happens . . . why, at this point, when they're well anticoagulated? Damned if I know.

Mr. P. did it. He wiped out his heart . . . . You know, there is no goddamn way on the face of the earth that you can prevent these things. He's on coumadin, bed rest, and what the hell can you do! It's so goddamn frustrating.

Mr. P. is said to be the agent of his own destruction "wiping out his own heart", despite all that was done. Most often anticoagulation works. Its failure coincides with Barry's self-asserted ignorance; he does not know why.

Barry is too often "surprised" by a patient's course. Even if the surprise concerns an unexpected improvement, it is of ambiguous worth. He remarks, for example, that a patient's course is, "just surprising as hell". While the patient may be much better off than expected, surprise in itself is an index of ignorance and impotence; this is the "hell" of the surprise. In this instance the patient has a cancer, and while this type of cancer is usually painful, this patient has no pain. Barry's own efficacy is vitally important to him, as is his effect itself, the result.

In response to his self-perceived inefficacy, Barry's notion of knowledge shifts from the realism of pictures, fixed Platonic "entities" which are more or less apt to patients' conditions, to a more and more stringent nominalism, in which medicine becomes a less and less useful tool, and medical practice becomes increasingly a matter of "what you believe", "what you like", that is judgment, beyond science. (While in the Western tradition of realism, 'pictures' or 'entities' are more real than our dimly experienced impressions of them, in the opposed tradition of nominalism, the experience is more real than the categories which capture this experience arbitrarily and transiently.) In Barry's thought, the collapse of rigorous science into subjective judgment takes place in three stages. (See Figure 2.)

Efficacious science of pictures ←————————→ Science fails

	Realism	Individualism	Uncertainty a property of events	Nominalism
Metaphors	Pictures Stories Things	Statistics don't apply to the individual. Avoid betting, become believer.	Nothing black or white. No such thing as black or white.	Medicine as what you think/ enjoy. Nothing written in stone.

Fig. 2. Idioms of potency and impotence, realism and nominalism.

The first stage might be described as "individualism" or "particularism". Here Barry denies that principles true of patient populations allow "prediction" of the courses of individual patients. For Barry, "prediction" is not simply an assertion of expectation about a future event, perhaps qualified with a degree of likelihood; "prediction" is *true* assertion, so that assertions which turn out false are not predictions. Barry is too rarely able to predict a patient's course and the spectre of his failure is always close by.

The statistics don't apply to the individual. If we are told that 5% . . . . What do we do? That's right. You're really in a squeeze. I think they all should be anticoagulated, because you can't tell which will get . . . . And once they die, they're dead.

That probably will never happen again, but it did happen once.

Barry reacts to this particularism, the failture of "predictions", the absence of "crystal balls" and "clairvoyance", with an idiom of gambling, an activity which he avoids.

I don't think he's had an MI, but I'd hate to bet his life. It's a pity we didn't know earlier.

First trimester, if you listen to people, they wouldn't even breathe air. If you think of all the possible risks of everything, you wouldn't do anything. You're betting her life on minidose heparin (an anticoagulant).

. . . Then we get a call from the wife, and she says, "Hey, he's dead". You know!
(*RAH*): Even after, even after . . .
You bet ya, even after you've done those things. And, ah, so you become a believer. It doesn't have to happen a hundred times, and it doesn't have to happen to you. You can hear about it happening to someone else. And the good Lord hopefully makes us wise enough so it doesn't have to happen to us.

Here again the event of focal interest is that which happens to Barry himself or his colleagues; the death which initiates this focus is set aside.

Barry's response to what he takes to be his failures and those of the field of medicine escalate to a second stage, in which the uncertainty of events is no longer a quality of the knower or his relation to the event, but rather a quality of the event itself.

I think nothing is true any of the time any more. (*Resident says, "Nothing's true all the time".*

Nothing is black or white. I'm beginning to think there's no such thing as black and white. When they're dead they're white.

When radiologists cannot clearly diagnose from an X-ray, Barry reports they say, "It's gray". In Barry's claim about himself, however, he makes the same and a more damning statement as well, an acknowledgment of sharp limits and incapacity. He confronts a horrid paradox, in which his own impotence may be pitted against the most potent issues of life and death: the non-existence of black or white (diagnostic indicators) and the consequently inevitable stark whiteness of death.

At the third and last stage in the collapse of Barry's science of pictures, some principles of medicine, or even all of medicine, become, in Barry's account, "what you think", what you want to believe", "what you enjoy". While such expressions may exaggerate Barry's own concern that his medical work is arbitrary and even frivolous, at least he clearly verbalizes a possibility. He evinces a bitter humor. Valid pictures, or even useful pictures have given way to a nihilistic vision in which nothing is secure or certain; there is no "thing" or "picture". Medicine is then anchored only in the fanciful thoughts and personal pleasures of the practitioner rather than in anything approximating lawful events of human physiology. There is profound irony in such "pleasures" or fancies.

I think the answer is still up in the air, and I think it depends on what you want to believe.

Which just proves that there are a lot of experts or authorities with different ideas about things . . . . You do what you enjoy.

Medicine is mostly what you think.

It's just that: There is nothing written in stone someplace.

Here it seems that medicine itself may be at heart founded in judgment, a realm in which no answer excludes another, and all are equally good (or bad). Judgment, too, is close to emotion and to what, in some patients, Barry calls "screwing around", a violation of Natural Order.

The opposition between science and judgment engenders a deep and troubling tension in Barry's work and his thought. For, while he is successful and at ease in the science of his work judgment hovers too close by, at an uncertain distance from his science, persistently threatening. Judgment is closely linked with a host of phenomena which not only signal failure and impotence, but which also in themselves bring out anxiety. Judgment is the indeterminate product of a disquieting realm in which darker sentiments lurk beyond awareness and nothing is clear, or controllable.

We have seen that this strained opposition breaks down at two crucial moments: first, when the knowledge of science indicates alternate responses which are equally promising (or unpromising) and equally dangerous; second, when the strategies of science fail utterly because they yield no solutions or because the "solutions" they yield turn out to be false. In the first event, judgment must be made, and science can give no further help. In the second event, the solid foundation of science dissolves entirely, and all medicine slips into what is for Barry a morass of judgment. Pandora's box has been opened.

E. "TREAT THE PATIENT, NOT THE LAB"

In the course of his work with residents, perhaps the predominant principle of Barry's teaching is "Treat the patient, not the lab". There are many variants of this epithetical remark, all permutations on a few themes. The remark is a complex one; alongside its explicit intent run several hidden agenda and implicit emotional undercurrents. Beginning with this epithet, and calling on others, I explore Barry's concept of patients and persons, and some of his attitudes toward medical practice and its limits.

Look at the numbers you're fed. Don't believe numbers.

Are we treating numbers or are we treating her? My word of wisdom today, as everyday, is 'Fuck the number'.

Screw the lab!

Screw this number. See, you're treating a number!

You treat the patient, and screw the machines, and, if you can catch them, the nurses.

We want to put everything into numbers. (*Smiles*) . . . How do we know he's in failure?

A lot of medicine is common sense. It just doesn't take an act of God or a laboratory to tell you these things.

You don't need a blood gas. She's dyspneic. She needs O_2.

Instead of killing him in the course of further study, this is enough to indicate renal insufficiency.

Barry makes such comments in response to the diagnostic recommendations of his subordinate apprentices — the students, interns, and residents on his service at the hospital and the physicians' assistants and nurses for whom he is attending physician at the Hypertension Center. Barry believes that these assistants employ a logic in many of their recommendations which approximates this (in my version):

The patient is sick and his/her this-or-that (*a physiological function, measured on some standardized scale*) is such-and-such a reading or "value". Therefore, if we bring this value back to normal, by whatever non-harmful means available, we also will remove the pathology and restore the patient to normalcy and health.

Almost without exception, Barry rejects this logic.

Barry believes that contemporary medicine emphasizes a reliance on technology which neglects the development of reasoning and the use of more palpable evidence. Technology distances from more direct knowledge of his patients' conditions. Yet contemporary students are taught to order "batteries" of tests, and to respond to their results in a reflex fashion, without broader, more systematic consideration. Neglected is information often more relevant and more readily available, namely the patients' presentation and history. Barry's epithetical remarks are intended as an antidote to the bad habits of his apprentices.

While his prescriptions suggest that Barry believes numbers (and labs) not to be the sort of thing which one does or should treat, this inference is misleading. The essence of these formulaic teachings is his insistence that patients' characteristics not be treated one at a time, in isolation. Treating single features is not treating the patient.

On another plane of meaning, Barry's remarks about the treatment of patients suggest agreement with the currents of contemporary public and practitioner attitudes which favor "treating the whole person", "treating patients as persons", "holism", "individualism", "patient rights", "the unity of mind and body", and so on. The apparent agreement expressed here and in other of Barry's statements, for example, "Listen to the patient", is only superficial. Underlying a thin rhetorical mask is a very different, far narrower conception of patients. It is one which may have emerged with the Biomedical ideology of this century, still predominant in Barry's thought and practice. There is further evidence for Barry's narrow, even apersonal vision.

There may also lie in his remark an urge for self-reliance – a desire both for the use of self as instrument of knowledge, and for an independence from other sources. Not that Barry is a "loner" in his work, but that he wishes to retain control – fostering knowledge as direct and unmediated as possible.

Barry is concerned with excessive technology in medicine not only because the information produced may be irrelevant, misleading, or superfluous, but also because of its cost to the bodies of patients, to their financial stores, and to broader social insitutions. He is persistently conscious of the side effects and expenses of laboratory procedures, therapeutics, and other medical events. He seeks economy, finanical and corporeal. His economic concerns may have led him to work with the PSRO, this work in turn leading to heightened awareness of costs.

Barry's recommended response to common abuse of costly and misleading machines and their investigative products is to "screw" or "fuck" them. The metaphor of condemnation is secondary to the primary sexual one, but here the sexual association hovers close by. Thus Barry jokes, ". . . and, if you can catch them, the nurses". Thus also, he uses alternately "screw" and "fuck" in the same syntactial position.

In Barry's usage, numbers and labs (like nurses, patients, and other physicians as well) may be encountered in at least two modalities: numbers, etc. may be treated or they may be "screwed". While "scewing" is an intrusive form of dismissal, treatment is a response to the characteristics of what is treated, toward some particular end. One screws a number by throwing it aside, a violent rejection. One treats a number by altering it so that it returns to its "normal", healthy state. Barry insists that treating (single) numbers is not treating patients.

Barry does not believe, however, that the treatment of numbers and other patient characteristics is incompatible with the treatment of patients. "We absolutely have to have the numbers", he says. *Rather, it is against the treatment of single features that he inveighs.* He expresses his response to this insufficiency in another epithet:

Treat them by the company they keep.

That's why we say, "Treat them by the company they keep".

The "them" to be treated are clearly not patients, but their signs and symptoms, patient characteristics which include numbers and labs. Numbers and labs are treated, then, and in a social manner, in a company, as they interact with one another.

The logic of Barry's treatment thus runs as follows: Patients become diseased and systematically manifest their pathology in a variety of characteristics, including those they themselves report and others which are measured by variously complex and distancing devices. Interpreting these characteristics and responding appropriately to the patient requires understanding the sources of knowledge themselves and the way in which patient characteristics operate together to produce the sensible disease. We don't or shouldn't treat single numbers, but rather patients. We treat patients by treating the system of their characteristics, their picture. Thus, if not identical, there is at least a very close approximation of patient and syndrome. *Treating a patient is treating a syndrome.*

Rarely Barry will tell a resident, "Treat the number", or in a persuasive suggestion, "I'd treat the number". Two occasions on which I heard this prescription concerned high blood pressures. Very high blood pressures may be fatal in a short time, and moderately high ones over longer periods. But Barry's prescription in these cases was not contrary to his more common one, for he was familiar with each patient, and thus knew of other features in whose "company" the blood pressure was treated. This striking contrast to his usual recommendation was thus a rhetorical insistence on the critical importance of this particular number.

The third (and last) occasion on which I heard Barry call for the treatment of a number concerned a dying patient. Barry had consulted a hematologist for advice on how to proceed. He tells the resident on his service:

Just call him up and ask him for numbers to treat with. I don't know why it takes three weeks to get a report from a hematologist . . . . I think I need a day off.

Here again, Barry will not respond simply to a single number, but to the patient's other features which he already knows to be part of the picture. Two other conditions make the number compelling here. First, Barry does not feel competent to decide what to do here on his own; he thus depends on a colleague's formula. Second, the patient is dying, and the number in question, one beyond his own full comprehension, may be the last hope.

The company kept by the patient's characteristics is clearly an exclusive one, bounded by sharp but troublesome limits which include many of the patient's physical or physiological features, while excluding almost all of the patient's psychological, psychiatric, and social characteristics. The latter enter Barry's consideration only for highly specific diagnostic and therapeutic purposes. The core content of the company kept are physiological features.

"Listen to the patient", Barry repeats emphatically to the residents. The members of "the company kept" can most often be ascertained from the patient him or herself. "Nine times out of ten the patient will give you the Diagnosis".

I don't know. I just don't try to explain it. The tenderness does not matter . . . . Listen to the guy. Listen to him. That'll tell you most of the diagnosis.

You don't make a diagnosis of obstruction . . . from a cardiogram. You make it from what the patient reports.

You have to judge by the way they feel. Treat them and not the X-ray some of the time, most of the time.

Part of what Barry listens to is current symptoms. The remainder is the patient's "history". "Your history is so damned important . . . . Take that history for what it's worth." The "history" is a chronology of the patient's symptoms, activities, and environment. The "worth" of this chronology, transformed from the patient's to a medical "history", is essentially diagnostic. The history is cast as an impersonal thing: it is "that" history and "your" (the physician's) history, and it is taken by the physician from the patient, medically transformed and medically used.

Again, "listening to the patient" and "taking the patient's history" have the appearance of conformity to contemporary concern with the whole person, the patient's interests, individuality, context, and so on. Again the appearance is deceptive. Barry redirects the sharply delimited information drawn from the patient to his physiological examination. "Listening to the patient" and "taking the patient's history" are not efforts to sympathetically comprehend the patient's life world, inner meanings, fears, or desires, but rather to diagnose disease conceived of by criteria independent of their personal features.

Barry by no means ignores the psychological characteristics of his patients, nor their pathological, psychiatric counterparts. Yet his encounter of these is highly ambivalent. On the one hand he employs these characteristics in his medical work. On the other, he anxiously avoids patients' troubles, "deferring" exploration, and "referring out" the patients themselves.

Barry uses patients' psychiatric characteristics in three distinct ways. Most basic is their diagnostic use as indices of physiological process or disturbance. The assumption justifying this usage might be described as "somatopsychic" — that physiological events have psychological consequences or concomitants, and that these may be used, like other clinical signs, to assess physiological process. In this form of diagnosis, it is more often the manner of the patient's presentation than the content of the presentation which is indicative. The content in itself is tangential, misleading.

So the sensorium isn't all that clear . . . . Her sensorium is altered from normal. She's confused.
What do you think of the affect? . . . . Not the sensorium, but the expression on the face. It's flat. It's just flat. What meds is she on? She's normally a very astute and alert gal. This is not like her at all.
Try to shrink his brain and see what happend to his sensorium.

Talk here is directed toward medical co-workers, and most often away from patients. It refers to the patient, sometimes attaching a description to the named patient, sometimes depersonalizing the patient, as in "*the* sensorium" and "*the* expression on *the* face". Such talk may be conducted in the patient's presence, especially if the patient is (seemingly) unaware (e.g., asleep, drowsy, or stuporous or deaf.)

Patients' psychological qualities are useful also in interpreting their behavior and their own accounts or reports of their conditions, that is, in "listening" and in "taking that history". Barry notes of a Black woman patient, "This woman feels pain very strongly, very deeply", and of another patient, a White man, "He's a very stoic guy". Barry interprets their responses accordingly: he may minimize the woman's responses and amplify the man's.

Finally, Barry makes use of his knowledge of patients' psychological styles to predict and perhaps to influence their compliance with some medical procedure he believes appropriate. Again, in none of his medical listening is there a direct concern for the patient's experience. Rather, Barry presumes that his own reality is, or should be, the correct one and the one followed.

Psychiatric Pandora's

When he encounters the more psychiatric issues of his patients, Barry himself is disturbed, his own anxieties aroused. In order to depict Barry's encounter with psychiatry, I begin by citing his commentaries on two patients with psychiatric difficulties.

The first commentary is Barry's report on the patient's initial visit. Barry dictates his note for her chart, and interrupts the dictation to make comments aside to me. (I present the whole dictation.)

S: (*dictating history and physical examination of new hypertensive patient.*)
Date of initial examination and dictation 8.10.78. Chief complaint elevated blood pressure 5 years duration . . . states that she was found to have an elevated blood pressure with a diastolic

of approximately 112 as well as quote borderline diabetes unquote approximately 5 years ago. She is not aware of the level of her blood sugar. Nor is she aware of the level of her systolic blood pressure. She was under a great deal of tension with a great deal of responsibility and initially was treated with a muscle relaxant and later with hydrochlorothiazide 50 mg. daily with apparently improvement in her Hypertension. Approximately 2 years ago she was instructed in home blood pressure readings, and was able to control her blood pressure over the past year with a diet alone parentheses (1200 calories, without awareness of sodium) without any hydrochlorothiazide. She has moved to Cartown within the past year and has continued to check her blood pressures, and states that with her new position she also is under pressure and has noted a gradual increase in her blood pressure. Presented in the Hypertension Center where she was instructed to restart her hydrochlorothiazide, period. She felt tired and exhausted and quote "supertense" unquote, not resting well, but better since her blood pressure has been controlled. New paragraph.

The patient appears to be very te, ah, very, very tense, very bright, very anxious, expressed a great deal of her emotion and of her job responsibility. Expresses a great deal of anxiety regarding her mother who is very depressed.

(*Stops dictation; aside to RAH.*) See, I get the, I get the picture of this gal not being the bright eyed cheerful good natured gal that she is. Underneath all that there's a great deal simmering. And I'm not so sure that this gal isn't exceedingly depressed herself and isn't exceedingly anxious about her self as she sees her mother, and I, you know, I've, there are a lot of things I didn't even get into with her. I'm just damned afraid of opening a Pandora's, and I wouldn't know how the hell to put the lid back on her, so I, I just circumvented a lot of areas.
RAH: You wouldn't want to suggest to her seeing a psychiatrist?
S: I'm sure reading this thing here that this has been suggested to her, and ah, no I don't, nah, I didn't, I didn't feel now, not the initial visit. It's pretty hard sometimes to come about this. Sometimes you can antagonize an individual by the way you approach that or by what you might suggest to him, and I think you could drive them off rather than helping them get into the hands of a good therapist. I think you can drive them further way from a good therapist. And I feel very insecure about her emotionally, and I just want to play it close to the belt. I'll see her again, and we'll talk some more and see what the heck we can come . . . (*RAH interrupts*).
. . . I'm not sure how she handles other people's problems. I'm not really sure in my own mind what this (her history) all means, and, and I'm not sure that I want to get involved in that. I'm not sure that I can handle what I come up with.
. . . (*returns to dication*) Systems review . . . .
. . . rectal and pelvic exams are deferred at this time . . . .

Barry circumvents "a lot of areas" because he is "just damned afraid of opening a "Pandora's" and wouldn't know how the hell to put the lid back on . . . ." Barry explains that he listens, but avoids getting into "a lot of areas", in order to engage the patient's trust, so that she will return for future visits. This may be a common and productive strategy. Deferral may have a deeper significance for him, namely the avoidance of work which is troubling to Barry himself. Barry's language here is highly ambiguous, referring to his patient and to himself in the same troubled phrases. Barry is susceptible to the effects of the patient's psychiatric condition, if not by some sort of contagion, then by a deep parallel sympathy.

And *I feel very insecure about her emotionally*, and I just want to play this thing cool.

I'm not sure how she . . . *I'm not really sure in my own mind* how she . . . *I'm not sure that I want to get involved in that. I'm not sure I can handle what I come up with.*

Grammatically, his word, "emotionally", refers to his own mode of feeling; he feels emotionally insecure. Yet I believe he intends to refer to the patient's emotionality. Then he is multiply insecure in his own mind how she can handle other people's problems, or how he can handle hers. His description places both the patient and himself in the same predicament. Finally, beyond wanting to postpone exploration of her psychiatric problems, he doubts that he wants "to get involved in that" at all.

A second commentary concerns an adolescent girl who has been Barry's patient for several years. Her medical problem is diabetes. Barry describes her psychiatric problems as "depression" and "suicidal tendencies", and he suggests factitious illness as well, that is, illness which the patient has deliberately induced in herself. The hospital rounds team has just visited her and talks in the hall. (I transcribed Barry's comments selectively at the time, without benefit of tape recorder.)

She's been hard to manage partly because of emotional problems. She's been depressed and has suicidal tendencies.

One of her problems is her mother.

I finally threw up my arms, and asked her to go somewhere else.

That's a mess.

And, in addition to that, they really like medications.

She's been seen by every psychiatrist in town, too.

The medications can't do anything for her. We're stuck with all her problems, and we can't do anything.

The only thing that's going to help this girl is letting her complete her suicide.

(*A medical student reports, "She lives with her parents".*) Which is part of her problems.

Maybe we're doing too much for her. Maybe we ought to let up on all her medications.

Knowing Mary, maybe she's got a bottle of milk of magnesia by her bed, and is taking it.

She has physical problems, too. She was depressed before she had her problems.

I don't know what the hell to do with her. I've told her. I've asked her who she wants to see.

If you want to try it (*some medications*) that's okay, 'cause all we're doing now is treading water.

And send her home. I don't know why the hell she's here.

As far as I'm concerned, this gal is totally hopeless.

(*Student asks if he can talk with her.*) Do it in a causal way. Bump into her in the corridor, 'cause she's been talked to by everyone.

And I tell her I can't help you. And she says, "Don't ever leave me, 'cause you're the only one who ever talks to me".

I'm impressed with these agents, that they don't help over the long haul, except in psychotics.

I want to send here home, cause I don't want to see her any more in the hospital.

Her mother called me and said that she felt that Mary should die so she wouldn't suffer. Her mother is a large part of the problem .... Her father is extremely passive .... Her mother is quite aggressive. But I don't know how I would act with a daughter like that.

This is a litany of impotence and frustration. Barry has had difficulty "managing" Mary's medical problems, principally those associated with her diabetes. He begins by noting that management of the diabetes is complicated by Mary's emotional problems: she is depressed and suicidal. Barry has a vague schematic theory of the etiology of Mary's psychiatric problems: Mary lives at home; her mother, and perhaps her father too, are "part of the problem". Barry seems to regard the parents' behavior as not only causative of, but also reactive to Mary's problems. Thus he says, after describing the parents' behavior styles, "But I don't know how I would act with a daughter like that". He condemns both Mary and her parents, and finds justification for both condemnations.

Barry regards Mary's depression as worsened, but not initiated by her physical condition. He suspects she may induce her own physical problems, for example, by taking milk of magnesia. He believes that no psychiatrist or psychiatric medication has done her any good. And, although she has gained admission to the hospital for his care, and has told him, "Don't leave me, 'cause you're the only one who ever talks to me", he insists that he can do and has done nothing for her problems. "Doing nothing" is a highly medical notion, one which seems to include talk.

Again, as might many other physicians, including psychiatrists, Barry attempts flight. He is unsuccessful. He has thrown up his arms and asked her to go elsewhere. He says he wants to send her home, at first because he doesn't know "why the hell she's" there, and then, " 'cause I don't want to see her anymore in the hospital". Nor, he hints, does he want to see her elsewhere.

His strong desire to rid himself of this patient follows his assumption of her problem: "We're stuck with her problems . . .". While her hopelessness, expressed by her in her presence in the hospital and by her plea to him, is not yet total, his hopelessness regarding her is total: "As far as I'm concerned, this gal is totally hopeless". It is he rather that she who is totally hopeless about her condition. He takes on himself the burden of her emotional problems, and strongly desires to cast off this weight. Emotionality not only complicates his work, but is contagious, and beyond his control.

More briefly I cite Barry's commentary on a young woman he was asked to see. The woman has a history of drug addiction. His response further indicates his fears. He "refers out" to a psychiatrist. The "deep involvement" which a psychiatrist may offer might provide relief not only for the patient, but for Barry himself.

I think she needs a therapist who knows what the hell she's doing . . . . Just taking her off drugs is not enough. She's got to have something to take its place. You put her in a vacuum. You don't leave anything to replace. I would be anxious about that . . . . I don't know enough about her to make any more comments about that. I'm scared of a gal like that. I'm scared 'cause I don't know what to do with her. I'd punt to a psychiatrist. I'd have a psychiatrist get deeply involved in her management . . . . If I saw her in the office I'd say, "Hey, baby, I can't take care of you . . . ." Some people, even Sigmund Freud couldn't help them. It's true they can't help everybody, like you can't help everybody.

Barry has no pretentions about being a psychiatrist. "I'm as poor a psychiatrist as I am a dermatologist". He tells me of a plan a psychiatrist colleague once proposed to him. While he explained the proposal as a joke, its appeal to him reflects his apprehensions and his troubled uncertainty in psychiatry. His colleague proposed:

That we ought to have, rather than diagnoses where there's so much overlap and so much uncertainty in psychiatry, that we ought to have functional diagnoses. For example, this person is emotionally ill to a degree of grade one. We know whatever that arbitrarily means, that means he can still work and earn a living and come home and stay out of the hospital setting, in contrast to an emotional grade five who is totally unable to work and totally dependent. And then you have grades in between. I think this tells you a whole lot more sometimes than "psychoneurosis". What does that mean you know, unless you go on . . . . Well, I don't know. That's just my own kind of thinking. Ah, it doesn't mean anything.

Barry's classification accepts social notions of functioning and utility, while ignoring the personal qualities in capacity and suffering. His classification is functional not only in the sense which he implies, that is, based on the degree of social functioning of which the patient is capable. It is functional to him also in reducing the fears of psychiatry's Pandora's. Barry suggests, unintentionally, his attitude toward psychiatric patients. He describes patients with grade one illness as person, yet he reduces grade five patients to the illness itself. The patient is described as "an emotional grade five who is totally unable . . .".

Of his understanding of patients' emotional and social problems, Barry told me once:

Our training and background in some of these situations are, ah, what we hope to think, or like to think of as common sense. Ah, or you know, answers or responses to 'em (these problems) or manners of dealing with 'em, and the ability hopefully to recognize that the problems exist in these other areas, to call for assistance where we need it – for some of the non-medical, non-physical things, situations. I think we're, our training and background is largely, deals with physical disease . . . . But out thinking isn't limited to that.

In contrast to his medicine, these issues are matters of common sense, taught incidentally and casually. While Barry is troubled by the uncertainty of psychiatric diagnosis and theory, the limited psychiatry which he practices is highly formular. The lack of black or white certainty which haunts his medical practice is absent here. Barry's psychiatric categories seem rigidly bounded, and patients fit or do not fit them. While Barry may have difficulty placing patients into these categories, as he admits he does not know them well, nevertheless he speaks of the categories as if they were solid and fixed. His approach is illustrated in a sequence of five diagnostic comments on a male patient whom we saw first on September 11. The last comment is made two and a half months later.

I think this guy, if he's not psychotic, is severely neurotic . . . (Sept. 11).

I don't know if you'd call him a conversion reaction or just a severe neurotic.

He's a conversion reaction. The psychiatrist said he was an organic brain syndrome.

I don't believe it . . . . I think the drugs played an important role, and whether there was a conversion reaction, I don't know (Sept. 15).

I still can't help the feeling that he's having a little conversion reaction, too . . . . He got an IQ of about fifty, too (Nov. 15).

There are two complementary understandings here: first the patient is said not to have these conditions, but to be them. Psychiatric conditions are closer to identities than to afflictions. There is a suggestion of this also in Barry's proposal for psychiatric grading. Here a patient may be *a* catatonic, or *a* conversion reaction, or *an* organic brain syndrome. Second is the apparent sharpness of the boundaries between these diagnostic categories. If a catatonic is a kind of person rather than something a person has or something that happens to a person, then any given person either is or is not a catatonic. In his psychiatry, Barry is at his realist, reificational extreme.

Medical – Non-Medical

A strong dichotomy pervades Barry's thought and his work: Medical versus Non-medical. This dichotomy defines the limits of Barry's field of work and his competence. It demarcates two domains of the universe which are assumed to be empirically separable, though sometimes only with difficulty. In one he works comfortably, in the other he is troubled. The division has many versions and associations. It is at once reinforced by associations, oppositions, and threatened by invasion. (See Figure 3.)

	Medical	Non-Medical
Problems and responses	Physical Organic	Just Social Non-Physical Functional
Knowledge – sources and processes	Objective Science	Subjective Emotional and social Judgment, philosophy

Fig. 3.

The dichotomy has several characteristics. Barry regards the two categories as mutually exclusive, so that a problem or some facet of it which is medical (or physical, organic . . .) is therefore not non-medical (non-physical, functional . . .) and vice versa. Thus Barry refers to emotional and social problems as ". . . some of these non-medical, non-physical things, situations". For example, he reports to his partners that a patient has "more subjective complaints than objective findings", and he notes to a resident that a patient has "really got nothing objective in his joints".

At the same time, Barry regards patients' problems to be often compounded by both medical and non-medical components, sometimes in a way which is difficult to disentangle. Problems vary in the percentage of each component present.

They overlap; a good many times they overlap. But very often you can pick out the individual components of the major problem.
RAH: You think there are, there are clear cut medical problems that have no, that aren't social? Yes, well I can, there are, there are clear cut problems that are 99% medical and 1% social, yeah. And there are clear problems that are 99% social and 1% medical. The guy, the person who's got a, who's got a marital problem, and needs counseling, she (*sic*) may have a headache as a result of all the, you know the problems she got at home, but I consider that 1% medical and 99% social.

RAH: What would the other end be?

Well, someone who's got a metastatic cancer, for example, and that has insurance to take care of their financial needs for their medical care. You know, they may have, I mean, their, their immediate problem is 99% medical. Sure they got a problem about their will and . . . going to look after the family when I'm gone and that kind of thing, and dispose of the cat, and whatever else. But, but, you know I think their problem is 99% medical and 1% social. Well, maybe not that much. Maybe it's a 90% and 10% or 80% and 20%. I think there's clear divisions where a majority fall in one sector or the other. I wish to hell I had answers. I wish to hell someone had answers. Not just . . . .

RAH: Those are often questions of value judgment rather than . . . there are no answers.

Yeah, that's right. You're absolutely right. They are. And, and, you know, you can talk to ten people, as you know, and . . . get twenty different answers, in a situation like that.

Barry's wish that "to hell I had answers. I wish to hell someone had answers", is directed to social problems which he says, are questions of judgment for which there are as many answers as answerers.

Though Barry does not do so in this fashion, we may divide causal relations to somato(cause)-somatic(consequence), somato-psychic, psycho-somatic, and psycho-psychic. (See Figure 4.) Somato-somatics is Barry's proper medicine: 100% physical, 0% emotional. Somato-psychics he employs for diagnostic purposes; a psychological event may be an index of physiology. But patients may also react psychologically to their disease in ways which do not directly indicate a physiological process; such reactions are peripheral to Barry's medicine.

Psycho-psychics is the realm of the "functional", socio-emotional, and falls within the domain of psychiatry. And Barry may think of psycho-somatic effects as short-lived; thus he tells me that psychic stress affects blood pressure only transiently.

It is likely that psycho-somatic conditions are rare among his diagnoses because they make less sense to him. He believes that psychological explanations mask ignorance, and that when we know what really occurs, our understanding will be couched in terms of organic process. For example, he talks of changes in the understanding of "ulcerative colitis":

They used to teach that ulcerative colitis, one of the diseases of the bowel, was an emotional disease, and was treated by psychiatrists. Well, you know, if you're shittin' thirty times a day, ah, what kind of emotional problem, what kind of emotional response would you have to this illness? It, you know, it can't be complacent. If you lost a hundred pounds shittin' 30 times a day, how would you feel? You see, and, and I don't know. I think we've, now if we coming around to thinking that it's, it's an organic, we don't understand it fully, but it's an organic illness to which people have an emotional response. And that makes more sense to me. Merely because we don't know what causes, we used to classify it as an emotional illness. And there was a period of time, merely because we don't know what causes it, we classify it as an allergic disease. Now we're getting another fad: If we don't know what causes it, we say it may be autoimmune, ah which is another thing.

I ask whether "the answers that are ultimately convincing are those that are biological in nature, that are microscopic — explain the small processes?" He suggests agreement, but does not commit himself.

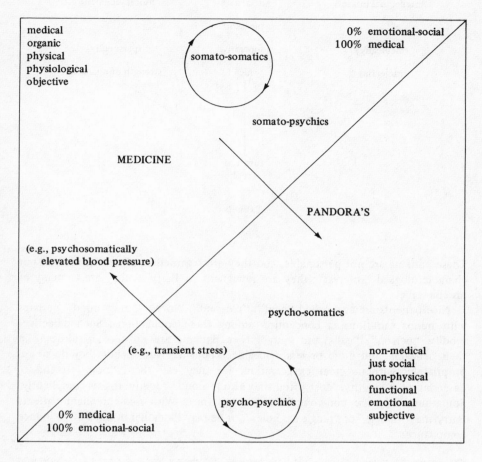

medical
organic
physical
physiological
objective

somato-somatics

0% emotional-social
100% medical

somato-psychics

MEDICINE

PANDORA'S

(e.g., psychosomatically
elevated blood pressure)

psycho-somatics

(e.g., transient stress)

psycho-psychics

non-medical
just social
non-physical
functional
emotional
subjective

0% medical
100% emotional-social

Fig. 4.

Well, this is more scientific, certainly. Ah, you know, how you explain what you see sometimes
can be a variable thing, too. So I don't think that always applies. But I think it's more likely
that's the case.

Patients and their Relations

Barry describes his various patients in strikingly different ways, and he responds
to them accordingly. I discern in his distinctions among patient three basic axes
or dimensions: one of medical interest, a second of personal pleasantness, and a
third of strength and interest of character (See Figure 5.) At the negative extreme
on all axes is the patient described as "a turd", "a nut", or rarely "a crock".

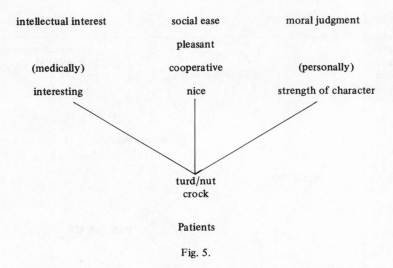

Fig. 5.

These patients are not personable, and they are regarded as of neither medical nor characterological "interest"; they are repugnant to Barry as they are to many of his colleagues.

Nice patients are also called "neat", "pleasant", "lovely", and "good", perhaps with minor variations in conception among these appellations. Such adjectives modify "person", "gal", and "guy". Nice patients are most often pleasant in their behavior, and more or less agreeable. They may suffer, but they do so appropriately, without great exaggeration. He may call them "poor" so-and-so, deserving of sympathy. Most often they also respond properly, that is compliantly. Sometimes they are non-compliant, but still nice. With non-compliant patients Barry may "tangle" or "tangle ass holes", or he may "kick her in the ass" to induce compliance.

She knows the whole bit. She's lost both her legs. But she's a lovely person. (*A diabetic who has lost her vision as well as her legs.*)

He's a nice guy. I'm glad he's doing well.

Don's a nice guy. What can you do with a guy with chronic pain. Do you give it to him or do you hold it? . . . And he's such a nice, pleasant fellow. (*He questions giving addictive pain-killers.*)

She's a nice person. I have to kick her in the ass every now and then, but she's a nice person.

He's a nice guy, God, he's a nice person. I often wonder how you yourself would respond to an illness like that.

That's too bad. What a nice guy he is. (*Patient just diagnosed with rectal cancer.*)

He's so sick, that poor guy. Why the hell doesn't the Good Lord take him?

Are you smoking again?
Patient: Yeah.
I can't understand you.
Patient: You got to smoke a little.
Don't smoke, man . . . (*Aside, away from the patient's bed.*) Every time I see his card, I say, "Oh, no, we're going to tangle again". But I like him, He's a nice guy.

Barry is pleased when nice patients do well, troubled when they suffer. He works for them with urgency.

Some patients are also described as "interesting"; these are not necessarily the same patients as the nice ones. Interesting patients may also be described as "fascinating", perhaps also as "good".

Just a horrendous mess . . . . Every metabolic problem he can have . . . . He's fascinating. He's got every metabolic failure known.

This guy is going to be real interesting . . . . It's an interesting differential. A guy, 80, insulin dependent. It's going to be fun.

Interesting! I wasn't prepared for him at the end of the weekend. But he's an interesting guy.

She's a good gal. I think you should get all the teaching we can out of her.

There are some interesting people (*in the hospital*). I can't think of a single crock.

These patients are interesting because they present problems which are sufficiently complex to be intriguing, yet probably soluble. (The patient described above as a "good gal" may be so classified because she is nice rather than because she is interesting. She turns out to be of interest also, however, and thus teaching is to be extracted from her difficulties.) Interesting problems (or patients) contrast with those which are simple and soluble, such as "nice juicy pneumonias" or "strep throats". They contrast also with those problems which are complex and insoluble by current means, such as sickle cell anemia and some forms of "terminal" cancer. With interesting patients, Barry and his followers test their medical abilities, with reasonable success.

Other patients are valued not because they are medically interesting, but because they have strong and striking, but not offensive personalities. These patients are "characters", or "real characters".

This guy's a real character. He's got emotional problems, he and his wife. He's hard to manage sometimes.

In contrast to all of these patients whom Barry values, though for different reasons, are "turds", patients for whom he has strong dislike. He calls them also "bitch", "nut", "son of a bitch", "a crock". One such patient he saw following a sleepless night on call. The patient complained of being tired, and Barry later told me:

This guy I tangled ass holes with . . . He's a real turd . . . . Last time he was here with his father, and they just rubbed me wrong . . . . That was just too much.

On another occasion, one day while on rounds, Barry was called from the Emergency Room (ER) regarding a patient of his who had just arrived there. "That gal in the Emergency Room, she really gets impatient. She's a nut". He mentioned to us her "semi-annual bath", and he complained that for three months she had had the same "belly pain" which now brought her into the ER. As the patient is impatient, Barry is impatient with her. As she has delayed coming in for her belly pain, Barry delays in going to see her in the ER.

Barry objects also to patients whom he finds morally or socially offensive. He objects to patients who abuse themselves and others at the same time, patients, that is, who seem to be the principal agent in their own disease. One patient had hepatic complications of alcoholism. Barry's anger is thinly veiled, and his medicine highly ambivalent, not "compulsive". He discusses forms of treatment with the residents.

And I wouldn't object to trying them on him. After all, we've, we've nothing in the world to lose, and if we bring this guy back, ah, I don't know if that's good or bad. It's probably not particularly good. But I don't know that it's bad necessarily either. That's a, that's a philosophical thing you can debate all you want. But my feeling about a guy like this is that I think he deserves the same kind of care as someone coming the first, the first crack. If he dies, well he dies, and you've tried. And I'm not just trying to obviate guilt. I don't have any guilt about alcoholics, oh, about, within reason I do have guilt, of course. But I don't feel that compulsive about alcoholics.

As another example of his moral repugnance, Barry saw a patient who was on welfare and had a number of "illegitimate" children. Barry was offended by her "promiscuity" and by his inability to do anything but offer her the option of contraceptive pills, and monitor her blood pressure. He wants her to take the pills to prevent conception. He wants her not to take them to avoid problems of hypertension. He talks about liberal reformers:

Unfortunately in people who are full of ideas as to what to do with them, with situations in regard to them. You know the person is well-intentioned, and said, "Well, it's her life. She can do what she wants to". Well, fine, sure she can go out and screw all she wants. That's her bu, it's her business. But do we have to support her mistakes, or do we have to support her in the process of doing that? And, do we have to pay her way, really, as a, as, as a non-compensated prostitute, or whatever? Really. Which is what we're doing . . . .

His moral certainty leads into his offer of contraceptive pills. He resents public support for this woman's "promiscuity" and her procreative "mistakes".

That's her decision. I don't know what you can do about that . . . . It's her decision, not to come, not to take her pill . . . . We're powerless. All you can do is beat your head against the wall.

Barry may turn violently angry also against the relatives of patients. One patient's diabetes was exacerbated when her husband left home for another woman. "Her husband. I would wring his balls off, if I could ever get a hold of him". He makes a similar remark about the daughter of the patient, noted above, who lost her legs, but remained a "lovely person". The patient's daughter has taken money from one man to abort the child of another. With morbid irony, perhaps unintended, Barry says, "Bitch, I'd like to wring her tits off, honest to God". Vengeance as well as healing are expressed in the corporeal idiom.

Alongside Barry's common sexual reference are occasional hints of a highly ambivalent attitude toward women. A resident showed him a series of small, graded holes drilled in a plastic sheet, used as a template for measurement. Barry joked, "Is that for cervical dilation?" On another occasion he was talking about problems of instructing patients, and he illustrated the difficulties with this example, quoted above,

You got to instruct people in really simple things. If you give a woman a vaginal suppository, you've got to tell her to take the foil off.

His examples are not randomly chosen. In them there is a bitterness; and thinly masked in humor, there is a strain of misogyny. The allusions are sexual, in stark, physical terms. They are at least suggestive of a lack of intelligence among female patients.

At the same time, Barry remarks often that his favorite patients are "little old ladies":

Little old ladies are so much fun. So much more than little old men.

Patients get older as I do. My favorite patients are little old ladies. I love them. They're just great . . . until they start spitting at you. (*Laughs*)

He notes their wisdom and the stories they tell. There are undoubtedly other qualities as well which personally attract him. The sexuality of these women is greatly diminished; yet they may remain maternal, and they require his close attention. I speculate, but leave full inference of these dynamics to other analysts.

Barry is a complex man, perhaps as much a comment on my representation of him as on the man himself. I attempt to portray him as human — as human as he is, neither super-, nor sub-human — as human as we all are. Like many of us, his different layers are difficult to discern. They are often indirectly expressed, they are often contradictory, ambivalent. I believe that his character fits well the educational system which has shaped it. It fits also, though uneasily, in the current setting of his practice.

F. FLOW AND OBSTRUCTION IN A CORPOREAL UNIVERSE

Two idiomatic strands, closely intertwined, connect Barry's expressions of the movement, intensity, and intimacy of his work: an image of the body, and another of the dynamic of flow and obstruction. Imagery of bodily structure and bodily function is widely recycled in Barry's expressions of this world. With these idioms he refers not only to the medical focus of his work, that is, his patients' bodies, but to the surrounding work as well — his own efforts of diagnosis and treatment of patients, his control of the hospital environment, and his sense of control in his own functioning. His own functioning as well as the workings of the world are spoken of as analogous to human physiological function. To be sure, most of the expressions he employs are not uniquely his, yet the intensity and persistence of his use of them, and their reflexive presence in a medical setting (where they are thus both subject and metaphor) are indicative of his own deep emotional involvement. His multiple physiological references would provide a rich mine for analytical digging, in which I have no expertise.

I am suggesting that as Barry moves, physically, intellectually, emotionally, through hospital corridors, his office, the administrative, social and economic "structures" of the circum-medical regions, and through his own thoughts and feelings about patients and their conditions — in this movement, as well as within his patients' bodies, Barry is perpetually concerned with the qualities of the channels of passage, with obstructions to passage, and with rates and regularity of flow.

The system of the human body, with its multiple, complexly related parts, is the center of Barry's medical attention. This corporeal focus is a passionate one. I have noted his fears and anxieties at patients' conditions, as well as his frustrations with his incapacities and his satisfactions in competence and effect. The flow of blood is a persistent worry. Barry runs scared of pulmonary emboli. He fears that clots of blood, dislodged from their vessels, may obstruct the vital passage of blood through the lungs, and thence of oxygen to the blood. Obstructed blood flow may effect "MIs" in the heart, strokes in the brain, aneurysms (blood vessel ruptures), ischemia (circulatory shortages), and infarction (complete obstruction and tissue death) in other organs and tissues as well. The only "number" which Barry ever advocates treating is that indicating severely high blood pressure, a precursor of many other complications, often lethal. Other systems of flow are also of concern: the flow of air in the respiratory system, passage through the alimentary canal, flow of hormones through the blood, urine production and excretion, and the horrid and often occult "metastasis" of cancerous processes from one body part to others.

The dynamic of events and contingencies in patients' bodily flow are recorded by all medical participants in what is referred to in another metaphor of movement as a "chart". This common medical idiom compares the patient to a ship at sea. The chart maps what is called the patient's "course". The patient is said to have this or that medicine "aboard". The patient's course may proceed straightforwardly, "without complication", following the normal picture of such conditions; or the course may deviate from normal, and is then said to be "complicated" by this, that, or the other further condition.

Barry speaks also of his medical actions in terms of movement and obstruction, applying bodily images to these medical manipulations of bodily events. Tests may be "run on" the patients; and when a test result contradicts is hypothesis, Barry may advise, "Fuck the lab, treat the patient". In diagnosing patients' conditions, he speaks of maintaining alternative pictures and of keeping an "open mind", perhaps also to allow proper flow of ideas and evidence. Barry may talk of the resident whose diagnostic or therapeutic acts or plans are unlikely to yield results as "spinning your wheels", or "treading water", rapid motion without desired effect.

Treatments as well are referred to as "courses" or "routes". Barry refers to one treatment in particular, intense anticoagulation, not simply as "*a*", but as "*the* route", promoting proper flow by this standard medical movement.

Within the hospital itself, the "rounds" move through the corridors at a pace which Barry monitors so that he may be at his office on time. The movement of patients is controlled as well; patients are said to be admitted and discharged, and in between they may be transferred to or from "the floor", and to and from different diagnostic and treatment locations within the hospital. Barry speaks of "cleaning house" and of "opening up beds with some of these folks", thus maintaining a good hospital circulation by effectively treating patients. Beyond his medical work, Barry monitors and certifies the circulation in his work with the PSRO.

Especially in situations of uncertainty, frustration, and conflict of purpose and action, where others interfere with his medical work, Barry may refer to the offending relations and persons — patients and their families, other physicians, nurses, and residents, in terms of physiological parts and functions. Patients or others may be "turds" or "shits", and Barry may "tangle assholes with them". Doctors and nurses may be "shitty" insofar as they are uncooperative in Barry's work and plans. They may be said to "screw", "fart", or "diddle around". They may be "a pain in the ass". He may recommend "pissing on them".

Other persons from the patient's milieu may be similarly indicated. In response to a resident's concern for the unborn child of a diabetic woman, near term, but with an as yet undiagnosed complication, Barry says, "Fuck the baby". And he may, as noted, vent his anger at patient's family members who aggravate the patient's condition or interfere with treatment by an expressed intent, as noted to "wring his balls off", "wring her tits off", "twist her legs off", strong physical, perhaps sexual revenge. All of these bodily citations are intended to be vulgar and deeply offensive. Patients, their relatives, and medical personnel not only produce filth, but may themselves be filth; and they may be its target.

These sexual and scatological references are not simple metaphors. Literal reference remains close by. A crude sexuality underlies his condemning urges to "screw" this or that. I have cited earlier the variant of his epithetical demand to treat the patient and not the lab, to which he added, in his wry humor, a remark about the nurses, "Screw the lab, and the nurses, if you can catch them". While his command to "screw" the lab rejects it emphatically and derrogatorily with a secondary metaphor (based on a primary sexual one), here, in Barry's additional remark about the nurses, the primary sexual reference returns to the fore.

Similarly, Barry once referred to a pen he was using, given him by a patient, as "stool brown". On another occasion he asks a clinic nurse if a patient had "brought in his bowel movements, any stool, has he?" The nurse answered that she didn't know, and Barry said, "Shit, literally shit". He then remembered the lab report from the patient's specimen, and he changed his mind, "Yes he did too. He brought 'em over to the lab. I take it all back. I take it all back . . .".

Engagement with his patients' bodies touches him in a personal, emotional way. Beyond his medical concern for proper flow within the body, Barry is troubled by bodily effluence and excretion. Here the concern is one of contamination — contamination not in a medical sense, but in a more generic sense of dirt and impurity. In introducing Barry, I noted his remark that from the outside of his medical career, "snot" was the only thing which he could not tolerate. His vulgarity here seems deliberate — an explicit repulsion, clarifying a boundary against filth. I have noted other similar references as well:

I think the emergency doctor would have the ability to tell people that it's not an emergency. "Look, if you've got a snotty nose . . . ."

It just keeps the snot and stuff from getting on my street clothing. (*His white coat.*)

The human body, its workings and its failings, is not only the literal object of Barry's work, but is widely disseminated in metaphorical reference to the world of his work itself, a means by which the work, participants in it, and its relations are experienced and expressed. The work is about the body, the body about the work. Nor is this recursion simply on intellectual exercise, but rather one which seems both to penetrate and to emerge from Barry's personal and emotional core. Corporeal images carry expressions of deep engagement and deep revulsion. Barry moves in a corporeal universe, as it lives in him also.

G. BARRY, ON HIMSELF

Barry's acts, including his speech, are all parts and indices of his self. In some of these acts Barry refers to himself explicitly, thus more deliberately representing his self-conception and attitude; other acts are unwitting self-representations. I conclude this portrait by examining these performances, mostly verbal in order to depict Barry's self-understanding, especially regarding his engagment and disengagement in relations with patients.

In a most direct medical fashion, Barry uses himself as a diagnostic device. Certainly he is always his own diagnostic instrument, combining all of his particular and general knowledge to make the final assessment. He uses himself also for a more unusual form of diagnosis in which he reads his own sensations, or "feelings", in order to achieve on intuitive diagnostic knowledge of the patient. I do not know how he believes such diagnosis to work — perhaps it is an unconscious calculus, the residue of his experience — what he was taught in medical school to be "the sixth sense".

There's no question in my mind what he's got, but I can't prove it to you.

He looks better, but I can't measure it.

I still can't help the feeling that he's having a little conversion reaction, too.

Barry looks inwardly to himself as meter of a patient's condition. He is intuitively impelled by his feelings, without rationale.

Barry uses his own sensations also to estimate the validity of a diagnosis or proposed therapeutic action. He speaks of fears and anxieties when things do not feel right, and of being comfortable when they do. Comfort is a measure of his proper place within the confines of his medical specialty, as well as in his particular assessment of the patient's condition.

Yes I think there's got to be some balance that, that the physician at least is able to feel himself comfortable with, 'cause if he's not comfortable in a given area, he's not going to do justice to anybody.

I don't feel comfortable . . . . It's nice to feel comfortable, and you often don't feel comfortable with a situation.

When he is not comfortable, Barry expresses fear and anxiety regarding both the conditions which may affect patients and his uncertain "knowledge" of this or that patient. Two common regions of fear and anxiety are obstructions of blood flow and psychiatric disturbances.

That's a frightening thing to me. I, I, I just, ah, I just don't know, you know, you just feel these people are sitting there with a guillotine blade hanging over their head, and, ah, if that thing is going to flop, I, I, I, tend to be more aggressive.

Everybody's got this damned residual anxiety about this guy . . . .

I just don't feel right about her. I just don't know her well enough.

I would be anxious about that . . . . I'm scared by a gal like that. I'm scared 'cause I don't know what to do with her.

Barry sometimes explicity imagines himself in his patients' situation.

I would be anxious about all those agents. I don't know about the combination . . . . I wouldn't want it on myself.

But I don't know how I would act with a daughter like that. (*See above, p. 94.*)

He may retreat from his imagined response by shifting from the close "I" who imagines to the more distant "you yourself" who is imagined ill.

He's a nice guy. God, he's a nice person. I often wonder how you yourself would respond to an illness like that. (*A kidney patient, now on dialysis.*)

Barry suggests experiencing medical procedures as a way of sympathizing with patients and restricting the uses of these procedures to a necessary minimum.

I think that everyone who wants to order a Levin tube down should have one down first. I think that everyone who thinks that an I.V. is non-invasive should have one done. (*The Levin tube is inserted through the patient's nostril to his stomach, nasogastrically (i.e., n.g. tube), for more direct feeding.*)

Barry sometimes talks in a way which represents either diagnosis or therapy as affecting or promoting his own well-being, in addition, perhaps instead of the patient's. Some of this talk is partly in jest.

Take a deep breath for me.

Please take your medications, just to please me if nothing else.

One patient is asked to take a deep breath, another his medications, for Barry's sake.

Likewise, relief of the patient's suffering or of the threat of disease brings relief and healing to Barry also. Very commonly Barry expresses in words and in comportment his own pleasure and release in his relief of patients' medical problems. Relief is thus "his" both as healing agent and as recipient. Success is a sign of self, its potency and livelihood.

You can breathe easier.

That's the big change in the past ten years, the survival rate of children of diabetic mothers. That was sad. The salvage rate of the infant is so much better. It's refreshing. Boy it's nice, because I think a third of them used to lose their babies. Now it's only five percent.

Barry thus suffers alongside his patients, and he is healed when they are. His response is a form of sympathy, a pathos in parallel, but separate and distant from that of his patients. It is a medicalized sympathy; Barry suffers not empathically, in the same form as his patients do, but in response to their medical conditions. Thus he may suffer when they do not, for some asymptomatic conditions; and when they do suffer, he may do so also, but for a different reason, a medical one. His response to the suffering of patients might be described as "allo-pathic", a tangential, alternative suffering. This response is consistent with his "treating the patients" and his "listening" to them, a response shaped by medical vision.

As noted earlier, Barry's anxiety at patients' psychiatric conditions emerges in ambiguous statements in which he refers to himself and to his patients at the same time. Similar ambiguous reference appears in his reflections to residents (and me) on a patient whose life has been full of tragic losses:

You know, when a patient loses a couple of kids, for whatever reason, I don't think you ever recover from it. And she's like an old Jewish mother. She'd come in, "Ach . . . ." You know, like this. And you know, you understand it. Shit, you know, you got any kids at all, and you think of what would happen to them, and how you'd react to that.

He suggests here that he himself does not recover from the patients' traumatic losses. Barry is cognizant of his emotional engagement in his patients' lives and deaths. The death of a "terminal" patient with unrelieved pain is both "a blessing" and a sorrow for him.

Sometimes it's a blessing, sometimes. They're always with some sorrow. They're more than patients. They're not close friends, but they're friends . . . . They're all different. It's hard to generalize. There are different attachments to people. They all leave their mark on you.

Barry talks as well of the more general and persistent effects of his work on himself. He talks in terms of his body and in more personal terms. He talks of "the firing line" which may summon the primary care physician at any hour of day or night. He notes the absence of "protection" from access which is afforded to specialists (who also earn more money, unjustly, Barry complains). In a personal mode, he talks of not wanting to read more journals because he is "so fatigued"; he "unwinds very easily" by jogging, putting himself "in a trance".

It's very demanding, unfortunately, not only of yourself, but of your family. They've got to be very understanding, very sympathetic. And it gets very depressing at times with the fatigue and sometimes the chaos that when you're almost, when you're asked to be in three different places at the same time. It's just impossible to do. It's very frutsrating too.

Work with colleagues is also felt in personal and emotional ways. Colleagues may help or hinder him in his work. Barry expresses satisfaction and pleasure in working with some colleagues, anger and frustration in trying to work with others. Again the sensation may be expressed in bodily and physical terms. While he says he has been "burned" by bad medical encounters and experiences, he describes the results of bad relations with colleagues as being "frosted".

That's communication again, with surgeons; we just don't get it. I get very irritated by that — by not knowing what's going on with patients.

We're the one she calls when she has problems, not X . . . . Sometimes it's very hard working with surgeons. It gives you a pain in the ass sometimes.

I get a little impatient with him. He does things a week behind. I think it's a serious thing to miss some of the things he misses . . . . He talks down to people. I don't like that. He puts himself on a throne and talks to his subjects. That frosts me.

A strong current runs through Barry's thought, linking his work and his self: a persistent need for evidence for and assurance of his efficacy, the powers of himself in the broad scope of his work. Once attempting to force a choice, I asked Barry if his satisfaction derived from "seeing improvements in people's lives or from knowing you had been able to influence these?" Barry replied, "I think both, Oh, I think both are very satisfying. It's ah, you have to experience it, I guess". It often seems that Barry is as concerned with his personal potency as with its positive results — the cure or palliation of his patients' medical problems.

There's such great satisfaction in seeing people benefit by what you do. There, there, there are very few areas in life that you can do that, and ah, where you can see good, and it, it, it's certainly rewarding . . . .

If she has pulmonary emboli, and you don't treat her for it and she dies, that's a catastrophe.

That's neat. That's neat. God! I'm pleased with her, that she can go home. She's so much better . . . almost came back from the other world. It's really a great feeling that you've done something like that — that you're able to do something like that.

Here it is not simply the death of the patient which would be catastrophic, but her death by untreated pulmonary emboli. Similarly he is both pleased that the patient can go home and greatly satisfied by his own abilities to so powerfully affect her life.

Barry's deeper personal motives in medicine are further indicated by his response to three situations, all mentioned above. Recall that in the treatment of an alcoholic patient, dying from his excesses, Barry was explicitly ambivalent, implicitly indifferent to the patient's impending death (p. 102). Any treatment which the resident wanted to try was all right with him.

If he dies, well, he dies, and you've tried. And I'm not just trying to obviate guilt. I don't have any guilt about alcoholics. Ah, about, within reason I do have guilt, of course. But I don't feel that compulsive about alcoholics.

Barry suggests here that compulsion entailing deep commitment to some goal, is a characteristic of his more common motivation, though not for alcoholic patients. He suggests also that guilt, perhaps from failure to act effectively, is a common motivational source. There are no further references to guilt in my notes, yet its companion, anger, is common.

Barry's response to questions about HMOs further indicates his motives. He imagines that working in an HMO his motivation would drop to the minimal standard of the organization. He thinks it a "human" reaction to work the minimal amount possible if on a fixed salary. There is an implication that what motivates his effort is some reward seemingly monetary, beyond that of his utilitarian goal of helping patients and the greatest number of patients possible.

On another occasion, also in response to my question about HMOs, Barry told me: "Physicians by and large don't like to work for someone. They like to be their own *macher*". Barry too likes to be his own *macher*, boss, agent, or authority. Barry dislikes having others controlling his work. Embedded here also is a strong sense of personal autonomy, control, and self-reliance. Working for himself, he has clearer evidence of his independence, perhaps loneliness, and nothing between his own powers and the vast forces of deified Nature.

Barry's self-expressions show him intimately engaged in the world of his work. Through medical channels, he enters and distances himself from the conditions of patients. He intuitively gauges both their conditions and the validity of his own judgments by reflexive examination of his own responses. He imagines himself in their medical place, and then observes this experience. He suffers also when his patients do, though still at a medicalized remove.

Barry is healed also when patients are. His role in affecting their "vital signs" is a felt sign of his own vitality. He heals himself, then, by healing them; or he fails in both. These powers are multiplied through a social witness to them. Barry is in great demand in the medical community, at once distracting him with the pressure "to be in three different places at the same time", yet also signalling his potency.

Oh yeah, I think there, there's, there's certainly some pride, there's pride in that. Ah, but I think the pride is overwhelmed by the fatigue sometimes, and the inability to do all that's required or requested of you, and sometimes not only that others request of you, but what you demand of your own body. It, it's overwhelming, you just want to give it all up and go away. Really. But, fortunately that idea ends when you have some rest, a couple of good hours sleep. But, ah, I don't know, there's such great satisfaction in, in seeing people benefit by what you do. There, there, there are very few areas in life that you can do that. There are very few endeavors that you can do that, and ah, where you can see good, and it, it, it's certainly rewarding. Where you not able to do good, it's ah, to help a person, it's, it's, it's very, it's very frustrating in that you can't . . . . You try hard not to become involved emotionally in these situations, and try to derive the pleasure that you can from what you can do, and not be knocked down too far by what you can't do. Ah . . . oh overall it's fairly rewarding in that regard, I think.

NOTES

1. This eassay is the first in a series of studies of internists at work, set in a cross-cultural, comparative perspective. I undertook the initial research as a Postdoctoral Fellow in Medical Anthropology at Michigan State University, under the guidance of Arthur Rubel. I continued the research as a Science Fellow in Clinical Anthropology, in Psychiatry and Primary Care at the University of Washington, with the luminary companionship of Arthur Kleinman. Since 1980 this work has been generously supported by the James Picker Foundation Program in the Human Qualities of Medicine, under the insightful and inspired leadership of Renée C. Fox. For this support, company and guidance I am most grateful. I am very grateful too, for the comments of friendly critics, especially Ronald Simons, Esther Brown, Deborah Gordon, Brigitte Jordan, Sarala Krishnamurthy, Atwood Gaines, Catherine Lutz and Py Bateman.
2. For characteristics and a cursory history of internal medicine among medical specialties, see Hahn (1982).

REFERENCES

DeTocqueville, Alexis
1966 Democracy in America. Garden City, New York: Doubleday and Co.
Devereux, George
1967 From Anxiety to Method in the Behavioral Sciences. The Hague: Mouton.
Fox, Renée
1979 Essays in Medical Sociology. New York: John Wiley and Sons.
Giddens, Anthony
1976 New Rules of the Sociological Method. New York: Basic Books.
Hahn, Robert A.
1982 "Treat the Patient, Not the Lab"; Internal Medicine and the Concept of 'Person'. *In* Atwood D. Gaines and Robert A. Hahn (eds.), Physicians of Western Medicine: Five Cultural Studies. Special Issue. Culture, Medicine and Psychiatry 6(3): 219–236.
Rosengarten, Theodore
1981 Stepping Over Cockleburs: Converstations with Ned Cobb. *In* Marc Pachter (ed.), Telling Lives; the Biographer's Art. Washington, D.C.: New Republic Books.
Taussig, Michael
1980 Reification and the Consciousness of the Patient. Social Science and Medicine 14B: 3–13.
Young, Allan
1980 Anthropological Perspectives in Medical Knowledge. Journal of Medicine and Philosophy 5(2):102–116.

SECTION III

MEDICAL SPECIALTIES

MARGARET LOCK

MODELS AND PRACTICE IN MEDICINE:
MENOPAUSE AS SYNDROME OR LIFE TRANSITION?

INTRODUCTION

Popular journalism in the last few years, directed primarily at women, reflects a new trend — an interest in the older woman, and in particular, her health, sexuality and her experience of aging. Titles such as 'Menopause: A Positive Approach', 'Good News About Menopause', and 'Breaking the Age Barrier', indicate that the older woman now has one foot, at least, out of the closet. There is a conscious attempt to create a new image in which the transition to and the last part of the life cycle are viewed as a time of growth rather than loss. One introductory paragraph to such an article reads as follows: "Menopause, the myth: a period of prolonged physical and mental anguish. The reality: a time for reassessing and rebuilding with the years to come filled with new meaning".

The majority of authors who write these articles support such claims by referring liberally to statements of practicing gynecologists. This contrasts with recent academic literature produced by social scientists, which implies that the management of the menopause in particular, and the problems of older women in general, are handled by gynecologists very poorly and certainly not in a positive fashion. Here, a brief review of the conclusions drawn by social scientists in connection with the practice of gynecology will be presented, followed by a discussion of some of the results obtained by social scientists doing research in connection with menopause. Medical attitudes towards menopause over the past hundred years will be presented along with the major controversies which appear in the current medical literature. The production of clinical models in general will then be discussed, followed by the presentation of some preliminary data on the application of medical knowledge to menopausal women in clinical settings by gynecologists, gynecological residents, and family practitioners.

This information will be analysed in order to promote a discussion of two issues: the relationship of the beliefs and practice of individual clinicians to knowledge contained in medical texts, and the "cultural construction of clinical reality" (Kleinman 1980) of menopause.[1] The results suggest that generalized statements about the medical profession or its related clinical fields are not appropriate at the clinical level, and that there are many different ways of shaping behaviors related to menopause in clinical settings.

GYNECOLOGY AND MENOPAUSE: THE SOCIAL SCIENCE PERSPECTIVE

Social scientists writing on menopause and its management by gynecologists have tried to demonstrate how in both historical and contemporary times, attitudes

115

R. A. Hahn and A. D. Gaines (eds.), Physicians of Western Medicine, 115—139.
© 1985 *by D. Reidel Publishing Company.*

toward women and their roles in society have affected the form of gynecological practice (Ehrenreich and English 1978; MacPherson 1981: Posner 1979; Smith-Rosenberg 1973). They have, therefore, taken a stance familiar to medical anthropologists in that the conceptualization of a disease is seen as a product of social values and perspectives.

But recent research into current gynecological attitudes towards menopause reaches several different and contradictory conclusions. MacPherson (1981), for example, points out that in nineteenth-century Western medicine, menopause was believed to *cause* disease, but that since the mid-twentieth century it has been redefined as itself a disease. She states, "Physicians (have) extended the boundaries of their roles beyond diagnosis and treatment of the usual diseases to include the definition and management of a heretofore normal female condition. Medicine also extended its power as an agent of social control by stating that physicians should care for all women in menopause" (1981:104). MacPherson calls for a "dismantling" of the present "metaphor" which is based upon the "particular economic, social, and political conditions" of the times and which has led to overmedication and iatrogenesis.

Posner (1979), in her study of the medical model of menopause, demonstrates a paucity of experimental and epidemiological research. She then cites gynecological textbooks from the 1960s and early 1970s to support her hypothesis that the medical profession downplays the physiological symptoms of menopause, regarding it as largely a "mind over matter" phenomenon. She points out that in several texts, statements such as the following are common in connection with menopause: "[t]he emotionally mature, busy and happy woman usually has few if any difficulties in adjustment" (Pettit 1962: 353). Posner asserts that there is a conservative attitude on the part of the medical profession which is both "condescending and paternalistic" towards the female patient, and that the significance of physical symptoms is denied by dismissing them in preference to psychological (and hence supposedly untreatable) explanations. In contrast to MacPherson, Posner believes that there is not enough medical care for this problem; she concludes that women are being left to "pull themselves up by their own bootstraps" (p. 186). Posner shows in addition that this is an attitude shared by many feminists who focus on social and psychological explanations for menopausal symptomatology while downplaying physiological factors. She suggests that while gynecologists tend to rationalize their position by stating that women with menopausal problems have not come to terms with their feminine role, feminists believe that social and cultural factors have shaped women's expectations and behavior so that they experience unnecessary psychological and somatic changes at menopause.

The studies cited above assume that a shared medical model is adhered to rather closely by clinicians, such that one can readily generalize about their attitudes. These studies also assume that the contents of texts for medical and lay audiences are closely allied with, or even synonymous with, the ideas and behavior of practitioners. While gynecological texts attempt to portray current ideas about biological structure, function and pathology of females in general, they have to be reinterpreted in a clinical context to fit a specific contextual situation. The problem is further compounded in the case of menopause since it is a topic which has been poorly researched and is politically charged. Thus, any of a variety of textual accounts might form the basis for clinical practice.

Mythology and the Menopause

Menopause is a subject which has encouraged the development of mythologies because it is associated with much ambiguity and paradox. One aspect of the menopause is the universal, biological event which, in theory, is marked clearly by the last menstrual cycle. However, the actual transitional period, the climacterium (see Townsend and Carbone [1980] for a complete definition), often takes several years during which time ovarian functions and hormone levels decline. Data are sparse, but it is known that while the decline in some women is steady, in others, hormone levels drop suddenly and precipitously, and in still others the decline is irregular (Green 1971). There is a direct relationship between the hormone estrogen and the menstrual cycle, so that while some women experience an abrupt end to menstruation, others experience intervals of unpredictable, heavy bleeding and/or times of scanty bleeding. An irregular menstrual cycle indicates to a woman and any doctor she might visit, the occurrence of several possible events: that she is menopausal, that she is pregnant, or that she has pathological changes. It can, therefore, be the source of recurrent anxiety of several years duration. According to biomedical diagnostics, the occurrence of the menopause can only be assessed in retrospect after an interval of 12 months of complete amenorrhea; this adds to the ambiguity, and possibly accounts for the universal lack of ritual associated with the biological event, as noted by Van Gennep (Kaufert 1982).

There is, in addition, a lack of concensus among doctors, social scientists, and the general population about the signs, biological and behavioral, which are associated with the menopause. While there is a general agreement that the hot flash is a "true", though not inevitable symptom (that is, it is generally agreed that it is a direct result of hormone decline), there is considerable disagreement about the incidence and significance of other symptoms which have been singled out: depression, irritability, tiredness, headaches, dizziness, loss of libido, dyspareunia and so on. Townsend and Carbone (1980:230) define menopausal syndrome as "the range of somatic and behavioral symptoms and complaints in women which are caused by or commonly attributed to the climacteric". They and Kaufert (1982) summarize the work on cross-cultural and intra-cultural variation in the form and incidence of changes reported at menopause. Despite the paucity of data, it is clear that there is enormous variation and that only the cessation of menses and decreased estrogen production are universal events, while hot flashes and sweats probably occur in all cultures but are by no means inevitable, and are not necessarily associated with menopause (Flint 1974). The conclusions drawn are that the experience of menopause is subject to considerable social and cultural conditioning. This variability in the experience and interpretation of menopause leads to the rationalization of different treatment plans and to a variety of expectations on the part of doctors, patients and the general public as to what exactly should be treated, if anything.

Physiological changes involved in menopause also act, of course, as a marker for the sociocultural event, the "change of life". At this sociocultural level, too, there is apparently a clear message; the end of fertility. But the meaning of this event is profoundly influenced by the status and roles of women in the society in question (Flint 1974; Kaufert 1982; Townsend and Carbone 1980), and by their personal life history and transitions through previous life-change events (Kraines 1963). It can be viewed predominately as either a positive or a negative event depending upon the social and cultural context.

Among the Rajput of North India, a woman who no longer menstruates can come out of purdah, visit other households more freely, and join the men of her own household without restrictions. Flint's (1974) Rajput informants described a symptom-free menopause which she believes can be linked to their increased social status at this time. Among the Gisu, in contrast, La Fontaine (1960) discusses the rejection of women by their own husbands and families once they can no longer give birth to children. She does not consider the relationship of this change in social status to the incidence of physiological symptoms during menopause, but does link it to the high suicide rate in this age group. Kaufert (1982) points out that the cultural construction of menopause becomes a stereotype for all members of the society; even the symptoms that one may expect are included in the stereotype. Thus, Rajput women expect no symptoms, while Manitoban women believe that most women will be depressed and irritable at menopause (Kaufert 1980).

Kaufert (1982) hypothesizes that women whose self-esteem is high will not be as susceptible to a negative stereotype as women whose self-esteem is low. She suggests that women of low self-esteem are more liable to psychological distress and possibly to fluctuating hormone levels during menopause in societies where there is negative stereotyping. Crawford and Hooper in their study of 106 middle and working class women in England concluded that there is "little evidence that supports the idea that by itself the menopause is a critical transition, unless it is associated in other ways with other life events" (Crawford and Hooper 1973: 480). This conclusion is reinforced by Fiske (1979), who found that in a non-clinical population, the majority of women stated that menopause is not a particularly difficult time.

The practicing clinician, of course, also holds a stereotype of menopause which is shaped by his or her culture and personal experiences. In an urban North American setting, this stereotype or model is unlikely to correspond with more than a minority of the patient population whose ethnic origins and social class are extremely varied.

Because the significance of the physiological event and the possible association of psychological symptoms are unclear and because the cultural stereotyping of the event is very varied, the possibilities for the shaping of behavior in a clinical setting in connection with menopause are numerous. Moreover, within the hierarchical relationship that obtains between doctors and patients in the usual medical setting, there is a great potential for recruitment of women at this stage of the life cycle into the sick role by doctors who expect that women will suffer at this time. But, there is equally a potential for clinicians to interpret the event as of little consequence and, hence, to dismiss potential patients rather hastily.

For the practicing clinician, the issues are compounded by numerous controversies which are debated in the medical literature on this topic. After a historical overview of changes in attitude by the medical profession towards menopause, some of the current controversies in medical texts will be presented.

MEDICAL EXPLANATIONS FOR MENOPAUSE

Nineteenth century medical attitudes towards "female complaints", including menopause, appear to be "decidedly unscientific and even obsessive to a modern observer", states Wood (1974:3). She goes on to quote a Professor Hubbard of New Haven who, addressing a medical society in 1870, said that it seemed "as if the Almighty, in creating the female sex, *had taken the uterus and built up a woman around it*". Numerous other disorders such as headaches and psychiatric problems were attributed to the uterus, and it was thought that women were subject to many more diseases than men as the result of being in possession of a womb. Attitudes towards menopause at this time reflect a biopsychosocial approach and provide a beautiful example of an extremely warped clinical construction of reality which places the responsibility for the occurrence of problems firmly at the victim's door. A woman who "transgresses nature's law" is likely to find that menopause is a "veritable Pandora's box of ills" wrote gynecologist John Kellogg in 1833 (quoted in Haller and Haller 1974:135). Smith-Rosenberg shows that "transgression" is synonymous with stepping outside one's accepted social role and included such things as use of birth control or abortion, undue sexual indulgence, a too fashionable life-style, failure to care fully for husband and children, and an interest in obtaining education (Smith-Rosenberg 1974:30). Treatment, unlike causal explanations, was limited to the somatic level, directed at the womb and often very painful (Woods 1974). But ambivalence associated with menopause on the part of both doctors and women has been documented at least since the middle of the last century, while some doctors associated every disease and negative emotional state imaginable with the cessation of menstruation, others noted "how fresh and lovely some menopausal women looked − with a lightness to their step and a countenance free from anxiety" (Smith-Rosenberg 1973: 32).

From the early twentieth century onwards, Freudian theory influenced the development of a new approach to menopause which is exemplified in the writings of Deutsch (1945), Bendek (1950) and Erikson (1968). Menopause, it is thought, is a time when repressed desires and unconscious fantasies are likely to be acted out. Freud noted that menopausal women "become quarrelsome and obstinate, petty and stingy, show typical sadistic and anal-erotic features which they did not show before" (quoted in Silberman 1950). According to Erikson a woman's grief for lost children is experienced at each menstruation and it becomes a "permanent scar" at menopause (1968:278). Psychosomatic explanations such as these interpret symptoms which are experienced at the time of menopause as largely the result of unresolved conflicts from earlier developmental stages, and in particular as issues revolving around the loss or rejection of femininity (Osofsky and Seidenberg 1970). Women at this stage of the life cycle are considered to be susceptible to "menopausal syndrome" or the "empty nest syndrome".

The preferred form of therapy is pharmacological, especially tranquilizers and anti-depressants. Deutsch believes that successful psychotherapy is difficult for women of this age, "for reality has actually become poor in prospects, and resignation without compensation is often the only solution" (1945:476).

As in the nineteenth century explanation, responsibility for problems at the menopause lie primarily with the woman herself and her attitude towards expected female social roles. More subtle than the nineteenth-century version which damns overt behavior, some of which is reasonably acceptable for the twentieth-century woman, the Freudians and their sympathizers locate the problem largely in the unconscious.

Since the 1930s synthetic estrogens have been available as a low cost substitute for the natural estrogen no longer produced in the ovaries of menopausal women. This availability has raised a number of complex issues in the medical profession about the nature of menopause itself, and the role of the doctor in connection with menopausal patients, including the type of medication, if any, that should be administered.

A Brooklyn gynecologist, Robert A. Wilson, has become the best known promoter of menopause as a "deficiency disease". In his numerous publications, including the popular book *Feminine Forever* (1966), he claims that menopause is a problem which threatens the "feminine essence" and he describes menopausal women as "living decay". Wilson claims that with the use of estrogen replacement therapy both menopause and the aging process can be subverted, and he advocates that women be given estrogens from "puberty to the grave".

The initial discovery and promotion of estrogen replacement therapy came at a time when antibioties began to be used most effectively against infectious diseases" was at its height and "the cure" for cancer was thought to be 'just around the corner'. Menopause, for the first time, could be defind as a named disease for which there was a specific cure. In this type of belief system "diseases" are entities for which patients are not responsible; they are "things" which can be conquered by the weapons of medicine, while the patient in whose body the battle takes place is neutral, uninvolved territory. The distinction is medicine versus microbiology, not medicine versus frustrated womanhood. In all of the above models women are seen as victims of their biology; but, whereas in the nineteenth-century and early twentieth-century versions there is a belief that the misdemeanors and conflicts of a lifetime cannot be undone and that medicine can only offer symptom relief, in the deficiency disease version, the medical profession offers the most control over and hope for potential patients by its claims of power over nature. None of these versions suggest ways in which the social roles ascribed to women might be changed or reinterpreted so as to avoid predisposing a segment of the population to problems thought to be associated with menopause.

It was not until the late 1960s that a competing explanation for menopausal problems emerged. In connection with the rise of the women's health movement, with a questioning of the biomedical approach in medicine (Dubos 1968), and especially with the reports of possible side-effects in connection with the use of estrogen replacement therapy (Horwitz and Feinstein 1978), an explanation which stressed menopause as part of the normal life cycle was promoted. This thinking has penetrated the medical profession, and is particularly evident in specialties concerned with primary care and community medicine. In this belief system, menopause is seen as an event which does not normally pose problems. But, if a woman has difficulties, then it is thought psychosocial as well as biological factors are involved. Overt moral condemnations are not made, but it is believed by many primary care practitioners that a good doctor can and should intervene in order to try to help a patient, and sometimes her family, to change and to adjust to psychosocial factors which are disorienting their lives.

A woman, for the first time, is not visualized as usually being dominated by her biochemistry, but rather as someone who is subject to a constellation of psychosocial and biological constraints to which she can adjust and adapt, or even, to some extent, change. This model accepts the multi-causal explanation for disease and is, in theory, flexible enough to explore many levels of causes contributing to menopausal problems. Responsibility for the origin of the problems can be attributed partly to social and cultural variables which lie largely within the domains of politics, economics, and religion, partly to the family and its dynamics, partly to the individual woman and her personality, and partly to the neutral domain of biochemistry. Professionally controlled therapy can take place at all of these levels and, hence, there is a potential for the medicalization of many spheres of life. But there is, at the same time, a tendency to encourage the thinking that a patient should be responsible for her own health.

Current Medical Literature

Current medical thinking incorporates the Freudian, the psychosomatic, the deficiency disease, and the life cycle explanations, although different medical specialities emphasize different interpretations. A survey of current gynecological textbooks reflects aspects of all these belief systems, and also confusion in connection with this topic. For example: should menopause be seen primarily as a normal process — another developmental stage, in which a biopsychosocial model is most applicable, as Fink (1980), Musaph (1979) and others suggest? Or should it be seen as a disease, as Barnes (1968:24) suggests when he states, "I would like to propose that these changes represent a disease — that this is a serious disease — a disease that requires treatment on the part of the medical professional".

With respect to treatment, should the biomedical model be firmly applied in order to avoid iatrogenesis, as Studd et al. (1979) appear to believe when they write that,

It is a truism to state that the best way to prevent complications of treatment is to withhold such treatment particularly in patients where this therapy is inappropriate. It follows that the correct selection of patients and a general agreement about symptoms which are due to estrogen deficiency, rather than the results of the many life stresses of the middle years, is vital. Any carelessness in the criteria for treatment will lead to the misuse of estrogen replacement therapy which will then be in danger of becoming the therapeutic crutch of stressed womenkind, such as has happened with tranquilizers in the last two decades (p. 23).

Although no clear connection has been established between psychological states and hormone changes associated with the climacteric (Crammer 1978), certain textbook authors emphasize the links between psychological and somatic symptoms. Green (1971), for example, says that attention to psychological components should take primacy in treatment and that this can frequently relieve physiological symptoms. Other authors state categorically that while psychological support is indicated, estrogen therapy should be used for treatment of symptoms which are characteristic of estrogen insufficiency — hot flashes, sweats, and vaginal atrophy (Kistner 1979; Utian 1979), but that estrogens are not indicated for any other problems. Greenblatt et al. (1980), on the other hand, cite numerous experiments to support their position that estrogens with and without the addition of an androgen often improve general well-being and, in addition to the complaints listed above, the following: arthritic discomfort, bone aches, myalgia, urinary incontinence, psychosexual disturbance and disorders associated with the mucus membranes, including those of the nose, eyes and urethra. These authors conclude, "Too many women in need of [hormone replacement therapy] have been neglected because of hesitancy by the physician to expand the goals of therapy. He fears the untoward consequences of estrogen therapy, nor does he wish to hear criticism from his more conservative peers. The physician's desire to do no harm is most commendable, but it is not a mandate not to try to do good" (p. 169).

Another area of dispute is the postulated connection between the use of estrogen replacement therapy and increased incidence in endometrial cancer. Jones and Kemmann (1980) point out the problems with clinical and epidemiological data obtained so far, studies are retrospective and poorly designed in terms of dosage sizes and control groups. Nevertheless, they state that there is, "a considerable amount of clinical and epidemiological data (which) have recently implicated estrogen intake in the development of endometrial carcinoma" (p. 185). But they also point out that there is little, if any, direct laboratory evidence that estrogens themselves are carcinogenic. Their conclusion is that estrogens should only be used very cautiously and in low dosage for a limited amount of time (p. 187). However, Greenblatt et al. in the *same book* (p. 161) quote the study of Horwitz and Feinstein (1978) which appeared in the *New England Journal of Medicine* in which studies previously published in that journal were resubjected to statistical analysis thereby "removing the element of bias" detected in the inital calculations. Horwitz and Feinstein conclude that there is no significant increase in endometrial cancer with the use of estrogen therapy. Greenblatt adds, "Forty years of experience with [hormone replacement therapy] ... in a university setting permits us to say that the reported risks of endometrial cancer are exaggerated" (p. 162). He claim also that limiting oneself to short term, low dosage therapy is "conservative" and "simply inadequate" (p. 152).

When the subject of menopause is so controversial (and there are other issues such as the postulated relationship of estrogen deficiency with the incidence of osteoporosis and various cardiovascular diseases [Green 1971; Kistner 1979]), what should clinicians do in actual medical practice? Furthermore, what is the relationship between a clinician's personal, working knowledge, cultural stereotypes of menopause, and medical texts?

The data presented below were obtained by interviewing twelve gynecologists, twelve family and general practitioners, and five residents in obstetrics and gynecology in the Montreal area. In addition, I participated in lectures, seminars and clinical rounds on the topic of menopause in three teaching hospitals and observed, wherever possible, the treatment of menopausal patients in clinical settings. The results may reflect only a current urban Canadian setting, and should be compared with other contexts.

Transmission of Medical Knowledge

All of the physicians interviewed in this study work in the city of Montreal and have some contact with the major teaching hospitals attached to McGill University. Several of the gynecologists teach their speciality to students, interns and residents in addition to running a clinical practice and doing research and/or administration. Their use of medical knowledge, therefore, may be different from that of clinicians who do not teach. Only two of my informants actually teach subject matter encompassing menopause. All of the informants read parts of one or more professional journals regularly but they also note that outside of their sub-speciality they limit their reading to review articles. There are four important additional ways in which they acquire new information in areas outside of their sub-speciality: by rapid "goal-oriented" reading for information on specific clinical problems and with which they are either out of date or unfamiliar; by taking part in clinical rounds and seminars inside the hospital; by asking colleagues for specific information; and, for those who teach, by interacting with residents who are assumed to be "on top" of the literature, unlike most practicing specialists. These types of information-gathering were described by more than one clinician as "learning by osmosis".

Although students are exposed to a few of the controversies in the literature on menopause during their first two years in medicine, their clinical rotations and clerkships emphasize the case history approach. Teachers do not presume to cover the literature, on the contrary, they expect, with the residents especially, to have a type of dialectical exchange in which the newest knowledge obtained from textual sources by the resident is tempered into working information for clinical practice through information drawn from the clinical experience of the specialist/ teacher. Clinical knowledge is retrieved from memory usually without reference to textual sources for verification, and at least in the teaching hospitals I have observed, is open to discussion and dissent. In practice, this means that the exposure of students, interns, and residents to ideas for clinical practice is arbitrary and subjective and depends upon the nature of the personal clinical practice of their particular teacher.

The gynecological residents, when interviewed, admitted that in the final part of their residency they make a point of questioning several specialists about actual clinical practice in order to solidify a working body of knowledge for themselves. In the case of outpatient problems such as menopause, with which they have had little experience, residents feel particularly lacking in expertise and rely heavily on advice from their chosen mentors. Knowledge obtained from medical texts, therefore, is not applied *in toto* or without modification in actual clinical practice and it cannot be assumed that medical texts reflect very closely what clinicians actually do.

Medical Models and Clinical Practice

Several recent articles which attempt to characterize contemporary medicine use the concept of a "model" in order to facilitate an understanding of the general approach adopted by medical practitioners (Engel 1977; 1980; Fábrega 1980; Leigh and Reiser 1980). The model which is generally accepted as dominant has been labeled "biomedical". More recently, as an interest in teaching about the psychosocial components of illness experiences has been promoted, an alternative concept has been developed and advocated, the "biopsychosocial" model.

In the teaching of medicine until recently the biomedical approach has been predominant; it has been defined by Engel (1977) as follows:

The dominant model of disease today is biomedical, with molecular biology its basic scientific discipline. It assumes disease to be fully accounted for by deviations from the norm of measurable biological (somatic) variables. It leaves no room within its framework for the social, psychological, and behavioral dimensions of illness. The biomedical model not only requires that disease be dealt with as an entity independent of social behavior, it also demands that behavioral aberrations be explained on the basis of disordered somatic (biochemical or neurophysiological) processes. Thus the biomedical model embraces both reductionism, the philosophic view that complex phenomena are ultimately derived from a single primary principle, and mind-body dualism the doctrine that separates the mental from the somatic (p. 130).

The biopsychosocial approach, in contrast, is derived largely from open systems theory and is thought by some to represent a new paradigmatic approach (in Kuhn's [1962] sense of that word) in medicine. According to Fabrega (1974: 214),

... since reversibility, modifiability, and compensability are hallmarks of the systems paradigm, we are forced to adopt a rather broad or inclusive view of what medicine and disease encompass. The systems view thus appears to require that equal emphasis be given to all the components or levels that appear to be implicated in an instance of what it terms disease as well as to matters currently viewed as external to and separate from disease.

In the teaching of students, interns, and residents in obstetrics and gynecology at all four of the McGill teaching hospitals, conscious attempts have been made to adopt a biopsychosocial approach. My informants who teach have developed these programs over the past ten years. Three of the specialists teach sessions in which psychosomatic medicine and a biopsychosocial approach are the principal topics. This situation, combined with the lack of agreement in the medical literature, suggests that the gynecologists in this study are unlikely to employ a highly biomedically oriented model in their clinical practice. I found this to be so (see below) but, despite this tendency, the family practitioners and general practitioners who were also interviewed (three of whom are associated with the university), work from a model which is more psychosocially oriented than that of all the gynecologists.

However, despite the more general psychosocial orientation of the family practitioners and general practitioners, there is, among all the clinicians of whatever speciality, a large degree of variation in the way menopause is managed. Sociologists doing research into professional organizations pointed out many years ago that it cannot be assumed that there is homogeneity within a profession. Bucher and Strauss (1961) state:

There are many identities, many values, and many interests. These amount not merely to differentiation or simple variation. They tend to become patterned and shared; coalitions develop and flourish – and in opposition to some others. We shall call these groupings which emerge within a profession "segments". (Specialties might be thought of as a major segment, except that a close look at a specialty betrays its claim to unity, revealing that specialties, too, usually contain segments, and, if they ever did have common definitions along all lines of professional identity, it was probably at a very special, and early period in their development.) (p. 326.)

What I suggest happens in clinical practice is that over the years, a physician develops his or her own working model for the problems that are encountered regularly. This model depends on numerous variables, and in the management of menopause the following are important:

(1)   The personality of the physician, and, in particular, attitudes towards women and their role in society, attitudes toward responsibility and towards sexuality. These attitudes are, of course, partially formed before entry into medical school, and are subject to modification.

(2)   The age, sex, and experience of the physician and his or her personal stage of development in the life cycle.

(3)   The sub-specialty selected for emphasis in research and/or clinical practice. (A physician who is known to specialize in oncological abortion, for example, may see very few menopausal patients.)

(4)   The type of training the physician was given — biomedically oriented or biopsychosocially oriented.

(5)   Isolation from or closeness to teaching hospitals, house staff, and medical library facilities.

(6)   The professional literature that is read — family practice journals or obstetrics and gynecology journals, for example.

(7)   The physicians' clinical population — their socioeconomic group, education, ethnicity and general expectations about treatment.

(8)   The mass media — impact on the physician, patients, or physician's spouse.

(9)   The economic and political organization of the health care system that the physician is part of.

Working clinical models of menopause (like those in psychiatry, see Gaines 1979) can best be described as folk models, since they are based on popular cultural principles and are very variable. Holy and Stuchlik (1980: 17) define a folk model as follows:

Every member of the society has a number of notions, conceptions, ideas, etc. which are somehow relevant, actually or potentially, to the conduct of his life. Their totality may be referred to as an actor's knowledge or stock of knowledge. Since the expressions of this knowledge, i.e., actions, are observable and understandable to others, this entails that his knowledge is to a large extent shared by others. It is intersubjective or public. However, his stock of knowledge, or any part of it, is not made available to other actors or to the observer in an amorphous or non-organized form: it is presented in more or less coherent structures of different generality, which can usefully be called models, i.e., folk models.

Moreover, these structures are not set and fixed, but are continually created and recreated on the basis of probably not a very high number of theoretical principles similar to those on which any philosophical or scientific theorizing is based (identity, correspondence, analogy, functionality, etc.)

A feature common to the knowledge subsumed under most folk models is that it is stored and retrieved from memory and used in oral transactions. Although clinical models are modified by textual sources, they are used almost entirely or predominantly in oral exchanges. As Goody and Watt (1963) state of oral and literate traditions:

Writing establishes a different kind of relationship between the word and its referent, a relationship that is more general and more abstract, and less clearly connected with the particularities of person, place and time, than obtains in oral communication (p. 44).

They also point out that oral communication is subject to a process of "selective forgetting" in that the participants will focus on and use what interests them most of the entire repertoire initially committed to memory. An oral tradition, therefore, while less subject to critical reflection, is more flexible than a written tradition, and open to numerous re-interpretations in light of specific contexts (see Bohannan 1953). This is essentially what happens in clinical practice. Information in medical texts is concerned almost exclusively with anatomical and cellular structures and processes, or with inferences based on statistical sampling. This information *must* be re-interpreted by a clinician to be relevant to individual patient care; an experienced clinician is inclined with time, to draw on empirical, clinical evidence which, because of its direct and immediate nature is likely to be more compelling than literate abstractions in justifying medical decisions (see Hahn, this volume). Becker (1961) showed how, in the teaching of medicine, the idea is encouraged that "book" and scientific knowledge are inadequate for the care of individual patients, and Freidson (1970) has commented that since the focus of medicine "is on the practical solution of concrete problems, it is obliged to carry on even when it lacks a scientific foundation for its activities: it is oriented toward intervention irrespective of the existence of reliable knowledge" (p. 172). Freidson summarizes "the clinical mentality" as follows:

Individualism is a dominant element in orientation and behavior. Each man builds up his own world of clinical experience and assumes personal, that is, virtually individual, responsibility for the way he manages his cases in that world. The nature of that world is prone to be self-validating and self-confirming, if only because by hypothesizing indeterminancy the role of scientific (that is, generally agreed or shared) knowledge and the role of others' opinions in practice are minimized (p. 172).

FOLK MODELS AND CLINICAL PRACTICE

There are certain characteristics which are generally associated with a biomedical orientation and which can be contrasted with ideas promoted in a biopsychosocial approach to medicine. When the clinicians in this study are classified according to these two orientations both groups of specialists in dealing with menopause fall predominantly into a biopsychosocial approach, although the gynecologists are the more biomedically oriented of the two groups.

In the present research the following pairs of characteristics were contrasted:

(1)   (a) a disease oriented approach or (b) a 'normal life-change' oriented approach.

(2)   interest (a) limited to physiological changes or (b) in the patient, her family, and social context, in addition to physiological changes.

(3)   therapy directed primarily towards (a) somatic changes or (b) somatic and psychosocial changes.

(4)   responsibility for restoration of health thought to lie principally (a) with the doctor or (b) with the patient.

(5)   concern for (a) immediate results or (b) long-term results and possible side-effects of treatment.

(6)   menopause viewed as a time of (a) loss or obsolescence or (b) for starting a new phase in the life cycle.

(7)   efficacy judged in terms of (a) scientific and empirical results or (b) scientific, empirical, and symbolic results, and patient learning.[2]

The responses of the clinicians to these paired contrasts appear in Table I. Although the results indicate a general biopsychosocial orientation, they minimize the considerable variation of response within that orientation. Part of the individual responses of several of the informants will be presented to demonstrate this variation.

TABLE I
Treatment of menopause: physician responses

	1			2			3			4			5			6			7		
	a	b	c	a	b	c	a	b	c	a	b	c	a	b	c	a	b	c	a	b	c
Gynecologists	2	9	1	8	4	0	5	7	0	2	9	1	2	8	2	4	8	0	5	6	1
Family and general practitioners	0	12	0	1	11	0	0	11	1	2	10	0	1	11	0	1	11	0	1	10	1

(a) Biomedical orientation.
(b) Biopsychosocial orientation.
(c) Response unclear or undecided.

Case Studies: Gynecologists

The most biomedically oriented of all the physicians interviewed in this study, informant *A*, is a gynecologist in his early sixties who describes menopause as a syndrome. He believes that "vasomotor and atrophic changes"[3] are the only "bonafide symptoms of menopause" and the only symptoms "which one can trust a patient to discuss in a reliable way". He considers that secondary effects caused by these symptoms such as irritability and tiredness are significant since they interfere with a patient's lifestyle, but that the role of a gynecologist should be limited to the diagnosis and treatment of specific physical symptoms in as "scientific" a fashion as possible. He performs an endometrial biopsy as a routine test on all peri-menopausal[4] patients since he believes that this is the only way to assess accurately the level of estrogens in the uterus. He bases his decision to administer estrogen on the results of the biopsy and says that of the 65% of his patients who still have a uterus at this stage of their life cycle, 50% need treatment.

He agrees that the data on a possible connection between estrogen deficiency and osteoporosis are controversial, but adds that alternative theories which hypothesize that exercise combined with a calcium enriched diet and supplemented with Vitamin D are therapeutic, are equally controversial. Of the two possible courses of action to recommend to patients, he thinks estrogen therapy is preferable since it is "much easier" for the patient to take a pill once a day than to exercise and take calcium and, he adds, the cost of estrogen is less than that of calcium.

Informant *A* views menopause as a time of loss. He states that "every patient has some kind of negative manifestation" and that sexuality and aging are big problems. He administers androgens (male sex hormones) to "some" of his patients in order to improve their libido and "energy levels and metabolism" and he stresses that it has been shown that androgens act as a protection against breast cancer. (There are several side-effects associated with androgen consumption described in the literature including "masculinization" and a possible increase in the incidence of atherosclerosis). This is the only informant who consistently objectifies his patients and who did not once present what he supposes is the patient's point of view. He also admits that with most of his patients he "doesn't always have time" to describe what he is doing and why he makes certain choices.

Informant *B*, a gynecologist in his late forties, describes menopause as a "natural" event, although when asked to elaborate he gives a biomedical explanation solely in terms of changes in ovarian function. He states that his patients only rarely see menopause as a time of loss, that most of them are pleased to be past both menstruation and the need for contraception, and that few of them have any sexual problems. He believes that only hot flashes and vaginal dryness are "true" menopausal symptoms. If patients with these symptoms insist on medication, he will prescribe low doses of estrogen, after describing its possible relationships to endometrial cancer. He estimates that about 15% of his patients who are at this stage of the life cycle receive medication. He believes that his role in connection with menopause is primarily as a source of biomedical information and that, since they are going through a normal process, patients should be largely responsible for their own health. His position is the same regarding child-birth, and he would like to see midwifery and home deliveries widely accepted. He acknowledges that some women may need psychological support at the menopause, but feels like a 'charlatan' if he enters this arena since he has no formal training in psychology.

Informant *C*, also a gynecologist, and in his fifties, describes menopause as "a change" and goes on to say that how a woman copes with it depends both upon her coping with other major changes in her life and upon her expectations. He says that many women do not need treatment, and that there is not necessarily a decline in physiological and psychological well-being, but that in his particular patient population *all* go through a "grey" period just prior to and during meno-pause in which they lose interest in sex. They also become anxious about their age at this time, he states, and very few say, "Thank God my periods are over". Unlike informants *A* and *B*, he takes a full social and sexual history of all his patients, and also asks them if they are happy and enjoying life. He refers what he considers to be "difficult cases" to a family therapist, and deals with more moderate cases himself. He has, in the past, given up Saturday mornings to help patients with psychosocial problems for which he does not receive payments. (The Québec health care system encourages gynecologists to use a biomedical approach since they are not allowed to bill the government for any type of psy-chotherapy or supportive therapy, in contrast to family practitioners and general practitioners who can and do so frequently.)

This informant says patients should not suffer at menopause, and if their hot flashes are incapacitating or markedly decrease the quality of their lives, then, after discussing side-effects, he will prescribe estrogens upon the patient's request. (Unlike informant *A*, informants *B* and *C* do not believe that it is always necessary to do a biopsy in order to ascertain uterine estrogen levels. These two informants make their decisions to prescribe medication in light of the patient's assessment of the severity of her problem.) Informant *C* states that every patient in his practice who has had cancer of the endometrium had been given long term estrogen therapy in the past, but that, of course, all patients who are given estrogen do not get cancer. He adds that, provided the patient receives regular six-monthly check-ups, the cancer could be diagnosed very early and easily stopped. He says that people are excessively frightened of cancer, and that the quality of life for women suffering hot flashes is so improved by estrogen, that the risk is well worth taking.

Informant *D* is a young gynecologist who has been in practice for five years and whose specialty is oncology. He believes that menopause is a "natural process, a fact of life", and estimates that only 10% of his patient population in the relevant age group need medical help during this time. He states that pre-menopausal women *may* experience any combination of the following symptoms: depression, hot flashes, palpitations, tiredness, loss of libido, and atrophic vaginitis but that hot flashes and palpitations are the only symptoms which he believes are directly related to lowered estrogen levels. However, he adds, one cannot separate out psychological and physical symptoms, and changes in hormone levels *do* have an effect on emotional states. And, he continues, there are implications associated with menopause – aging, no more children, a time for reassessment – which need to be discussed. He says that during the physical examination he brings these topics up with a patient, but that he has no time to get involved with "empty nests" and divorces, and that he only acts as an agent to "point people in the right direction". He adds that in Québec he receives $10 for an office visit, and is only reimbursed in addition to that basic fee for any physical procedures that he performs.

He discusses "a woman's options" with her if she comes to him seeking help for physical problems around menopause. He says that the body will adjust itself in the post-menopausal years to lower estrogen production and that hot flashes and palpitations will cease. One option, therefore, is to "tough it out". A second option is to use estrogen which will mean regular visits to the doctor and careful monitoring. The medication will relieve hot flashes but probably not affect feelings of tiredness or depression. He does not discuss the possibility of contracting cancer while taking estrogens because he believes that the statistical data are "terrible" and "trash". He explains to a potential user that his aim will be to try to prescribe estrogen for as short a time as possible; that after a month or two be will reduce the dosage to once every two days, and then to one in three, and then, by nine months to a year, he will try to stop it altogether. He says this takes up more of his time than patients with cancer since the situation has to be continually monitored. A third option is to take another medication (either bellagal or dixarit) which, the gynecologist believes, can provide symptom relief, but is not always effective. (Nine out of the twelve gynecologists reject these medications as totally useless.)

Informant D has worked with the Inuit in northern Québec, who, in his experience, do not suffer from hot flashes. He links this primarily to the high proportion of body fat common among Inuit; estrogen is produced by adipose tissue. In his experience thin women have more problems with hot flashes and he believes that excessive concern with slimness in North American culture may have exacerbated the problem.

There are, therefore, marked differences in attitudes held by the gynecologists in connection with menopause, so that a woman who goes to informant A, for example, has a much greater chance of being recruited into the sick role and being placed on medication than one who goes to informant B or D. This may be partly a function of the patient populations which are of different ethnic compositions but it also appears to be linked to physician attitudes. Informant A views menopause as an event which should be controlled professionally and "scientifically" while the majority of other informants say that they try to discourage a woman from taking estrogen replacements and put more responsibility into the patient's hands.

In the practice of gynecologists there are two other major areas where patient treatment may vary considerably. Several informants believe that they should try to pay attention to more than physical symptoms at the time of menopause, but rather than enter the realm of family dynamics they have decided to focus on sexual problems alone and to spend considerable time questioning the patient on this topic, particularly on her attitudes towards aging and sexuality. The patient is then counselled on sexual behavior, but not usually on family problems or larger social issues; the husband is not involved. There is a tendency among these gynecologists to medicalize sexual behavior.

Other gynecologists, although often very sensitive to possible psychosocial components in connection with menopause believe that they are incapable or unqualified to deal with more than symptoms which they can readily diagnose as physical. These practitioners, in their helplessness, tend to avoid discussing psychosocial components with their patients, although some are willing to refer patients to family therapists. (The two female informants fall into this category.) The Québec health care system, as noted, reinforces this attitude by penalizing specialists who spend time giving "supportive therapy". However, these specialists do not appear to be handing out medication in lieu of more comprehensive treatment and cannot be accused of "medicalizing" the problem.

Case Studies: Family and General Practitioners

Informant E is a 44 year-old family practitioner who states that menopause is a "physiological change of minor proportions that has been blown up by our culture for various reasons, and because of the way our culture is geared there are drastic life changes around that time". She says that most women have no physical symptoms and rarely make a medical problem out of this event. She will give estrogens at a very low dose if the hot flashes are incapacitating, and she then sees these patients every three months; but she says that patients on estrogen replacements comprise only about 2% of her patient population in this age group. She states that menopause is the "ticket of admission" for most patients, and she looks for their "hidden agenda" which is usually part of a "mid-life crisis". She says she has probably never seen pure, independent physiological changes, and that she asks many questions about the patient's family in order to try to get a complete picture. This practitioner makes it a rule to see only whole families, either separately or together; only very rarely does she make exceptions.

She has noticed that once she focuses on life cycle changes, the physiological symptoms are usually forgotten, and patients discuss, instead, their concerns about the adolescent children, the marital relationship, the husband's retirement or the death of parents. Informant *E* states that with three sessions on family problems she can work through some realistic options for changes within the family. She will refer patients to self-help groups, but never to groups limited to women which she thinks tend to antagonize marital relationships. She believes in anticipatory guidance prior to menopause because she sees this transition as a symbolic marker for a time of loss. She believes that a woman should go through a type of grieving process, that she should talk about it, mourn a little, and then move on to a period in the life cycle when freedom of choice is increased.

Informant *F*, a general practitioner of forty-six, also states that age 40–55 is a crisis time, but for both sexes. In his experience the patients who complain of hot flashes are few in number, and almost all of them are on anti-depressives which he believes are causally implicated in their physiological changes. He says that many patients are unwilling to deal with life crises, and like to avoid psychological issues by focusing on physical factors. He takes a social history on all his patients because he is interested in finding out why they have come to him at this particular time. He says, "people who are getting on well with their life do not come to doctors with a few hot flashes". Informant *F* has taken extra training in psychotherapy because he says that 75% of his patient population needs good psychological support. This clinican sees himself first and foremost as an educator and tries above all else to encourage self-reliance. He sees menopause as a time when women are suffering many losses – their parents' death or their children's departure – and these losses must be explored by the patient. The doctor's role is simply to initiate the process. He uses estrogen reluctantly and very rarely, and tries other types of medication if the hot flashes are severe.

The final informant whose ideas on menopause will be presented is a general practitioner, aged 32, who works in a store front clinic. She believes that menopause is a natural process. If a patient comes to her with hot flashes or atrophic vaginitis, she will prescribe estrogens for a few months. She says that since her patients are very poor and have numerous social problems, they would not come to her unless they were suffering badly. She is, therefore, willing to give estrogens very readily but does describe the possible side-effects to her patients. Unlike all the other informants, this physician finds that her patients can be "weaned off" estrogen replacements rather easily.

This informant does not see menopause as a time of loss since the majority of her patients are single mothers with between three and seven children. By this stage in their life cycle, they are usually grandmothers. The "empty nest syndrome" is not applicable to them and their worst problem, their financial burdens, may be somewhat relieved as the children grow up. This physician states that she is not "psychologically" inclined but that she is "biosocially" oriented since she is concerned about her patients' social problems which she analyses in terms of class conflict. She recommends a women's group to her patients and she says that for those of her patients who do have husbands, this group often causes much family conflict.

In summary, the family and general practitioners without exception view menopause primarily as a life cycle event about which, they believe, there is usually little concern on the part of most women. They treat proportionally fewer of their patients in the relevant age group with estrogen replacement therapy than do the gynecologists, but they, of course, see patients with many medical problems, not only gynecologically related problems.

These practitioners all consider their role as a doctor to be one of an educator in addition to that of a therapist but they are not equally interested or willing to educate or treat people in connection with psychosocial problems. Some limit their role to the dissemination of biomedical information while others try to help their patients and families manage many areas of their lives. There is a fine line here, for these latter physicians, between the medicalization of the whole life cycle and family system, and the judicious encouragement of growth, learning, and self-responsibility in a needy patient and family.

SUMMARY

Inconclusiveness of research evidence on menopause, and ambiguity associated with the meaning of the event, leave the subject open to numerous interpretations. The above case studies demonstrate how the "construction of clinical reality" is shaped in many ways which have implications for patient care. The variety of approaches used in clinical practice may account, in part, for the disagreements among social scientists and feminists as to the exact shortcomings in the practice of gynecology. Those social scientists who claim that the biological reality of menopausal symptoms, dysmenorrhea and similar problems, are prematurely dismissed in favor of psychogenic explanations (Lennane and Lennane 1973; Posner 1979) would be likely to criticize practitioners who view menopause as a life change event, and who try to avoid giving medication for physiological changes by focusing on the psychosocial aspects of the event. (A similar ideological stance was taken by Susan Sontag [1977] in her study on contemporary approaches to cancer.) Such social scientists and writers adhere to an essentially reductionist, biomedical approach in which there is an emphasis on the idea that biological differences between the sexes can lead to special medical problems for women. This stance is also taken by Kistner (1979) and Utian (1979) in the medical literature. As Utian suggests, if the benefits can be shown to outweigh the risks, then some women will opt for medication to remove the organic symptoms associated with menopause.

It is clear from the present study, that the biomedical information available on menopause is open to numerous interpretations, and that in the clinical situation, depending upon the attitudes and values of the physicians, *either* the benefits *or* the problems associated with the medication may be emphasized, or not discussed at all. Is informant *A*, for example, "over-medicalizing" the problem and "recruiting" women into the sick role under the pretext of scientific precision? Is informant *B*, for example, leaving women to "pull themselves up by their own bootstraps" by strongly encouraging independence and stressing the possible negative consequences of medication?

Other social scientists regard menopause in a way which is different, and often opposed to the biomedical approach cited above. Townsend and Carbone (1980) call this second group "the social role school", in which, if symptoms are present at menopause, they are thought to be largely a response to psychosocial factors: to sex-role conditioning, decreased status at this stage of life cycle, and to a lack of role alternatives (Flint 1975; Griffin 1977). This group shares with MacPherson (1981) (see above) the belief that the medical profession tends to medicalize menopause which should be seen rather as a larger social problem.

Social scientists who take this viewpoint criticize both a biomedical and a biopsychological approach such as that used by informant *C* which focuses on psychodynamics and sexuality but ignores the social implications of the problem. It is possible that this physician is "organizing amorphous complaints into (a) menopausal syndrome", as Townsend and Carbone (1980: 241) suggest. The family practitioner, informant *E*, could also be criticized by the group, for her "medicalization" of normal life change events since, even though she avoids over-medication, she uses her role as a physician to justify providing family therapy in connection with life cycle transitions.

Further research along the lines suggested by Townsend and Carbone (1980) may well provide clearer evidence that menopausal symptoms are frequently a response to psychosocial factors. This then raises the very difficult question of what a physician should do when patients ask for help in connection with such problems. Should the physician's role become one of family therapist or psychological counsellor; should they refer patients to professional counsellors, or should they send all such patients to whatever support groups are available in the local community? How does one best foster enlightened independence in the context of a brief medical consultation?

CONCLUSIONS

Research on menopause is sparse. As far as symptomatology is concerned, three hypotheses still stand: that all climacteric symptoms are cultural artifacts (Flint 1975) and, therefore by implication, should not be medicalized; that some symptoms are due to hormonal deficiency, but that others, the psychological and psychosomatic symptoms, are due largely to social and cultural factors (Maoz et al. 1977), a third possibility is that there is a direct relationship between hormone production and psychological/social variables. In addition, as Kaufert (1980: 192) cautions, "all studies concerned with ascertaining the presence of subjective symptoms face a problem of bias".

A woman does not enter and pass through this period of her life in a cultural vacuum. What she experiences is mediated and interpreted through the filter of her expectations, her stereotype of the climacteric and its symptoms (p. 193).

It follows, therefore, that women, if they consult a doctor at all, do so with different expectations and needs. In North America today these expectations are partly shaped by the current medical models, the deficiency disease explanation, the Freudian-based psycho-sexual explanation, and the life cycle explanation. If a woman wishes to avoid any interruption of her life at the time of menopause, then she may eagerly request medication. Her children may not be leaving home, her parents may not be ill or dying, and her professional life may be busy. On the other hand, a woman may use the experience of menopause as a time for reevaluation of some family matters; she may wish to avoid medication but would appreciate some psychosocial support.

Doctors, if they know and acknowledge each other's biases and explanatory models, and those of their patients, can refer patients to colleagues if they think it would benefit the patient. In fact, referrals are already being made among some of the Montréal gynecologists. Such an arrangement is only likely to take place regularly in a truly socialized medical system (of which Québec is not an example — the majority of doctors are not salaried, but are reimbursed by the government according to the procedures which they perform).

Analysis of the data presented above is preliminary, but nevertheless indicates shortcomings in previous research on the medical profession. It appears to be important, when analyzing medical traditions in literate societies, to make a clear distinction between textual knowledge and clinical practice. A closer analysis of their relationship would be a major contribution to medical anthropology and to anthropological theory in general. Furthermore, general statements about the beliefs and praxis of the medical profession, or even segments of it, cannot be made without careful statistical sampling, since, because of the very nature of clinical practice, individual physicians are inclined to work from folk models which form the basis for their decision-making. The contents of the folk models are very rich and subject to change. These models should be the object of close ethnomedical analysis in order to do justice to their complexity, and to demonstrate the modification of their biomedical or biopsychosocial bases (themselves culturally constructed), by further cultural and economic variables.

NOTES

1. An earlier version of this paper appeared in Gaines and Hahn 1982. The first version was read at the American Anthropological Association Meetings, December, 1981.
2. Allan Young (1979; 1980) distinguishes between empirical, scientific and symbolic efficacy. He states "a proof (of efficacy) is *empirical* when it is confirmed through events in the material world and explained by coherent sets of ideas .... Scientific proof sets more stringent standards for confirmation (e.g., hypotheses must be falsifiable) and specifies appropriate and inappropriate classes of ideas .... 'Symbolic' can be defined broadly as referring to the ordering of what would otherwise be adventitious collections of objects and events .... (Symbolic) practices persist because they enable people to *manage* sickness episodes and *orient* themselves to threats of sickness" (1980: 103–104).
3. "Vasomotor changes" is a term for hot flashes, and "atrophic changes" or "atrophic vaginitis" are terms for changes in the vagina leading to vaginal dryness and possible pain during intercourse.
4. "Peri-menopausal" is a medical term which refers to that period of time in the female life cycle from which menstrual bleeding becomes irregular until two years after menopause has taken place. Alternatively, the end point of peri-menopause can be defined loosely as that time when a patient no longer experiences "symptoms of menopause".

REFERENCES

Barnes, A. C.
    1968 The Long-Range Problems of the Postmenopausal Woman. Ayerst Symposium: Ayerst Laboratories.
Becker, Howard S., et al.
    1961 Boys in White: Student Culture in Medical School. Chicago: University of Chicago Press.
Benedek, Therese
    1950 Climacterium: A Developmental Phase. Psychoanalytic Quarterly 19: 1–27.
Bohannan, Paul
    1953 Concepts of Time among the Tiv of Nigeria. Southwestern J. of Anthropology 9: 251–262.
Bucher, R. and Anslem Strauss
    1961 Professions in Process. American Journal of Sociology 66: 325–334.
Crammer, J. L.
    1978 Psychiatric Aspects of Endocrine Disorders. Irish Medical Journal 71(8): 268–273.
Crawford, Marion P. and Douglas Hooper
    1973 Menopause, Aging, and Family. Social Science and Medicine 7: 469–482.
Deutsch, Helena
    1945 The Psychology of Women: A Psychoanalytic Interpretation (Vol. 2). New York: Grune and Stratton.
Dubos, René
    1968 Man, Medicine and Environment. New York: Mentor Books, New American Library.
Ehrenreich B. and D. English
    1979 For Her Own Good: 150 Years of the Experts Advice to Women. New York: Anchor Books.
Engel, George
    1977 The Need for a New Medical Model: A Challenge for Biomedicine. Science 196: 129–196.
Engel, George
    1980 The Clinical Application of the Biopsychosocial Model. American Journal Psychiatry 137: 535.

Erikson, Erik
  1968 Identity, Youth and Crisis. New York: Norton.
Fábrega, Horatio
  1974 Disease and Social Behavior. Boston: M.I.T. Press.
  1980 The Position of Psychiatric Illness in Biomedical Theory: A Cultural Analysis. The
         Journal of Medicine and Philosophy 5: 145–166.
Fink, Paul J.
  1980 Psychiatric Myths of the Menopause. In B. A. Eskin (ed.), The Menopause: Compre-
         hensive Management. Pp. 111–128. New York: Masson Publishers, Inc.
Fiske, M.
  1979 Middle Age: The Prime of Life. New York: Harper and Row.
Flint, Marsha
  1974 Menarche and Menopause of Rajput Women. Unpublished Ph.D. dissertation, City
         University of New York.
Flint, Marsha
  1975 The Menopause: Reward or Punishment. Psychosomatics 16.
Freidson, Eliot
  1970 Profession of Medicine: A Study of the Sociology of Applied Knowledge. New York:
         Dodd, Mead and Co.
Gaines, Atwood
  1979 Definitions and Diagnoses: Cultural Implications of Psychiatric Help-Seeking and
         Psychiatrists' Definitions of the Situation in Psychiatric Emergencies. Culture,
         Medicine and Psychiatry 3: 381–418.
Gaines, Atwood and Robert Hahn (eds.)
  1982 Physicians of Western Medicine: Five Cultural Studies. Special Issue. Culture, Medicine
         and Psychiatry 6(3).
Goody, Jack and Ian Watt
  1963 The Consequences of Literacy. In J. Goody and I. Watt (eds.), Literacy and Tradi-
         tional Societies. Pp. 27–67. Cambridge: Cambridge University Press.
Green, T. H.
  1971 Gynecology: Essentials of Clinical Practice. (Second Ed.) New York: Little, Brown
         and Co.
Greenblatt, R., B. Nezhat and Anthony Karpas
  1980 The Menopausal Syndrome Hormone Replacement Therapy. In B. A. Eskin (ed.),
         The Menopause: Comprehensive Management. Pp. 151–172. New York: Masson
         Publishers, Inc.
Griffin, Joyce
  1977 A Cross-Cultural Investigation of Behavioral Changes at Menopause. Social Science
         Journal 14: 49–55.
Haller, John and Robin Haller
  1974 The Physician and Sexuality in Victorian America. Urbana: University of Illinois
         Press.
Holy, Ladislav and Milan Stuchlik
  1980 The Structure of Folk Models. In L. Holy and M. Stuchlik (eds.), The Structure of
         Folk Models. New York: Academic Press.
Horwitz, R. I. and A. R. Feinstein
  1978 Alternatives Analytic Methods for Case-Control Studies of Estrogens and En-
         dometrical Cancer. New England J. of Medicine 299: 1089.
Jones, James R. and Ekkehard Kemmann
  1980 Estrogens and Cancer. In B. A. Eskin (ed.), The Menopause. Pp. 173–193. New
         York: Little, Brown and Co.
Kaufert, Patricia
  1980 The Perimenopausal Woman and Her Use of Health Services. Maturitas 2: 191–205.

Kaufert, Patricia
    1982 Anthropology and the Menopause: The Development of a Theoretical Framework.
        Maturitas. (Nov.)
Kistner, R. W.
    1979 Gynecology: Principles and Practice. Year Book Medical Publisher, Inc.
Kleinman, Arthur
    1980 Patients and Healers in the Context of Culture. Berkeley: University of California
        Press.
Kraines, R. V.
    1963 The Menopause and Evaluations of the Self: A Study of Middle-Aged Women:
        Unpublished Ph.D dissertation. Department of Anthropology, University of Chicago.
Kuhn, Thomas
    1962 The Structure of Scientific Revolutions. Chicago: University of Chicago Press.
LaFontaine, J.
    1960 Homicide and Suicide among the Gisu. In P. Bohannan (ed.), African Homicide and
        Suicide. Pp. 94–129. Princeton: Princeton University Press.
Leigh, Hoyle and Morton F. Reiser
    1980 The Patient: Biological, Psychological and Social Dimensions of Medical Practice.
        New York: Plenum Publishing Corp.
Lennane, J. K. and J. R. Lennane
    1973 Alleged Psychogenic Disorders in Women: A Possible Manifestation of Sexual Pre-
        judice. New England J. of Medicine 288: 288–292.
MacPherson, Kathleen L.
    1981 Menopause as Disease: The Social Construction of a Metaphor. Advances in Nursing
        Science 3(2): 95–113.
Maoz, B., A. Antonovsky, A. Aperter and N. Datan
    1977 The Perception of Menopause in Five Ethnic Groups in Israel. Acta Obstet. Gynecol.
        Suppl. 69–76.
Musaph, H.
    1979 The Trigger Function of the Menopause. In A. A. Haspels and H. Musaph (eds.),
        Psychosomatics in Peri-Menopause. Pp. 83–100. Baltimore: University Park Press.
Osofsky, J. and R. Seidenberg
    1970 Is Female Depression Inevitable? J. of Obstetrics and Gynecology 36: 611.
Pettit, M. D.
    1962 Gynecologic Diagnosis and Treatment. New York: McGraw-Hill.
Posner, Judith
    1979 It's All in Your Head: Feminist and Medical Models of Menopause (Strange Bedfel-
        lows). Sex Roles 5: 179–190.
Silberman, Isidor
    1950 A Contribution to the Psychology of Menstruation. International Journal of Psy-
        choanalysis 31: 266.
Smith-Rosenberg, C.
    1973 Puberty to Menopause: The Cycle of Femininity in Nineteenth-Century America.
        Feminist Studies 1: 58–72.
Sontag, Susan
    1977 Illness as Metaphor. New York: Farrar, Straus and Giroux.
Studd, J. W. W.
    1979 The Climacteric Syndrome. In P. A. Van Keep, D. M. Serr and R. B. Greenblatt
        (eds.), Female and Male Climacteric. Pp. 23–33. Baltimore: University Park Press.
Townsend, John M. and Cynthia L. Carbone
    1980 Menopausal Syndrome: Illness or Social Role – A Transcultural Analysis. Culture,
        Medicine and Psychiatry 4: 299–248.

Utian, W. H.
    1979 Estrogen Replacement in the Menopause. Obstetrics and Gynecology Annual 8:
          369–391.
Wilson, Robert
    1966 Feminine Forever. New York: M. Evans.
Wood, Ann Douglas
    1974 The Fashionable Diseases: Women's Complaints and Their Treatmentss in Nineteenth-
          Century America. *In* Mary Hartman and Lois Banner (eds.), Clio's Consciousness
          Raised. New York: Harper and Row.
Young, Allan
    1979 The Dimensions of Medical Rationality: A Problematic for the Psychosocial Study
          of Medicine. *In* P. I. Ahmed and G. V. Coelho (eds.), Toward a New Definition of
          Health: Psychosocial Dimensions. New York and London: Plenum Press.
    1980 An Anthropological Perspective on Medical Knowledge. The Journal of Medicine
          and Philosophy 5: 102–116.

WILLIAM RITTENBERG

MARY; PATIENT AS EMERGENT SYMBOL ON
A PEDIATRICS WARD: THE OBJECTIFICATION OF
MEANING IN SOCIAL PROCESS

INTRODUCTION

In each clinical situation the participants engage in a collaborative process of defining their situation as it unfolds. They jointly develop an answer to the question, "What is happening in this situation here and now?"

In most cases actors conduct the work of defining the situation habitually, without conscious reflection, and the result of their work is to see the situation as basically unremarkable and routine (Garfinkel 1967; McHugh 1968). However, in a minority of cases, special problems or serious troubles may develop which prevent the actors from seeing their situation as routine. Then the work of defining the situation becomes more self-conscious and deliberate, and there may occur an active process of "negotiating clinical reality" (Edgerton 1966; Kleinman 1980).

Regularly we find in these circumstances that collective attention will focus on certain actions which have special significance for the negotiating process. Normally social actions do not receive this kind of attention and are soon forgotten after they occur. But because these actions become the object of intensive public notice and comment, their meaning has the chance of entering collective memory and thereby of becoming part of the larger fund of shared meanings which actors have available for use in their social field.

This paper is a case study of this process by which the meaning of particular actions gets captured and preserved in collective memory. The case to be considered concerns "Mary", a rebellious 15-year-old girl with cystic fibrosis. I examine the course of events which occurred when Mary was hospitalized in December, 1980, on the pediatrics ward of a large metropolitan hospital in the western United States. My data on this hospitalization include over 120 pages of written observations, interviews, and medical records.

Figure 1 sketches the hierarchy of personnel on the ward. Independent pediatricians are on top, next in rank are the residents, and then come the ward nursing and social service staff. Within this setting, the hospitalization of a particular patient forms what Schutz calls "a project of action" (Schutz 1967).[1] At the time of a patient's admission, the ward staff develops certain plans about the future course of care for the patient. At the outset, however, it is always uncertain whether their plans will be realized. For one thing, the patient's medical condition or the caretaker's understanding of it may change and force change in their initial intentions. For another, the group of caretakers may have difficulties in collaborating and coordinating their work, and this too may force changes in the original plan of care. So that in the end what happens in the hospitalization depends not

141

R. A. Hahn and A. D. Gaines (eds.), Physicians of Western Medicine, 141–153.
© 1985 *by D. Reidel Publishing Company.*

```
Community Pediatricians
– – – – – – – –
Teaching "Attending"
Residents
– – – – – – – –
Nurses
Social Worker
Pediatric Psychologist
– – – – – – – –
Ward Clerk
Janitors
Housekeeping Staff
etc.
```

Fig. 1. Hierarchy of ward personnel. This is a very simplified model of the ward hierarchy. Its members are grouped according to their affiliation. The community pediatricians are independent entrepreneurs. The residents and teaching "attending" (i.e., the physician who supervises the residents' work) are affiliated with a university residency program. The nurses, social worker, and pediatric psychologist are employees of the hospital pediatrics department.

only on the initial intentions but upon an unfolding process of collaborative work to deal with medical and social contingencies and realize those intentions.

In this kind of process the caretakers have an intricate, normatively organized division of labor.[2] Each of them, therefore, is implicated in the patient's fate but no one of them alone can determine what that fate will be. To succeed in restoring the patient's well-being, they are collectively dependent on each other. Under such conditions, when trouble arises which seems to threaten the process of care, the caretakers will develop an increased, reflexive interest in the group process on which their response to the trouble depends. Critical actions will become the object of intensified collective interest and public commentary, and the meaning of those actions will then have the chance of becoming established in public memory.

So this is the kind of process I want to trace in Mary's hospitalization. As mentioned, Mary has cystic fibrosis, an incurable hereditary disease with a life expectancy of between twenty and thirty years. Patients with cystic fibrosis suffer from impaired ability to digest fat and gain weight, and also from secretion in the lungs of thick mucous, whose accumulation leads to chronic lung infections in turn causing lung deterioration and eventual death. On the ward where Mary was admitted there is a special treatment protocol for cystic fibrosis. The protocol prescribes a ten-day course of care called a "pulmonary clean out" whose purpose is to clear the patient's lungs of infection and mucous. It involves intravenous antibiotics for the infection and daily systematic physical and respiratory therapy to loosen and drain the mucous from the lungs.

Altogether over forty medical staff were involved in Mary's hospitalization. Figure 2 identifies the main characters in the drama, who included Mary, Dr.

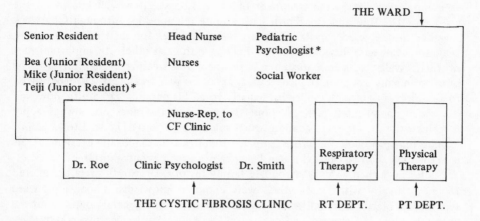

Senior Resident   Head Nurse   Pediatric
                                             Psychologist *

Bea (Junior Resident)   Nurses
Mike (Junior Resident)   Social Worker
Teiji (Junior Resident) *

Nurse-Rep. to
CF Clinic

Dr. Roe   Clinic Psychologist   Dr. Smith   Respiratory   Physical
                                                   Therapy   Therapy

THE CYSTIC FIBROSIS CLINIC   RT DEPT.   PT DEPT.

* No substantial history of working together.
** Each enclosed space represents a distinct institutional arena. Overlapping spaces represent situations in which the staff primarily associated with one arena participate in the affairs of another.

Fig. 2.   Medical staff involved in Mary's hospitalization **

Smith, Dr. Roe, the head nurse, and the residents. All the persons in the Figure, except those starred, had a substantial history of working together. Each of them, therefore, was acquainted with the personal background and social relationships of the others.

First of all, they were well acquainted with Mary from many previous hospitalizations. Mary comes from a very troubled family situation. Now 15, she is the product of a rape, and has a 13-year-old sister who recently had a child after several abortions. Her mother has had three violent husbands, the current one a police officer who is suspected of abusing Mary. Mary herself was also married, but the marriage was annulled at the request of the husband. Mary is notorious on the ward for being an extremely uncooperative patient. Also before the admission, several ward staff were aware that chronic infections had largely destroyed the right upper lobe of Mary's lung, so that it consisted mainly of infected, dead tissue.

Dr. Smith has been Mary's physician since childhood. He is a 60-year-old community pediatrician who had educated himself about cystic fibrosis and has treated children with this disease for over 20 years. Among the residents and university pediatricians involved with the hospital ward, Dr. Smith has a reputation for lacking up-to-date medical knowledge and for being easily manipulated by his patients. His relationship to Mary is a case in point. Ward personnel can cite many occasions in which Mary's objections, complaints, and anger succeeded in getting him to change or eliminate treatment that Mary did not like. They say that Mary has manipulated Dr. Smith all her life.

Dr. Roe is another physician regularly involved with patients on the ward. He is a 40 year-old clinical professor of pediatrics at the university who was trained as a lung specialist in the treatment of cystic fibrosis. It is well known on the ward that Dr. Roe and Dr. Smith have a tense relationship. Although they work together in the ward's cystic fibrosis clinic and cover for each other's patients, they are rivals who dislike and often disagree with each other. An important part of their rivalry concerns the clinic's protocol for treating cystic fibrosis. The protocol mainly contains Dr. Roe's ideas about correct treatment. Dr. Roe, therefore, approves of it and applies it regularly to all his patients. Dr. Smith, however, has more complicated feelings about the protocol and does not always apply it to his patients. On one occasion, when somewhat irritated, he said to residents, "I hate that protocol! We wrote it up five minutes after clinic, and everyone treats it as the bible. Got to think through [each case]. Each patient is different".

Such things then — Mary's troubled family history, Dr. Smith's reputation, and Dr. Roe's rivalry with Dr. Smith — were common knowledge among most ward staff before Mary's hospitalization. Figure 3 depicts some general points about the hospitalization. It lasted sixteen days from December 5th to December 21st. Mary was not severely sick at first but on the 10th became much worse and gradually improved after that. The persons who had formal responsibility for her care in the hospital were Dr. Smith, her pediatrician, and Teiji,[3] the pediatric resident who was assigned to manage her care under Dr. Smith's supervision. However, as line 4 summarizes, from the 7th through the 10th, Dr. Smith was out of town at a conference, and at this time Dr. Roe covered for him in caring for Mary.[4] Also, as line 3 shows, from the 7th through the 9th, Teiji was not much involved with Mary's care, and at that time Bea was Mary's de facto resident. True to her reputation from previous hospitalizations, throughout her care in the admission Mary resisted her treatment (through hostility, complaints, lies, outright refusals, begrudging acceptance with physical non-cooperation, and so on).

Now let me consider the sequence of events in the case and the way its meaning unfolded. When Mary appeared at the hospital she wanted treatment for vomiting and painful coughing. She was said to be "sick but not real sick". Over the phone Dr. Smith told Teiji to admit her in order to check whether anything medically serious was going on. The following morning, on the 6th, Dr. Smith came to examine Mary. But rather than order the full ten-day pulmonary clean out following the clinic protocol, which required the intravenous medication disliked by Mary, he told Mary she would be on oral medication and would only stay in the hospital "a couple of days". Dr. Smith gave almost no explanation of his plans for Mary's care to the others on the ward. After examining Mary, he noted "oral medication if possible" in the medical record, wrote orders for minimal treatment, contacted Dr. Roe about covering for him, and left town for his conference. As of Dr. Smith's departure, it was easy for anyone with background knowledge to see that his ordering minimal treatment, rather than full pulmonary clean out, was simply a standard expression of his relationship with Mary. At this point in Mary's hospitalization, therefore, the situation was a familiar one which had no special visibility on the ward.

Then, on the 7th and the 8th, Dr. Roe started covering the case. It was at this

December 1980	T 5	W 6	Th 7	F 8	Sat 9	Sun 10	M 11	T 12	W 13	Th 14	F 15	S 16	S 17	M 18	T 19	W 20	Th 21
Resident call schedule	T*	M*	T (sick)	B*	M	T	M	T	T	B	M	T	B	M	T	B	M
Main resident involved	Teiji		Bea	→		Teiji	Bea	Teiji	→								→
Attending physician	Dr. Smith		Dr. Lung		Dr. T?	?	Dr. Smith	→									→
Medical condition	Somewhat sick			→	↑	Worse	→	Improving	→								→
Patient response				Continuous resistance to therapy													
Major developments	1. Minimal therapy		1. Discharge ordered 2. Surgery recom. for future		1. Discharge not implemented		1. Minimal therapy for worse condition 2. Residents force more vigorous therapy	1. Conf. to insist on continuing vigorous therapy								1. IV out 2. Ethics conf. re: Mary	1. Discharge

Fig. 3.   Mary's hospitalization.

* T = Teiji; M = Mike; B = Bea.

point that Mary's hospitalization started to become less routine and more publicly noticeable on the ward. First of all, Mary was offering resistance even to the minimal therapy Dr. Smith had prescribed, refusing some treatment, saying Dr. Smith would not permit other treatment, and so on. This resistance drew attention to her case and to Dr. Smith's involvement in it. Secondly, Dr. Roe did not approve of the minimal therapy ordered by his rival, Dr. Smith, but his hands were tied from initiating more rigorous therapy by Dr. Smith's orders for oral medication only. What Dr. Roe did instead was to declare publicly at rounds, in the medical record, and to Mary herself that Mary would need lung surgery to remove her right upper lobe after Dr. Smith came back. By publicly insisting and documenting his case of the need for surgery, Dr. Roe drew attention to the discrepancy between the minimal care Mary was getting and the "aggressive" care she needed. Still, at that point on the 7th and 8th, not many people on the ward were listening closely to the dialogue of actions in the case, and had Mary been discharged on Saturday the 9th, as Dr. Roe ordered, her four days in the hospital might have left hardly a trace on the collective understanding and memory of the ward.

Due to confusion, however, Mary's discharge was not implemented as ordered, and then on Sunday, when she was still in the hospital, her medical condition deteriorated rather dramatically. It was these developments that brought the meaning of her hospitalization into full public view. By Monday Mary was running a 101°–103° fever, coughing up purulent sputum streaked with blood, and experiencing obviously very severe chest pain over her right upper lobe. Having returned from the conference, Dr. Smith came in very early to examine her and decide what to do. Again, as at the beginning, he did not explain his reasoning about the case to the residents. In the medical record he ordered some tests to assess the functioning of Mary's lungs (while suggesting to the head nurse that he didn't think surgery would be necessary). However, despite Mary's qualitatively worsened condition, Dr. Smith ordered no change in her minimal course of therapy, and he left the ward before the residents' morning rounds began.

At rounds the residents first of all had the job of unraveling their mutual confusion over Mary's missed discharge. Secondly, they had to consider the alarming deterioration in Mary's condition, emphasized for them by the sound in the hall of her painful coughing. And most importantly, they were confronted with the fact that Dr. Smith had apparently just reaffirmed a minimal treatment regime for Mary despite her deterioration. The spotlight was now definitely focused on Mary's case, and the discrepancy between the care she had been receiving since admission through Dr. Smith's orders and her current medical needs was apparent. In this situation the head nurse, who makes morning rounds with the residents, intervened in their discussion on Mary. The discussion went as follows:

Senior Resident: Okay: Mary
Bea: How come Mary didn't go home Saturday?
Mike: I figured someone was gunna discharge her. But she's worse now.
Head Nurse: Smith doesn't think she needs the operation. When's she gunna get a clean out?

Bea: I don't know, I don't know what the real game plan is.

.
.

Head Nurse: So is she gunna get a real clean out?
Mike: Probably not.
Head Nurse: She's manipulated Smith all her life.
(then somewhat later)
Senior Resident: I think we all agree she needs to be on a good clean out. We've gotta talk to Smith and then tell her . . . . Who will talk to Smith? Teiji?
Teiji: Better you talk to Smith.
Head Nurse: You gotta treat him like a child.
Senior Resident: Okay, next case, Claudia Hepler.

Here, under the prodding of the head nurse we can see the group collectively affirm an interpretation of the situation that had previously been implicit for some and explicit for others, and we can see the group publicly commit itself to a course of action based on this interpretation. Mary, the interpretation went, was not getting the medical treatment she needed because of her manipulative relationship with her physician. Her condition was much worse, so the residents had to pressure Dr. Smith to implement the necessary treatment: a full pulmonary clean out.

Having established agreement on this interpretation, the residents called Dr. Smith to get his go ahead to start the pulmonary clean out. Mary was going to get IV antibiotics for her infection along with systematic physical and respiratory therapy to loosen and drain the mucous from her lungs.

That night there were two major developments which reinforced the meaning and urgency of the projected ten-day pulmonary clean out. First, Mary's medical condition continued to deteriorate, and X-rays came back showing that her lung infection had spread from the right upper lobe to other previously healthy parts of her lungs. Secondly, in reaction to her new therapy, Mary called both her mother and Dr. Smith to try to cancel the clean out; she refused specific treatment to ease her worsening condition; and, in agitation, unable to sleep and afraid of dying from surgery, she kept the night nurse and resident on call up until 2:30 in the morning until she was finally sedated with chlorohydrate.

The next morning the head nurse acted again. Faced with staff frustration that Mary was deteriorating yet unmanageable, she called a nursing care conference with Teiji and Dr. Smith. At the conference the ward nurses tactfully confronted Dr. Smith with Mary's manipulations (with her refusal of treatment and her excuses that "Dr. Smith says I don't need it"), and then in front of all the nurses and also the resident, Teiji, as witnesses, the head nurse prodded Dr. Smith into publicly committing himself to carry out the full ten-day clean out for Mary. In this way, the head nurse later explained, if Dr. Smith had later tried to cancel the clean out she could hold him to his public commitment.

The resident's rounds occurred after this conference. The head nurse apparently had the social worker attend the rounds on her behalf. Like the nurses, the residents also repeated how Mary had been refusing treatments and trying to manipulate

Dr. Smith into cancelling the clean out the night before. The senior resident commented on the need for the residents to stay united. At that point, the social worker said, "What about Smith? How can we impact on Smith when he decides to pull the IV?" And in response to this prodding, originating indirectly from the head nurse, the residents vowed that they would be firm with Dr. Smith if he tried to cancel Mary's treatment.

There are many further details to the story. But the account given so far illustrates our main points. Based on an intricate division of labor, the care of ward patients requires on-going collaboration between ward staff. In this setting, a routine process of care for Mary became threatened by alarming medical and social problems, centering on the actions of the attending physician. In response to these threats, the other caretakers formulated an interpretation of what had happened and what should happen in Mary's care. And precisely because this interpretation arose through a team effort to deal with shared work problems, the meaning expressed in the interpretation was publicly emphasized, propagated, and agreed upon among the caretakers. In a nutshell the emergent meaning was this: Mary's manipulative relationship with Dr. Smith was threatening and undermining Mary's medical care, and this situation had to be reversed.

By the end of the nursing conference and rounds on Tuesday the 12th, Dr. Smith's strategic position vis-à-vis Mary's care had radically changed, due in considerable degree to the initiatives of the head nurse. He was publicly committed to a course of action which everyone agreed was needed, but which everyone expected him to reverse under Mary's pressure. In this context, his behavior was in the public eye. Contrary to expectations, however, he acquitted himself subsequently in a way the head nurse and others approved. For the first time, for example, he leveled with Mary about her prognosis and about the life threatening consequences of refusing care. Also he explicitly affirmed in the medical record the orders for a ten-day clean out. As the Senior Resident said toward the end of the clean out,

This time Dr. Smith has done pretty well. In the past Mary could come and go pretty much when she pleased. Not good for her psychologically or emotionally. This time she's gunna finish.

Finally at noon on the day before Mary's discharge, the 9th day of the pulmonary clean out, a public Medical Ethics Conference was held about Mary's case at which half of the audience of 40 were persons who had been involved in her hospitalization. Given the placement of the conference at the end of the hospitalization, these persons were almost forced to evaluate the things said about Mary in light of what had just been happening. In this regard perhaps the central tension or irony of the event, suggested in comments to me afterwards by members of the audience, was the contrast between the authoritative role Dr. Smith played in presenting Mary's case to the public and the rather less authoritative role he had just recently played during her hospitalization. This raises a number of final questions about how the meaning that had emerged in the middle of the hospitalization had changed by the end, and what its long term consequences might be in its social setting. These questions cannot be pursued in depth here.

On the following day Mary completed the ten-day pulmonary clean out, the first ever in her fifteen years with cystic fibrosis. At discharge she was basically asymptomatic, and X-rays showed that while some of the acute deterioration in her right upper lobe had been reversed, in other sections of her lungs damage from the new infection remained. All the staff I subsequently spoke with stated their evaluation in retrospect that Mary would have been better served, and probably would not have contracted the new acute infection, had she been placed on a full pulmonary clean out at the beginning. Perhaps ironically, because Dr. Smith's personal accomplishment in sticking with the full ten-day course of therapy produced sufficient improvement in Mary's condition, it showed he should have started out with that plan of therapy in the first place. In any case, Mary went home on a detailed regime of drugs, exercise, and diet with orders to return to the hospital in a month in order to assess her need for surgery.

Two contrasting categories of meaning from social theory are related to the process we have traced in our narrative of Mary's hospitalization. Though the categories are associated with different research traditions and different conceptions of social order, for our purposes they can be used to define the opposite poles on a single continuum of public meaning. The continuum represents the different degrees of stability and strength with which meanings can be established in the social process, ranging from weakly established, short-lived meanings at one end of the continuum to strongly established, long-lasting meanings at the other. For us, Mary's case illustrates a process of transformation along this continuum, in which social meanings which are weakly established and transitory become better established in social life.

At the first pole of the continuum are meanings that are established in broad consensus — the meanings seen in fuctionalist theory as the core of the social order — such as religious symbols, schemes of social classification, systems of spatial and temporal reckoning, and many others. These are the "collective representations" of classical theory, recognized by the members of societies as having an existence external to their own thought processes and actions (Durkheim 1938, 1961). Meanings of this kind are established in existence as part of the social world before given individuals are born. Knowledge of them is distributed, however unevenly, throughout the community. These meanings are used in countless social actions and situations. They persist after particular individuals die.[5] They are institutionalized in social life and have a stable existence.

At the other pole of the continuum are the situated meanings of social action — that is, the public meanings given to actions in the situation of their occurrence.[6] When social actions occur, others perceive and respond to them, and through their response display a public interpretation of what the actions mean then and there in the unfolding situation.[7] These situated meanings are social realities (being both communicated and socially consequential), and yet they normally have a highly circumscribed and short-lived existence. Unlike collective representations which have a history prior to particular usages and occasions, these meanings are created and come into existence in the situation of action itself. Rather than being distributed generally among entire communities or classes of persons, they are usually perceived and known only by the actors in the situation. Rather than being remembered by these actors and communicated again on other occasions, they are usually forgotten when the situation passes. Their social existence is confined to the fleeting situation.

So normally there is a world of difference between the social existence of collective representations and situated meanings — the reference points at the poles of our continuum. Yet sometimes in special circumstances the gap between the two categories can be bridged, at least partially, by a process in which particular situated meanings get captured from the passing flow of events and become consolidated as more stable parts of the social world. I call this process "the objectification of situated meanings".[8]

How does the situated meaning of a passing action become consolidated as part of social life? Normally social actions get little or no attention as they occur, being perceived by habit and taken for granted. No one consciously or clearly *notices* them, so they are quickly forgotten. To escape this fate the key requirement is that an action must become an object of vivid collective attention. It must stand out in the social process. When an action gets collective attention, then several individuals will notice its situated meaning. They will then become aware that others have noticed that meaning. And they will therefore remember the meaning not merely as a personal recollection but as something they know in common.[9] In this way, by the mechanism of attracting vivid collective attention, the meaning of a transitory action may get established as part of public knowledge: as something which individuals know that everyone knows.[10]

Compared to the enormous number of social actions which are continually being performed, escaping conscious notice, and being forgotten, only a small number of actions attract collective attention and have their meaning transformed into public knowledge in this way. This transformation of ephemeral meanings into stable public knowledge — which we are calling the objectification of situated meaning — is a recurring and fundamental process of social life. It is found occurring in social groups from the most humble to a historical scale, from local groups to empires. Through it, actions become consequential deeds in their context, new collective representations may emerge, and the moral order can change.

By tracing how ideas about threats to Mary's care first emerged and then became publicly established among ward staff, our account of Mary's hospitalization illustrates how the objectification of situated meaning occurred in one hospital situation. More significantly, the account also suggests that Mary's case is not unique. Due to conditions which this case shares with many others, it seems safe to predict that similar objectifications of meaning will occur repeatedly on hospital wards across the country, as well as in other institutional settings.

What are these conditions? First, typically on hospital wards there is a division of labor which requires that ward staff must collaborate if patient care is to be effective. Second, on these wards the caretakers can handle most hospitalizations as routine, but inevitably, given medical and social contingencies, a certain number of hospitalizations will be disrupted by unexpected, serious threats to patient care. It is in these recurring hospital situations — where an interdependent work group is faced with unexpected and serious threats to its work — that the objectification of situated meaning becomes likely.

To respond to the threats to patient care, the caretakers will need to create a shared interpretation of the situation that can serve as the basis for collaborative action. Both the extraordinary nature of the situation and the work required to achieve consensus will focus their collective attention on the interpretation they create. As a result, the interpretation will stand out for them as a group, and, standing out, it will be noticed and remembered as something they know in common.

Once objectified, shared meanings emerge in a troubled patient hospitalization, their fate depends on how they are used subsequently in social interaction. It is through use in interaction that they can be kept alive in collective memory and maintained in consensus. In Mary's case, for example, not long after Mary left the hospital her caretakers scattered to other situations. The publicly objectified interpretation of her case was no longer used in their communication and probably began to decay in their memory. Though it had been a prominent social fact during the hospitalization, the interpretation began to pass out of social existence when the hospitalization ended. In other cases, however, different outcomes are possible. After a shared interpretation emerges from a troubled patient hospitalization, the meaning pattern may get swept into use in a larger social arena, for instance, by becoming embroiled in the courts and propagated over the media to a larger audience, as occurred in the recent case of "Baby Doe". Then, rather than decay, the social existence of the emergent meaning would become further consolidated, to the extent that, from the standpoint of the original caretakers, it would have become an alien and constraining force, truly a social fact in the Durkheimian sense.

Thus we can see that hospital wards are a particularly fruitful arena for studying the objectification of situated meaning. By carefully documenting the varying forms which cases of objectification take on these wards, and by analyzing the similarities and differences between them, it should be possible to clarify the character of a fundamental social process.

ACKNOWLEDGEMENTS

The research reported in this paper was supported by a Postdoctoral Fellowship in Medical Anthropology at the Department of Anthropology, Michigan State University, MH 151132. Thanks are also due to the Kantor Fund for a travel stipend to the research site, and to Robert Hahn and Atwood Gaines for helpful criticism of earlier drafts.

NOTES

1. A project in Schutz's sense is a process which opens with the formulation of an intention to perform a future course of action and then proceeds with the pursuit, reformulation, or abandonment of those intentions amidst practical contingencies in real time. Whether a project will be realized is always uncertain at the outset and only decided subsequently through an unfolding practical decision-making process.

2. A great many types of normatively expected collaboration and interdependence exist within the group. For instance, senior residents are expected to supervise the work of each junior; juniors are expected to trade off taking call at night when they must care for each other's patients; and the entire group is expected to consult together about the patients of each at morning rounds.

3. On the ward, attending physicians are referred to with a title and last name or with the last name only, but residents (such as Teiji and Bea) are referred to by first name.

4. To complicate matters further, Dr. Roe himself went out of town on the 9th and 10th, with the understanding that Dr. T. would cover for him in supervising Mary's care, but Dr. T. was not properly informed of this second transfer of responsibility for Mary. As of the 9th and 10th, therefore, the allocation of responsibility for Mary's care among ward staff was ill-defined and confused. This state of affairs is summarized by the notation "T?" and "?" in line 4 of Figure 3.

5. In my view, the proposition that definite and stable consensual meanings exist should only be regarded as a plausible hypothesis. There are enormous methodological difficulties in demonstrating empirically that it is true.

6. That social actions have meaning for actors is of course the starting point for all interpretive social science (see Weber 1964; Schutz 1967). That such meanings are situated, in other words created and defined in the unfolding situation in which the action occurs, is a point emphasized in several traditions in the social sciences, such as symbolic interactionism, ethnomethodology, and contemporary sociolinguistics (e.g., see Frank 1979; Gumperz 1982; Maines 1977; McHugh 1968; Moerman 1969).

7. Situated meanings, as here defined, are interpretations of actions that are publicly available to members of the interacting group. These meanings must be regarded as fluid rather than static entities that may get reinterpreted and negotiated as the situation unfolds. Moreover, the relation between these public interpretations of action and an action's "subjective meaning" (i.e., the meaning personally intended by the actor or the inner reaction by others in the situation) may be exceedingly complex. However, both the private and public aspects of an action's meaning in its situation will tend to be perishable.

8. The phrase "the objectification of situated meaning" suggests, on the one hand, the generally fleeting meaning of social action, and, on the other, the possibility that from these fleeting materials socially stablized objects of public knowledge may sometimes be created. Seen in one way, this process of objectification speaks to the contemporary interest in how transcendent order can emerge from particular historical events and, by implication, to the interest in how historical events may dialectically reorganize present structure (see Giddens 1976). Viewed from a slightly different angle, the process exemplifies how social creations of the moment may acquire a social existence which transcends individuals and constrains their will (see Berger and Luckman 1967).

9. Along with actions which are forgotten and actions which are collectively remembered, we should also mention actions which are "individually remembered". When an action is remembered by a single individual only (not others), then its situated meaning may serve in his or her memory as an object of thought (in daydreaming, reflection, etc.), as a grounds for judgment, and as an influence on future action. Such meanings have a continued existence that is basically of a personal nature. In general, the most common fate of social actions is to be forgotten and to have their meaning pass out of existence soon after the actions occur. The next most common fate of action is to be individually

remembered and to have its meaning continue with a personal or mainly psychological existence. The least common outcome to action is to be collectively remembered and to have its meaning continue in social existence as an object of public knowledge.

10. The term "public knowledge", as used here, presupposes three broad levels of knowledge. First are things that only one individual knows. Second are things that several individuals all happen to know without being aware that they share that knowledge. Finally, there are things which several individuals are aware that they know in common. To qualify as part of "public knowledge", a meaning must fall in this third category of things which "everyone knows that everyone knows". Meanings which have become public knowledge in this sense are socially established and stable.

REFERENCES

Berger, Peter L. and Luckmann, Thomas
  1967 The Social Construction of Reality: A Treatise in the Sociology of Knowledge. New York: Anchor Books, Doubleday and Company, Inc.
Durkheim, Émile
  1961 The Elementary Forms of the Religious Life. New York: Collier Books.
  1938 The Rules of the Sociological Method. New York: The Free Press.
Edgerton, Robert
  1966 Conceptions of Psychosis in Four East African Societies. American Anthropologist 66:408–425.
Frank, Arthur
  1979 Reality Construction in Interaction. *In* Annual Review of Sociology, 5:167–191. Palo Alto: Annual Reviews, Inc.
Garfinkel, Harold
  1967 Studies in Ethnomethodology. Englewood Cliffs: Prentice Hall, Inc.
Giddens, Anthony
  1976 New Rules of the Sociological Method. New York: Basic Books.
Gumperz, John J.
  1982 Discourse Strategies: Studies in Interactional Sociolinguistics 1. Cambridge: Cambridge University Press.
Kleinman, Arthur
  1980 Patients and Healers in the Context of Culture. Berkeley: University of California Press.
Maines, David
  1977 Social Organization and Social Structures in Symbolic Interactionalist Thought. Annual Review of Sociology, 3:235–260. Palo Alto: Annual Reviews, Inc.
McHugh, Peter
  1968 Defining the Situation: The Organization of Meaning in Social Interaction. New York: The Bobbs-Merrill Company, Inc.
Moerman, Michael
  1968 A Little Knowledge. *In* S. Tyler (ed.), Cognitive Anthropology. New York: Holt, Rinehard and Winston.
Schutz, Alfred
  1967 The Phenomenology of the Social World. Evanston: Northwestern University Press.
Weber, Max
  1964 The Theory of Social and Economic Organization. Talcott Parsons (ed.). New York: Oxford University Press.

PEARL KATZ

HOW SURGEONS MAKE DECISIONS

INTRODUCTION

This paper examines surgeons in the process of making decisions. The analysis focuses on decision-making occurring in the course of the surgeons' professional clinical activities. This paper examines non-medical criteria entering into medical decision-making among surgeons and their influence on medical outcomes. It also examines the situations or contexts in which these non-medical criteria play an instrumental role in medical decision-making.

Three clinical cases are described in which surgeons, in their multiple roles as clinicians, researchers, teachers, colleagues and income earners, made decisions which had serious implications for their patients. In this paper, I will be concerned to point up those aspects of decision-making which are clearly non-medical, and which are influenced by the culture of surgery and the social organization of the hospital (see Katz 1984).

The analysis of the clinical cases indicates that surgeons obscured the decision-making process in a variety of ways. These included: (a) denying that they were making a decision; (b) denying that they had the option of making a decision; (c) embedding decisions in irrelevant information; (d) making a series of small decisions which led to major decisions; (e) passing the decision-making buck; (f) representing complex decisions as simple ones; and (g) representing simple decisions as complex ones. When thus obscured, decisions are made based on non-medical criteria.

DECISION-MAKING IN SURGERY

> Surgeons make decisions. They don't just put
> their hands in their pockets like internists.

With this statement, the Chief of Surgery at Southern University Hospital[1] expressed both the high value surgeons place upon decisive action by surgeons, and the low value they place upon thoughtful, hesitant consideration by other medical practitioners. An article on surgeons by a leading surgeon further illustrates the value placed on active decision-making: "A surgeon knows nothing, but does everything. An internist knows everything but does nothing. A psychiatrist knows nothing and does nothing. A pathologist knows everything, and does everything, one day too late" (Schwartzbart 1982: 22). The article ends with the observation that a surgeon is "above all else a soldier. For this healer greets every day as a day of battle" (p. 22).

155

R. A. Hahn and A. D. Gaines (eds.), Physicians of Western Medicine, 155–175.
© 1985 by D. Reidel Publishing Company.

The surgical literature emphasizes the active posture of decision-making. It is a primary skill to be mastered and valued. In an article on surgical education and surgical competence in the *Bulletin of the American College of Surgeons*, three basic skills were emphasized, "capacity for deductive reasoning and decision-making", "emotional characteristics", and "dexterity" (Spencer 1978: 9). Foremost under the emotional characteristics the article emphasized that "a surgeon must have the capacity to make consecutive decisions under stress" (p. 9).

Surgeons make a large number of decisions in the course of a working day. And although they place a high value upon the ability to make decisions, their perspective of their actual decision-making activities is limited. Some of the surgical literature emphasizes that "a major portion of decision-making occurs in the operating room" (Spencer 1978: 9). Most of the medical decision-making literature emphasizes the exclusive medical grounds for making medical decisions. The focus upon the medical auspices for decision-making neglects the examination of the multiple conditions under which physicians actually make decisions. It ignores the social and cultural bases and contexts which influence decision-making, the consequences of the decision-making process upon the welfare of patients, and the implications of the decision-making process for the practice of the medical profession.

Actual medical decisions are made in situations in which multiple variables coexist. Examining solely the medical bases for medical decision-making limits the variables to be studied. By examining medical decision-making in the natural setting in which it occurs, we can begin to understand the ways in which medical considerations are influenced by non-medical variables.

This study presents an anthropological perspective on decision-making among surgeons. It is based upon anthropological fieldwork among practicing surgeons. It examines the ways in which surgeons actually make decisions in the course of their daily professional activities. As an anthropological study, it does not examine decision-making in a simulated environment (see Kleinmuntz and Kleinmuntz 1981). It is not restricted to surgeons' normative perspective of how they think they *should* make decisions. Nor is it restricted to surgeons' retrospective view of how they made past decisions. The study examines the contexts in which they actually make decisions and their ongoing perspective about that decision-making process.

The anthropological perspective not only refers to the ethnographic *methodology* of observation in natural settings. It also refers to a particular *theoretical* orientation embodied in that methodology. The theoretical anthropological perspective assumes that *the social and cultural world of the surgeons plays a significant role in the way in which surgeons behave*, such as the ways in which they make decisions.

MEDICAL DECISION-MAKING

An increased interest in medical decision-making in the past decade has two American cultural roots. One is the questioning of established authorities, such as physicians, and asserting or reaffirming the rights of the 'underprivileged', such as patient-consumers. The second is believing that scientific, empirical knowledge will eventually eliminate uncertainty; that if we understood rational cognitive processes, such as medical decision-making, uncertainty in medical treatment and outcome will be eventually eliminated. These cultural beliefs have resulted in a concerned, scholarly literature on decision-making in medicine that ranges from statistical, computer-based information-processing models (see Williams 1982; Sherman et al. 1978) to psychological models based on behavioral and cognitive concepts (see Elstein et al. 1982; Kassirier 1976; Kassirier and Gorry 1978).

The major part of the literature on medical decision-making concentrates on the role of biomedical variables (see Lusted 1968; Ledley and Lusted 1959; Weinstein et al. 1980; Krischer 1980; Feinstein 1974). Even when the psychology of the doctor or the patient is examined, it is restricted to those *cognitive* psychological variables, such as reasoning processes, which analyze only the biomedical data.

Some of the medical decision-making literature deals with the *ethics* of medical decision-making as a goal for humanizing medical care. This literature focuses upon the moral choices that physicians face in interpreting biomedical data (Bursztajn et al. 1982; Israël 1982; Brett 1981).

Two excellent sociological studies on the behavior of surgeons in the course of their daily professional lives are Millman's *The Unkindest Cut* (1977) and Bosk's *Forgive and Remember* (1979). They discuss decision-making in the context of managing surgical mistakes.

A much smaller body of literature on decision-making examines the social and cultural influences upon medical decision-making. Eisenberg (1979), who critically reviewed the sociological literature on medical decision-making, pointed out that most of that literature focused upon the influence of *specific* social variables, such as patient characteristics. Eisenberg noted that most of these studies were based upon simulated, not actual, clinical cases or upon questionnaires. They contained "normative descriptions of how a physician should behave" (1979: 963). Eisenberg concluded by suggesting that "further investigation is needed into how the clinician does behave" (p. 963).

ANTHROPOLOGICAL METHODOLOGY

This research was conducted in a hospital affiliated with a medical school. I have called it Southern University Hospital. The method consisted of accompanying six senior, experienced surgeons, one at a time, while they went about their work, for a continuous period of several weeks each.[2] I accompanied each of them throughout a day, from the time each came to the hospital in the morning (about 7:00 am) until each left the hospital in the evening (about 7:00 pm).

The surgeons in this study were exceedingly accommodating to my research and trusting of my promise of confidentiality. Their responses resulted in an unanticipated dilemma for me; they allowed me unlimited access to themselves, their colleagues, decisions, concerns, mistakes, patients and files. They trusted me to maintain confidentiality and not to harm them when I published my data. Their openness, candor and trust had the consequence for me of an unprecedented "block" about writing about them which might reveal their frailties. This concern has been exacerbated by my present research involvement in an anthropological study of psychiatrists. I finally resolved this conflict through discussions with some colleagues[3] who suggested that I both carefully alter some information about the identity of the hospital, department and surgeons, in order to assure confidentiality, as well as incorporate these methodological concerns into the text. I also learned from my data, by making my criteria for decision-making more explicit.

Some sociocultural factors in the anthropological field-work situation contributed to the acceptance and candor of the surgeons. These included: the surgeons' initial evaluation of me as "just" a woman and a non-M.D., who could not possibly critically understand them; their isolation from their colleagues and their patients, which resulted in their wanting to talk to someone who was interested, but who appeared non-judgmental and non-threatening. Their acceptance for these reasons was illustrated by the comment of one surgeon to his colleague soon after beginning the study, "Look, I've got a girl following me around all the time, taking down everything I say!"

As an anthropologist, I attempted to understand their 'culture', i.e., their world-view, ethos and their conscious (and unconscious) understandings of their own activities. However, I did not enter culture-free. It was easier for me to identify with the patient than with the surgeon. At first, I was appalled at the disregard the surgeons showed for the emotional and social situation of the patient. I cringed as I dutifully recorded their references to patients as "the breast", "the colon", "that messy, end-stage patient" (see Johnson, this volume). After a few weeks, I was equally horrified to discover that I had begun to recognize patients post-operatively by their operative site, even patients I had seen several times in the surgeon's office before the operation, discussing their symptoms and expressing their concerns. This transformation allowed me to understand some of the psychological, sociological and cultural mechanisms by which the personal and social identities of patients could be ignored. And it raises important questions about anthropological objectivity, identification and countertransference reactions. (See Good et al. and Gaines, this volume.)

CASE STUDIES IN SURGICAL DECISION-MAKING

This paper presents three different situations[4] in surgery in which particular aspects of decision-making are emphasized. The first case involves a decision about how to operate on a hiatus hernia and who is to operate. The second case involves a decision about participation in clinical research. The third case involves a decision about whether to refer a surgical cancer patient to an oncology specialist.

These cases were selected because they illustrate (a) different roles that surgeons assume, such as diagnostician, researcher, colleague and therapist; (b) difficult decisions in which a large number of options exist; (c) decisions which resulted both in unanticipated as well as undesirable consequences;[5] (d) representative decisions which bear much similarity to decisions faced by most surgeons and other medical practitioners. The ways in which these surgeons' decisions are made may apply to decision-making in other, non-medical, contexts.

Case One: The Hiatus Hernia

Mr. *G*, a fifty-eight year old male, presented to the Department of Surgery at Southern University Hospital with symptoms of gastric reflux and heartburn of many years standing. In recent months Mr. *G*'s symptoms worsened. His family physician referred him to Dr. Schneider, a general surgeon at Southern University Hospital. Clinical and radiological (X-ray) examination of Mr. *G* indicated that he suffered from a large hiatus hernia. A hiatus hernia is a condition in which part of the stomach, which is normally exclusively in the abdominal cavity, extends through a hiatus through the diaphragm into the thoracic cavity. It is rarely a life-threatening disorder. Most hiatus hernia repairs can be performed equally successfully by either a general surgeon operating through the abdomen or a thoracic surgeon operating through the thoracic cavity (see Mustard 1970). In a small minority of cases a hiatus hernia should be performed thoracically to insure success.[6]

In most hiatus hernia cases, the pattern of referral to a surgeon determines the kind of operation to be performed. If the family physician or internist refers the patient to a general surgeon, the hiatus hernia will be repaired abdominally. If the referral is made to a thoracic surgeon, the repair will be made thoracically.

Mr. *G*'s hiatus hernia was one which would be more likely to be successful if it were performed thoracically, and unlikely to be successful if it were performed abdominally. Neither Mr. *G* nor his family physician knew that he had the type of hiatus hernia which should be repaired thoracically. Mr. *G*'s family doctor referred him to Dr. Schneider, a general surgeon. He had referred many patients to Dr. Schneider in the past and had been satisfied with the results.

Dr. Schneider was a senior surgeon on the staff of Southern University Hospital. In recent years his referrals had not increased as fast as those of some of his colleagues. He often complained that the proliferation of surgical specialists took away much of the business that had previously been the exclusive domain of the general surgeon. "We used to have most of the body, but the head and neck surgeons took away the upper part, the urologists and gynecologists took away the lower part, the cardiac and thoracic surgeons stole our chests, and all we have left are the guts and breasts." Dr. Schneider complained frequently of financial problems. He was then struggling to finance a new summer house.

The referral of Mr. *G*'s hiatus hernia presented Dr. Schneider with the following situation:

(1)   As a general surgeon, he was able only to perform a hiatus hernia repair abdominally; he was not trained to operate thoracically.

(2)   Mr. *G*'s hiatus hernia should be performed thoracically to insure success. However, the probably of failure if it were done abdominally, although great, was not inevitable. And failure was not likely to be detected immediately. The hernia would probably reappear within a period of weeks or months. Failure of hiatus hernia repair was not life-threatening.

(3)   Dr. Schneider was experiencing financial problems at the time.

(4)   The patient and the referring family physician did not know that the operation should be performed thoracically.

Dr. Schneider was faced with a decision about whether to perform the surgery himself through the abdomen, or whether he should refer the patient to a thoracic surgeon. He avoided making that decision by *consulting* a thoracic surgeon in his department, Dr. Pullman. Dr. Pullman was a personal friend of Dr. Schneider, as well as a colleague, and he knew that his colleague was worried about decreasing referrals in recent years and about his current financial problems. By asking Dr. Pullman for a consultation, Dr. Schneider avoided making a difficult decision himself. He turned the decision over to Dr. Pullman.

Dr. Pullman examined the clinical and radiological data on Mr. *G*'s hiatus hernia in the absence of Dr. Schneider and in the presence of the anthropologist. He explained his decision-making process in the following way:

This hernia will probably not hold if Jeff (Schneider) does it. If he's lucky, it may hold until the patient goes home. It should be done thoracically. But Jeff is terribly worried about his income. That summer house means a lot to him, but it's above his head. He needs money now. He is my friend. It's a tough decision. But if I take it from him (i.e., decide that it be done thoracically), he'll think twice about consulting me again, knowing I'll take his patients. And he's a friend who's in financial trouble . . . . I'll let him do it.

Indeed, Dr. Schneider performed the hiatus hernia repair abdominally. During the surgery it became evident to him and to the surgical staff that his operation was not likely to remain successful, to "hold". It became clear to them that the patient would have to return for a thoracic hiatus hernia repair within a year after surgery. But they did not reverse their decision once this information became more glaringly apparent during the operation. The patient was open and the repair was in process; most of the surgery had been performed. After the surgery Dr. Schneider met Dr. Pullman in the surgeons' lounge and said, "Whew, that was tough. I don't know how long it will last!" By hoping that the surgical repair would last beyond the immediate post-operative period, Dr. Schneider could hope to avoid facing the full consequences of his decision.[7]

This example of decision-making illustrates how *responsibility for decision-making may be passed from one person to another, with neither person defining the decision involved, nor considering the implications of that decision.* Dr. Schneider refused to make a decision, even though he was aware of the decision that should have been made for the patient's best interest. He asked Dr. Pullman to make the decision for him, through the mechanism of requesting a consultation. Had he acted solely on the medical information available to him, he would have referred the patient to Dr. Pullman, and not asked for a consultation. He confused the nature of the decision, e.g., that it was based on medical grounds, by referring it to his friend who was aware and concerned about his financial problems. In turn, Dr. Pullman decided to "return the patient" to Dr. Schneider not for medical reasons, but (a) on the grounds of friendship (he did not want to "take away" the patient of his friend); (b) on the grounds of money ("He's terribly worried about his income. That house means a lot to him"); and (c) on the grounds of encouraging subsequent referrals to him by his colleague ("He'll think twice about consulting me again.").

Yet, all the discussions and data exchanged between the two surgeons about the patient, his hiatus hernia and the auspices for surgical consultation and decision-making, were discussed in the language of medicine. Notwithstanding the medical language, the actual grounds for the decision-making which both the surgeons shared were non-medical. They were concerned about Dr. Schneider's financial troubles. They were concerned about his decreasing referrals. And they were concerned about maintaining their personal and professional relationship, including the expectation of subsequent referrals.

Both surgeons shared a common medical and sociocultural environment. And both made medical decisions which had serious and predictably detrimental consequences for their patient, but profitable consequences for their financial and professional relationship. They chose not to make the criteria for their decision-making explicit to each other; they pretended the criterion was medical.

Case Two: Participation in Clinical Research

The Chief of Surgery at Southern University Hospital decided to initiate a research project in the Department of Surgery. He chose a project which could be easily implemented in the routines of the general surgeons. It was a prospective clinical trial of breast cancer patients who were to undergo mastectomies.

The Chief had read about two different diagnostic procedures for assessing the stage of development of breast cancers. He decided to compare the two procedures. In order to implement the research he needed the support and active participation of the general surgeons in the Department of Surgery. Although Southern University Hospital was a university-affiliated teaching hospital, and the surgeons were university surgeons who taught medical students and residents, few surgeons had training, experience or interest in research. Their main interest was in operating on as many patients as possible as well as possible, and in teaching surgical skills. Yet, the members of the Department of Surgery knew that their department could gain prestige through participation in research. And increased departmental prestige promoted patient referrals as well as opportunities for teaching. These professional priorities of the university hospital surgeons influenced their decision-making activities about research.

The research compared two diagnostic procedures for determining the cancerous involvement of internal mammary lymph glands for the staging of breast cancers. The cancerous involvement of internal mammary lymph nodes indicates a metastatic stage that is more widespread than that which involves axillary lymph nodes. One method of diagnostic staging was a radiographic procedure in which the internal mammary nodes were X-rayed.[8] The other was a histological procedure in which the internal mammary lymph nodes were removed and examined in the laboratory.[9] The Chief of Surgery proposed a clinical research trial which compared the radiological diagnostic procedure with the histological diagnostic procedure, for the staging of breast cancer of patients undergoing mastectomies in the hospital.

The Chief of Surgery first mentioned the idea of participation in the clinical trial to the general surgeons[10] in his department as he met them in the hallway[11] in the course of two days. The Chief said to each of them, "How'd you like to participate in research on your breast patients?" He described the research in extremely general terms, "We'll see if histological involvement of internal mammary nodes gives us an indication of stages". The question was asked in an informal manner in an informal place. The description was general, no details were offered. The informality and generality of the presentation influenced the informality and generality of the responses: "Yes, it sounds okay"; "Well, I get a lot of breasts". Each of the surgeons that the Chief approached indicated generally that it was a good idea. They knew that the Chief wanted the department members to become involved in research. They also believed that their research involvement would be minimal. They believed that the Chief would write up the protocol and tell them of a few extra procedures they would have to follow.

Because the Chief mentioned the idea in such a general and casual manner, the surgeons did not ask questions. The context of the informal chance meeting in the hallway conveyed both a message that he merely wanted the surgeons' tacit approval before proceeding further, as well as a message that serious questions belonged in another context. As a result, none of the surgeons made more specific inquiries about the research. They did not ask whether the research was invasive, how the patients were to be selected, nor how they would obtain informed consent.

The Chief mentioned the research in a manner and context that communicated to the surgeons that he was asking their opinion about their interest in that research. He did not communicate that he wanted them to make a decision. As a result, none of the surgeons realized at that moment that they were making a decision about their active participation in research.

During the following two days, the Chief wrote a three-page 'protocol' for the research. The protocol included a paragraph citing the original references about the substantive issues of the internal mammary lymph nodes as histological and radiographic markers for staging breast cancer. The remainder of the protocol dealt with details about the research population (e.g., pre- and post-menopausal women with no previous history of breast cancer who were provisionally diagnosed[12] as having breast cancer), procedures for obtaining the radiological diagnoses by having patients check into the hospital a day early to be injected and X-rayed by the Department of Nuclear Medicine, procedures for obtaining the histological samples at the time of the mastectomy, and procedures for sending the histological slides to the pathology lab so that the surgeons, the pathologists and the radiologists did not know the others' diagnoses. The protocol also stated that informed consent must be obtained from the patient prior to the date for the operation and the clinical trial. The protocol stated a starting date for the clinical trial to begin. That date was the week following the meeting of the Hospital Human Research Committee. The Chief anticipated no problems in obtaining approval. And, indeed, the committee approved the research.

The Chief sent the approved protocol to each of the six general surgeons, accompanied by a memo which stated, "Enclosed is the protocol for the Internal Mammary Node Biopsy Trial. We will begin on April 12. I'll be glad to offer every assistance in this research". The letter did not ask for their formal approval. Their informal approval had already been obtained in the hallway.

One of the six surgeons involved, Dr. Pectin, conducted a breast clinic weekly. Dr. Pectin only worked part-time in Southern University Hospital. He depended upon the Chief of Surgery for his operating privileges, referrals and the use of the examining room and receptionist during his outpatient clinic. Dr. Pectin was one of the surgeons whom the Chief originally consulted casually in the hallway. He never realized that that casual encounter in which he said that he thought the research sounded like a good idea, constituted a decision to participate in the research.

In the breast clinic, Dr. Pectin examined fifteen to twenty women a day who were referred by their primary physicians for suspected breast cancer. On the day in which the clinica trial was to begin, Dr. Pectin encountered his first problem. He found it difficult to persuade the patients who were to undergo a mastectomy to agree to enter the clinical trial and sign the informed consent form.

In usual circumstances, Dr. Pectin, in common with most other surgeons, found it difficult to inform his patients that they probably had breast cancer. Even though most of the surgeons admitted that they were correct more than ninety percent of the time based upon outpatient examination and even more frequently correct with diagnoses based upon mammograms and needle aspirations, they found it extremely difficult to communicate a diagnosis of cancer to their patients. Many surgeons typically told the patient that she had little to worry about, but nevertheless, just in case, they would book them into the hospital for a biopsy under general anaesthetic. Other surgeons suggested to their patients that there was a real possibility that there was a "malignancy", but they were optimistic in this particular case. For example, in one situation a surgeon at Southern University Hospital told me that he was 99.9 percent sure that his patient had a malignancy; she was a patient with a visible tumor in her breast and armpit and whose needle aspiration biopsy specimen appeared positive. Yet this surgeon told the patient that she had little to worry about. However, he acted on his suspicions and reserved a bed and operating-room time.

These routine ways of not communicating positive cancer information to patients were not possible with those breast cancer patients whom Dr. Pectin wanted to have participate in the research trial. In order to obtain their informed consent, Dr. Pectin was required to inform his patients not only that they probably had breast cancer, but also that he wished them to agree to undergo both a diagnostic radiograph and biopsy of their internal mammary lymph nodes for research purposes to determine the stage of their cancer.

On the first day of the clinical trial, Dr. Pectin found that he was unable to tell his patient that she had cancer and to explain to her that he would like her permission to have her undergo tests for research purposes. He came into the Chief's office to back out of the research. "I can't do it", he said to the Chief; "Do I have to tell them everything?" The Chief answered, "Just give them a very general idea. Don't worry them. Don't go into the specifics".

This exchange illustrates the way in which Dr. Pectin, who did not even realize that he had made the decision to participate in the research, again avoided making a decision about informing his patients. He turned the decision about informed consent over to the Chief. It was as if he believed that because he had no say in the original research decision, it was the Chief's research that was being carried out in the Chief's department. Therefore the Chief should obtain informed consent.

Indeed, the Chief had an interest in getting the cooperation of his staff to carry out the research. He made a decision that the patient need not be adequately informed. But he avoided the immediate implications of that decision by not facing the patient himself. He told Dr. Pectin to carry out the decision that he, the Chief, had made. Dr. Pectin, who was dependent upon the Chief for the use of his office for referrals and for operating-room privileges, continued participating in the research, but accepted the Chief's decision about not adequately informing his patients. This division of labor between Dr. Pectin and the Chief permitted the decision to be divided so that no one person was responsible for making the decision.

Dr. Pectin explained to his breast cancer patient that although he did not think that breast lump was malignant, it may be malignant. He suggested it would be necessary to have a biopsy under general anesthetic, as well as a nuclear medicine diagnostic test and a histological examination of the internal mammary lymph node, to determine her status. He informed her of the day she was to book into the hospital and presented the informed consent form to her to sign, which he said explained these procedures.

Dr. Pectin explained the information about the clinical trial at the same time that he told her that she may have breast cancer. The research trial was presented to her as if it were the regular diagnostic procedure. After all, it was her first breast cancer! The explanation of the research procedure was included both in the general explanation of the hospital procedure, such as when to check in and where to go and when the tests will begin, and in the announcement about the likelihood of cancer of the breast.

The information about the research trial was not seen in any way as separate either from the hospital procedure or from the information about her disease status. It was embedded in an announcement of the presence of possible cancer and the hospital procedures to be followed. The patient was presented with information overload exacerbated by the distress that accompanied the announcement of the possibility of breast cancer. This created a situation in which the patient could hardly distinguish between diagnostic procedures, surgical intervention and research activities. Nor was the patient made aware that she had the option of making a decision, including refusing to participate in the research trial.

The clinical trial involved a number of procedures in addition to the usual ones for suspected breast cancer. These included obtaining informed consent about participating in the research, having the patient sign into the hospital one day earlier than she would otherwise have had to enter. This was done in order for her to be tested by nuclear medicine procedures. This process involved injection of radio-active dye and exposure to radiation. Finally, there was the removal of additional lymph nodes, involving invasive cutting of pectoral muscles and other internal tissues.

The surgeons were required to make decisions about the additional procedures. How should they tell the patient that she has cancer and will probably undergo a mastectomy? How should they tell the patient that she has the option of participating or refusing to participate in the clinical trial? How should the surgeon tell the patient that the research is invasive and causes additional trauma to her body, which is likely to result in a longer recovery time and increased possibility of post-operative infection? How should the surgeon tell the patient that she has the option of not entering the hospital one day earlier or being injected with dye and subjected to radiation exposure and an additional invasive procedure?

When the first research patient at Southern University Hospital booked into the hospital a day earlier, according to the research protocol, the surgeons became aware of the fact that none of them had ever seen or carried out this procedure before. Indeed, none of the six surgeons were certain that they would be able to recognize the internal mammary lymph nodes. Although the Chief of Surgery initiated the research, wrote the protocol, presented it to the hospital committee, and arranged the organizational details for carrying out the clinical trial, he did not know how to identify nor excise the internal mammary lymph nodes. He had given no thought to the operative procedure, its feasibility with the surgical staff, nor its risks to the patient.

When the Chief of Surgery realized that neither he nor the surgeons on his staff knew how to excise an internal mammary node, they began to make discrete further inquiries. They discovered that one of the senior residents at Southern University Hospital had seen the procedure performed a year earlier at another hospital when he was a junior resident. Upon hearing this, the Chief asked him, "Do you want to show Chris (Pectin) how to do it?" The resident agreed to perform that part of the operation and to teach the senior surgeon, Dr. Pectin and the Chief, how to do the procedure. It was observed during the course of fieldwork among the surgeons that the residents not infrequently performed surgical procedures for senior surgeons who were not familiar with particular procedures.

Three surgeons were present in the Operating Room for the mastectomy and internal mammary node biopsy on the first research patient. Dr. Pectin performed the mastectomy (and the original breast biopsy to verify the malignancy). The Chief observed the operation to insure that the clinical research went smoothly and to learn how to perform the operation. And the resident excised the internal mammary lymph nodes, and taught Dr. Pectin and the Chief how to identify and excise them.

The resident had difficulty in locating the nodes. He explained to the other surgeons that he was looking for the internal mammary artery which indicated where the internal mammary lymph nodes would be. Until they observed this procedure, none of the surgeons had been aware of the difficulty in locating the nodes, their depth and the resulting injury to tissues.[13] During the operation Dr. Pectin exclaimed, "I wouldn't want my mother to go through this!" The Chief of Surgery commented, "We're going to have an increase in post-operative infections with these patients. If we get too many, we'll have to look into it".

The surgeons only became aware of the increased risks to the patients after performing the operation, after having made the decision to operate. No one previously had even questioned the risks. And when they became aware of the risks of, for example, post-operative infections, they did not consider stopping the trial, but only considered stopping *after* "too many" post-operative infections appeared.

This case illustrates ways in which surgeons made decisions without realizing at the time that they made them.

The Chief did not make them aware that they were making a decision about participating in research. He obscured the options for the surgeons by presenting the information in an informal manner in an informal place that discouraged questions or review of the options, or serious consideration of the value and consequences of the research. The surgeon, in turn, obscured the information about research participation for the patient by announcing it at the same time as the announcement of breast cancer, and at the same time as he explained the regular hospital procedure for a mastectomy. He embedded the information about the research participation in information about the forthcoming cancer operation. The surgeon seemed to present an "overload" of information to the patient so that she had to be selective in her understanding, acceptance and active participation in decision-making about the information. It is of considerable interest that in a completely different context, the Chief of Surgery explained to me, "You first get them to agree to the principle, and the details will come later". Through this incremental process (see F. Katz 1982), the surgeons made a decision which had serious implications for themselves and their patients. Moreover, this incremental process obscured the implications until after a major commitment had been made.

Case Three: Referring to Specialists

Cancer patients typically consult with a number of specialists for the diagnosis and treatment of their disease. The cancer patient usually has little knowledge of the range of specialists available, the appropriateness of the specialist's field for their cancer, or the limits of the expertise of the specialists. Most patients are simply referred by the first doctor who suspects or diagnoses their cancer, to another doctor whom the first believes is the cancer specialist. Thus, the referral may be to a surgeon, an internist, medical oncologist or a radiation oncologist. This pattern of referral based on the knowledge and network of the first doctor and his recognition and williness to refer, and the second doctor's knowledge, networks, recognition and willingness to refer, determines the type and quality of treatment and care of the cancer patient.

Most of the surgeons in Southern University Hospital were concerned about increasing the number of their surgical patients and increasing their income. Cancer patients comprise a large proportion of patients for surgeons and therefore a substantial proportion of their income. Usually the surgeons' responsibility, knowledge and training about cancer patients is limited to specific surgical interventions and follow-up during the immediate post-operative period, until they refer their patients to the oncologists.[14] It is often difficult for physicians to refer their patients to specialists. By referring, they "lose" their patients. The loss includes the emotional bond with the patients, control and management of them, and the income from treating them.

Some of the surgeons at Southern University Hospital were concerned about "losing" their cancer patients after surgery to the oncologists in the hospital. In order to keep their surgical cancer patients, the Chief of Surgery and some of the surgeons began to initiate clinical trials in the follow-up treatment of specific kinds of cancer patients. They were able to recruit breast cancer patients into the breast cancer trials, in addition to referring them to the medical or radiation oncologists. They recruited most of the colon and rectal cancer patients for participation in a colo-rectal clinical trial conducted by one of the surgeons. The Chief attempted to recruit the lung cancer patients into a clinical trial under the senior thoracic surgeon. However, the senior thoracic surgeon, Dr. Chestnut, decided to refer all his lung cancer patients, including those who were inoperable as well as those who underwent surgery, to the medical oncologists. Dr. Chestnut made that explicit decision because he knew that the medical oncologist was a specialist in the diagnosis, care and management of cancer patients, and that his own knowledge of oncology, except for surgical oncology, was less than that of the medical oncologist. In spite of the pressure of the Chief, and in spite of his wish to increase his income, he made a concrete decision to refer his patients to the oncologists.

Dr. Tushnet was the general surgeon who was conducting the colo-rectal clinical trials of the surgical patients who had colon or rectal cancer. In this trial one-half of the patients received a drug having some immunological properties and one-half of the patients received a placebo. The patients were randomly placed in either group. The surgeon did not know in which group the patients were placed.

Dr. Tushnet was also aware of the fact that he knew less about the treatment, care and management of colo-rectal cancers than the oncologists. Yet the number of patients and his income had increased significantly since he began to participate in the colo-rectal cancer patients were referred to him post-operatively. He not only could "keep" his own patients, but he could also obtain the patients of the other surgeons. Yet, because he was aware of his limited knowledge about oncology, and because he was both a colleague and a friend of Dr. Chestnut (who chose not to participate in oncology trials), he was uncomfortable about his role in treating and retaining these cancer patients and in his participation in the colo-rectal oncology trial.

The following verbatim conversation took place between Drs. Tushnet and Chestnut:

Dr. T.: You know the Chief asked me to be in charge of the whole colo-rectal program at the hospital?
Dr. Ch.: What's in it for you?
Dr. T.: I'm involved in research .... But I have a problem. A patient of Jim's (a colo-rectal surgeon who refused to conduct the colo-rectal clinical trials) with colo-rectal cancer, who comes to me for oncology (i.e., the clinical trial), called me several times this weekend. He's in bad condition – liver metastases, ulcerated mouth, pain. I told him, 'Why call me? Call your surgeon. I'm just the oncologist.' He said that his surgeon was not capable of handling his problem and had told him to call me. He was admitted to Emergency. Should I take him? Should I be the oncologist for colo-rectal? Why didn't Jim take him?
Dr. Ch.: Jim wants a clean practice. No cancer. Hemorrhoids and taking colons out, that's all. No messy end-stage cancer. You have to decide whether you want to continue oncology. What's in it for you to accept that you are the colo-rectal expert? Warren (the Chief of Surgery) suggested it because he wants oncology for surgery. You know we have an excellent medical oncologist on staff. He's good, but he's got no practice. You're taking his colons and rectums, Chris is taking all his breasts. All he's got are some lymphomas and my lungs. He may leave.
Dr. T.: I'll have to think about that. I figure I've got four options. Leave this region for the mid-west; go to a small town; stay at Southern (University Hospital) and fight; or stay at Southern and join the system.

The day after having this conversation, Dr. Tushnet met Dr. Chestnut and said, "I've been thinking about our discussion. I didn't realize that Davis (the oncologist) had so little practice that he may leave. I've decided to share some of my patients with Davis, especially the ones who need palliative care, like Jim's patient last weekend".

Dr. Tushnet made a decision. His decision was, at best, a compromise. He would share some of his patients with the oncologist, particularly the difficult, complaining, "messy end-stage" patients. Of course, this decision did not tackle the major problems that Dr. Chestnut clearly presented to his colleague. He did not question whether he was qualified to treat oncology patients, whether it was ethical to keep them from being treated by the medical oncologist. He did not explicitly examine the substantive medical issues regarding the range of treatments that may be available to the colo-rectal cancer patients.

Since Dr. Tushnet and Dr. Chestnut made completely different decisions about the same kind of problem, it is of interest to examine the components of their decision-making process, particularly the way in which each of them defined the problem, the decision and the options available to them. Most importantly, the surgeon who had already made the decision not to participate in the cancer trials, Dr. Chestnut, was aware of the decisions to be made, the options available and the consequences of the decisions for himself, his colleagues and his patients. In contrast, Dr. Tushnet, the surgeon who was not prepared to make the decision, not only refused to acknowledge to himself, his colleagues nor his patients which options were available to him, but he also confused them.

How did he confuse his options? First, he introduced the subject matter in an indirect manner: "You know the Chief asked me to be in charge of the whole colo-rectal program?" In this statement, he presented himself as the passive object of someone else's decision. Then he discussed a patient with "messy end-stage cancer", as opposed to the other surgeon's "clean" practice. The conversation does not suggest that there is a substantive medical issue involved, for example, should a surgeon rather than an oncologist be treating cancer patients. It suggests that the issue is one of convenience (messy versus clean), or professional loyalty (to the surgeons or to the medical oncologist) or one of personal concern for a colleague, (such as the oncologist who was losing so many patients to surgery that he may be forced to leave).

He confused the options by not referring to the welfare of the patients, nor to the options that were potentially available to the patients. He was not concerned about the patients who were deprived of their options to be treated by the better qualified specialist. He did not clarify that the patients had the option of having medical treatment based on informed knowledge of a wide range of treatment options available. Instead, the patient was not aware of the decisions which had been made for him and which could have serious consequences for the duration and quality of his life. Dr. Tushnet's decision took the decision-making away from the patient by not informing the patient of the choices he potentially had available to him. In fact, the entire discussion between the two surgeons about their participation in clinical oncology trials had no mention of the medical implications for the patients and the patients' families.

Dr. Tushnet confused his options by referring to highly generalized alternatives. When he actually attempted to make his options explicit, they took the generalized forms of flight or fight or joining the system — "go to the mid-west, a small town, or join or fight the system". In generalizing his options he did not deal specifically with the major decision, namely, what were the pros and cons of assuming expertise and responsibility for colo-rectal oncology. He confused his options by changing the subject. He seriously considered whether he should have extended palliative care to the end-stage cancer patient, but neglected consideration of whether he was qualified to make treatment decisions about salvageable cancer patients.

The way in which each of the surgeons made or did not make the options explicit, affected their decisions. The decision-making options were made explicit by the surgeon who was willing to make a difficult decision. The decision-making options were made confused by the surgeon unwilling to make the difficult decision. He misrepresented and obscured the relevant components involved in the decision-making. He did not clarify the major decision, whether he should continue to practice medical oncology, when he was qualified to practice surgery and there were highly qualified medical oncologists on the hospital staff.

By not clarifying the options available, Dr. Tushnet avoided making medical decisions according to medical criteria. By obscuring the components of the decision-making process, he made medical decisions on the basis of his social and financial exigencies. By confusing the decision-making process, he avoided the implications of his decision, namely that he deprived a large number of cancer patients of the opportunity to receive specialty care and treatment that may have prolonged their lives. The fact that other surgeons in his department made their options clear and decided not to participate in the post-operative treatment of cancer patients demonstrates that other viable options were available for decision-making.

SUMMARY AND CONCLUSIONS

This paper has examined surgeons in the process of making decisions in the course of their daily professional lives. It examined the ways in which non-medical criteria entered into medical decision-making and influenced medical decisions and medical outcomes. It examined the situations in which these non-medical criteria played an instrumental role in medical decision-making. Three clinical cases were described in which surgeons, in their multiple roles as clinicians, researchers, teachers, colleagues and income earners, made decisions which had serious implications for their patients.

Analysis of these clinical cases led to the following conclusions: (1) *surgeons obscured the decision-making process in a variety of ways* and (2) *as a result, non-medical variables influenced that process*. Below, I will briefly illustrate these points.

1.1. Surgeons obscured their decision-making process by not acknowledging that they were making a decision. A decision may be so obscured in its formulation that action is taken without the realization that a decision is being made. When the surgeons responded favorably to the Chief's informal statements about their possible participation in a clinical trial (Case Two), the surgeons did not know that they were making a decision. When the familiy practitioner referred Mr. *G* (Case One) to a general surgeon, he was not aware that he was making a decision about the kind of hiatus hernia operation his patient would be likely to undergo.

1.2. Surgeons obscured their decision-making process by denying that they had an option in making a decision. Decisions are frequently made in such a way that the person making the decision believes that it is the only decision option available to him. The patients in the colo-rectal trial (Case Three) were not made aware that they had the option of being treated by a medical oncologist rather than a surgeon Although the surgeon, Dr. Tushnet, was diligent in carefully explaining the content of the informed consent form to the patients, thus giving them the option of not participating in the colo-rectal trial, he did not let them know they had the option of being treated by a medical oncologist.

The perception of absence of decision-making options can frequently be inferred from an examination of the linguistic presentation of the decision-making situation (see Weintraub 1982). The person making the decision may describe the process in a syntactically passive manner: he is the object of the decision made by someone else. He is not the subject who actively makes the decision. For example, Dr. Tushnet claimed (Case Three). "You know the Chief asked me to be in charge of the whole colo-rectal problem at the hospital?" He implied that he had no choice and that he did not make the decision.

1.3. Surgeons obscured their decision-making process by embedding the decisions in irrelevant information. The surgeons in the breast cancer trial (Case Two) wanted their patients to agree to the research, but feared if they knew about the research they might not agree to participate in it. They obscured the information about the research by presenting it at the same time as they announced the possibility of the patients' having cancer and that the latter would be booked into the hospital for an operation a day earlier. The research information was embedded in the other emotionally-laden clinical information. As a result, the patients did not know they were making a decision about research.

When the Chief presented the idea of research to the surgeons in the hallway (Case Two), he embedded the decision about research in the context of informality in place of a formal presentation.

1.4. Surgeons obscured the decision-making process by making a series of small decisions which led to major decisions. When the Chief decided to participate in a research trial (Case Two), it appeared to be a small, limited decision. He knew he would have to write the protocol and arrange the X-ray and histological testing. But he believed that the other surgeons would carry out the research with few problems. This seemingly minor decision led to a series of other decisions that had major implications for the general surgeons and their patients. They included obtaining informed consent and coping with the realization that no staff surgeon had seen or done the operation, as well as how the patients and the research trial should be managed when post-operative infections increased. The significance of that small decision became obvious when one surgeon commented, "I wouldn't want my mother to go through this".

1.5. Surgeons obscured the decision-making process by passing the decision-making buck. For example, the surgeons who did not realize they had made a decision about research in the hallway (Case Two), in turn, obscured the decision about informed consent to the patients. Similarly, Dr. Schneider (Case One) passed the decision regarding the kind of hiatus hernia operation onto Dr. Pullman, by asking Dr. Pullman for a *consultation*. If he were prepared to take the responsibility for the decision-making, he would have referred the patient to a thoracic surgeon, or dealt with the patient without a consultation. Instead, he passed the decision-making buck to Dr. Pullman.

1.6. Surgeons obscured the decision-making process by representing complex decisions as simple ones. The decision to participate in the breast cancer trial (Case Two) was presented to the surgeons as a simple decision: "How'd you like to participate in research on your breast patients?" Yet, the decision was complex, because participation in the research involved a number of other considerations, including responsibilities to the patients about exposing them to risks, the meaning of informed consent and lengthening their hospital stay.

1.7. Surgeons obscured the decision-making process by representing simple decisions as complex ones. When Dr. Tushnet (Case Three) was making a decision about continuing to participate in the colo-rectal trials, he obscured the options by saying he had four choices, e.g., "move to the mid-west, move to a small town, stay and fight the system and stay and join the system". He did not clarify the actual options about a simple decision — whether he should continue to act as a colo-rectal oncologist or to refer the patients to a trained oncologist on staff.

2. In all the situations in which the decision-making options were obscured, non-medical criteria influenced the decision-making. The clinical cases indicated the ways in which variables such as colleagueship, hospital organizational structure, departmental hierarchy, the influence of the Chief, competition (such as that between medical oncology and surgical departments), increased referrals, and conceptions of appropriate income played significant roles in the medical decision-making. In surgery, the differences in incidence of specific surgical procedures in different geographic and cultural areas suggest that non-medical factors influence the decision to operate (see MacPherson et al. 1982).

When medical decisions are discussed, for example, during rounds or informal discussions with medical colleagues, they are discussed exclusively in medical terms. The language used is that of medicine. The criteria *acknowledged* are medical criteria. However, sociocultural variables are *embedded* in the terminology of the medical variables. For example, in the case of the hiatus hernia (Case One), although the criteria for decision-making were virtually entirely non-medical, e.g., potential for continued referrals, maintenance of colleagueship and friendship, increasing the income of a financially burdened surgeon, the entire written and verbal communication between the two surgeons referred exclusively to the medical domain.

Perhaps representing medical decisions exclusively in medical terms has led many researchers examining medical decision-making to assume that medical criteria are the only relevant ones. However, it may be that ignoring the influence of non-medical criteria in medical decision-making increases the non-medical influence on decision-making precisely because it further obscures awareness of the decision-making process.

Understanding the dynamics and principles of the *actual* decision-making process among medical practitioners is important because decisions affect medical outcomes, the quality and cost of medical care. In an article in *The New England Journal of Medicine*, Eddy suggests that a "better description of clinical decision making might assign a prominent role to clinical policies – guidelines . . ." (1982). Indeed, guidelines, policies and protocols must be based upon substantive knowledge of the way that medical practitioners actually make decisions. Such procedures may increase the autonomy for all the participants, including the physician, his colleagues and the patients. An article on ritual in the operating room suggested the ways in which autonomy was increased by ritual (P. Katz 1981). This paper suggests that autonomy and the understanding of medical practice may be increased when the components of the decision-making process are made explicit. We "need to make explicit the assumptions that guide our thinking in medicine. In making these assumptions explicit, we have the opportunity to change them" (Bursztajn et al. 1981).

NOTES

1. A pseudonym for the university-affiliated hospital in which the anthropological field-work was conducted. I wish to thank the anonymous surgeons for their generous support and help.
2. I wish to thank F. E. Katz for suggesting this methodology to me which is based upon the model of his work with pathologists (see F. Katz 1968).
3. I wish to thank Joan Cassell, Atwood Gaines and Robert Hahn for their suggestions and support.
4. I wish to thank John Singer, M.D., F.A.C.S. for help in reviewing the medical-surgical aspects of these cases.
5. Most of the decisions made by the surgeons in Southern University Hospital were highly responsible ones, based upon high standards of medical-surgical knowledge and practice. The decisions selected for this study were those in the minority which did not meet the usual standards. They were selected *because* they were problematic in their execution.
6. Most of the cases in which the hiatus hernia must be performed by a thoracic surgeon are those which repair previously unsuccessful operations. Occasionally, an unusual (stomach) angle requires the operation to be performed thoracically (cf. Mustard 1970).
7. Much of the data on surgical mobidity and mortality refer to the immediate post-operative period. The failure to examine beyond this period in many studies may significantly affect data upon which surgical decisions are based.
8. This was not a routine procedure of diagnosis.
9. The histological procedure was a routine procedure for medical breast lesions in some hospitals.
10. General surgeons operate on breasts.
11. The hallway was a usual and predictable place for communication of information. Meetings were likely to occur during the course of each day while "chancing" to meet in the hallways. They were predictable in that they were likely to occur, although the exact time was not predictable. The advantage of these meetings were that they appeared to be unplanned. They allowed flexibility in discussions.
12. Most of these women in Southern University Hospital had had positive clinical signs and positive histological signs (e.g., needle biopsy) of breast cancer. Nevertheless, definitive diagnosis of breast cancer was undertaken by frozen section in the laboratory near the operating room.

13. Increased trauma to tissues increases the likelihood of post-operative infection.
14. Surgeons continued to care for their surgical cancer patients who did not need treatment from an oncologist. Many surgeons prefer to follow their patients to coordinate their care even after referring to an oncologist.

REFERENCES

Brett, A. S.
    1981 The Hidden Ethical Issues in Clinical Decision Analysis. The New England Journal of Medicine 305:1150–1152.
Bosk, Charles
    1979 Forgive and Remember. Chicago: University of Chicago Press.
Bursztajn, H. et al.
    1981 Medical Choices, Medical Chances: How Patients, Families and Physicians Can Cope with Uncertainty. New York: Delacorte Press.
Eddy, David
    1982 Clinical Policies and the Quality of Clinical Practice. The New England Journal of Medicine 307:343–347.
Eisenberg, John M.
    1979 Sociological Influences on Decision-Making by Clinicians. Annals of Internal Medicine 90:957–964.
Elstein, A. S. et al.
    1982 Psychological Approaches to Medical Decision-Making. American Behavioral Scientist 25:557–584.
Feinstein, A. R.
    1974 An Analysis of Diagnostic Reasoning: III/The Construction of Clinical Algorithms. Yale Journal of Biology and Medicine 46:5–32.
Helfer, R. E.
    1971 Measuring the Process of Solving Clinical Diagnostic Problems. British Journal of Medical Education 5:48–52.
Israël, Lucien
    1982 Decision-Making: The Modern Doctor's Dilemma. New York: Random House.
Kassirer, J. P.
    1976 The Perception of Clinical Decision-making: An Introduction to Decision Analysis. Yale Journal of Biology and Medicine 49: 149–164.
Kassirer, J. and G. A. Gorry
    1970 Clinical Problem Solving: A Behavioral Analysis. Annals of Internal Medicine 89: 245–255.
Katz, F. E.
    1968 Autonomy and Organization: The Limits of Social Control. New York: Random House.
    1982 A Sociological Perspective to the Holocaust. Modern Judaism 2:273–296.
Katz, Pearl
    1981 Ritual in the Operating Room. Ethnology 20:335–350.
    1984 The Scalpels' Edge: Surgeons' Rituals and Decisions (ms).
Kleinmuntz, D. N. and B. Kleinmuntz
    1981 Systems Simulation Decision Strategies in Simulated Environments. Behavioral Sciences 26:294–304.
Krischer, J. P.
    1980 An Annotated Bibliography of Decision Analytic Applications to Health Care. Operations Research 18:97–113.

Ledley, R. A. and L. B. Lusted
1959 Reasoning Foundations of Medical Diagnosis. Science 130:9—21.
Lusted, L. B.
1968 Introduction to Medical Decision-Making. Springfield, Illinois: Charles C. Thomas.
MacPherson, Klim, et al.
1982 Small-Area Variations in the Use of Common Surgical Procedures: An International Comparison of New England, England and Norway. The New England Journal of Medicine, Nov. 18, 1982:1310—1314.
Millman, Marcia
1977 The Unkindest Cut: Life in the Backrooms of Medicine. New York: William Morrow.
Mustard, R. A.
1970 A Survey of Techniques and Results of Hiatus Hernia Repair. Surg. Gynec. Obst. 130:131—136.
Schwartzbart, A.
1982 The Romantic Aspects of Being a Surgeon. A.M.A. News.
Sherman, H. et al.
1978 Clinical Algorithms and Decision Analysis. Proc. 4th Illinois Conference on Medical Information Systems. Regional Health Resource Center, Urbana, Illinois.
Spencer, Frank Cole
1978 Teaching and Measuring Surgical Techniques: The Technical Evaluation of Competence. Bulletin of the American College of Surgeons 63:9—12.
Weinstein, M. C. et al.
1980 Clinical Decision Analysis. Philadelphia: Saunders.
Weintraub, Walter
1982 Verbal Behavior: Adapatation and Psychopathology. New York: Springer Publishing Co.
Williams, Ben (ed.)
1982 Computer Aids to Clinical Decisions. Volume III. Boca Raton, Florida: CRC Press.

WILLIAM RITTENBERG AND RONALD C. SIMONS

GENTLE INTERROGATION: INQUIRY AND INTERACTION IN BRIEF INITIAL PSYCHIATRIC EVALUATIONS

INTRODUCTION

Often in hospital emergency rooms, clinics and private offices a psychiatrist meets a new patient with potentially urgent problems. Sometimes only a short time is available before he or she must make decisions about management and initial treatment. In this circumstance the psychiatrist needs to gather relevant information rapidly from a patient who may be confused, distraught, and guarded. To accomplish this he or she needs a method of interviewing specific for this situation which differs both from ordinary social conversation and also from most forms of therapy talk (Turner 1972).

This paper examines the method by which an experienced psychiatric interviewer (RCS) conducts these brief initial evaluations. It is based on direct observation and on the study of videotapes of psychiatric interviews which he conducted as demonstrations for medical students and psychiatry residents. Some of these interviews were performed before a student audience and followed a student interview with the same patient, others did not. Some were as brief as ten minutes, others as long as forty-five. The patients interviewed were of both sexes and of various ages and ethnic backgrounds. Yet in spite of these differences, all interviews employed the same information-gathering strategy and techniques.

THE DEFINITION OF THE SITUATION AND INTERVIEW STRATEGY

Guiding the interviewer's strategy are his assumptions about first encounters with psychiatric patients. For a new patient, he assumes, meeting with a psychiatrist is an extraordinary life event. It is a sign that life has been disrupted by trouble, trouble so serious that the patient or others believe themselves unable to deal with it unaided and have instead turned to a psychiatrist for help. Thus in the interviewer's understanding the very fact that a patient has appeared before him poses the question: what kind of trouble has brought this person here for help at this time? How the psychiatrist answers this question will largely determine his initial management and treatment and his justification of his actions to others: the patient, his family, and the professional colleagues to whom he is accountable.

To answer this question, the interviewer's basic strategy is to elicit stories about salient events in the patient's life. First he attempts to get the patient to recount the happenings which led to the present contact.[1] The story which he seeks will tell in psychiatrically relevant detail who did what to whom in what order, and how the patient was involved. It will be a story which the patient could properly end "and so I decided to come here for help", or "and so they decided to bring

177

R. A. Hahn and A. D. Gaines (eds.), Physicians of Western Medicine, 177–191.
© 1985 *by D. Reidel Publishing Company.*

me here for help". As the interviewer is eliciting the story of this event, he attempts to identify other events in the patient's life relevant to the present contact, and he attempts to get the patient to tell the stories of those events also.

INITIATING ELICITATION OF A STORY

By virtue of the culturally special character of a patient's contact with a psychiatrist, the story which recounts the happenings leading to the contact becomes a relevant topic for discussion immediately after the opening introductions of the interview. Most patients acknowledge the pertinence of the topic at this point, and regularly this is where the interviewer brings it up. To start discussion, he usually employs a stock phrase such as: "Can you tell me what happened that led to your being here today?" For such openings the interviewer prefers questions which steer the patient toward describing the happenings which led to contact, rather than phrases such as "Why are you here?" which suggest a request for an interpretation or justification of events.

Save for the happenings leading to contact, it is impossible to anticipate in advance of the interview what other life events may be relevant for the purposes of initial assessment. The interviewer must identify these other events during the interview itself from things mentioned in the patient's talk. Since a patient's references to other potentially significant life events are often made in passing, within talk about other matters, the interviewer must listen actively for them or they will slip by. Once such a reference occurs and is noticed, the event's being mentioned provides the interviewer with an opening, albeit a fleeting one, to initiate discussion about it. If it should seem advisable to discuss some other matter before dealing with it, the interviewer may flag it in his mind for bringing up later; otherwise he will initiate discussion on the event immediately. Whether initiation is delayed or not, the interviewer usually begins discussion by employing an utterance which has a standard form. It begins by indicating that he is quoting the patient, it then repeats or paraphrases the patient's mentioning of the event, and it ends by asking the patient for information.

Some Initiating Utterances

Framing Statement	Quotation	Request
A moment ago you said	[Repetition or paraphrase of	Tell me about that.
A little while ago you said	patient's words]	Can you tell me about
You said		that?

In this manner the interviewer extracts the mention of an event from its intended function in the patient's developing pattern of ideas and identifies it for special attention in its own right. He legitimizes his interest in the event by presenting it explicitly as something the *patient* brought up. By using the patient's own words, he prevents the patient from claiming confusion about what he wants to know. He wants to know just what the patient was referring to.

Just as the interviewer proceeds at the earliest possible relevant point to initiate discussion on the process leading to contact, in this way too he is able to initiate discussion of other potentially significant events in the patient's life which the patient had not necessarily intended to explore. In both cases, by suggesting topics the interviewer makes explicit his preference about what the patient will discuss.

LISTENING TO THE PATIENT'S STORY

As the patient tells his story, the interviewer must first of all fulfill the social obligation of an ordinary listener to reconstruct the narrator's intended meaning (Moerman and Sacks 1974; Garfinkel 1967; Schutz 1971). To accomplish this, the interviewer, like any listener, must conduct an extremely rapid analysis of the unfolding talk. Because such analysis is habitual, unreflective, and almost instantaneous, it yields an apparently spontaneous and definite perception of what a narrator means by his talk. What is thus perceived is the patient's version of the targeted event. This version is useful and informative, especially since it is possible to infer from it how the patient would prefer the interviewer to construe the happenings he is relating. However the interviewer also wishes to consider how certain of the other participants might construe those happenings, and he must ultimately arrive at a construction of his own. Therefore, as he listens to spontaneously offered stories, the interviewer must subject what he hears to an additional special kind of analysis in order to extract from it those points and possibilities which he can then use to suggest alternative constructions.

To begin with, as he listens, the interviewer must identify and deliberately bracket the story's point of view, its implicit moral and motivational judgments. Concurrently, he must identify and carefully notice whatever bare facts about the event it may contain (for instance, *who* was present, *what* happened, *when* it happened) while extricating those facts from the moral, motivational, and affective weighting assigned them by the patient narrator. The aim of his analysis is to suggest a number of alternative constructions and to open up the possibility of discovering information which discriminates between these alternative constructions.

NARRATIVE ORDER AND INQUIRY: ELICITING MORE INFORMATION ABOUT THE EVENT

To elicit more information about the targeted event, the interviewer usually begins by attempting to establish agreement with the patient about the event's time frame, e.g., in what year or month it occurred and from what day to what day. Two illustrations of this are given in Example 1 and Example 2. (The appendix contains the conventions used in the transcription of these and later examples.)

Example 1

I   /*Interviewer starts the first topic of the interview*/
      Uhm can you tell me how come you're in the hospital?
P   Well uhm (   ) I took an overdose of pills. I'm in for observation.
I   /*establishing time frame*/
      I see. Can you — can you — When was that?
P   The last time was the second of December.

Example 2

P /*Patient ends her initial story about being depressed and taking pills*/
I mm Tell me about that.
P Well what else do you want to know, Doctor?
/*establishing time frame*/
I How long have you been feeling that bad about things?

1.0

P Over the past several months
I Past several months
P mmhm
I So this is now:: the middle of October.
P Yeah right
   [
I   middle of September. Sometime in the summer?
P mmhm
   [
I   Like in August? How did it start?

By this process of establishing agreement about an event's gross time frame, the interviewer orients the patient's attention to the familiar idea that the targeted event in the patient's life followed an objective and definite course in time which anyone, properly situated, could have witnessed. With the patient thus oriented, the stage is set to introduce the format that will guide the subsequent inquiry.

The basic convention guiding the inquiry is that the happenings in the event under consideration should be discussed in order in which they occurred. This familiar rule, which eschews literary devices like flashbacks, shifts in consciousness and changes in narrative viewpoint, is the simplest possible way of aligning the sequence of discussion with the sequence of happenings. In the present context, this convention of simple narrative order is an extremely useful device for organizing and controlling the interviewer's inquiry.

First of all, the narrative format provides a familiar and clear definition of the situation. Rather than suggest, "I (the interviewer) am gathering information to make a judgment about your (the patient's) character", it projects a more neutral and simpler definition of the situation, namely "We are describing how a sequence of happenings took place in your life".

Second, the narrative format can be consistently maintanined while the interviewer pursues the description of any particular happening in the event in however much or little detail its significance warrants. It allows him to vary and control the level of detail in considering the current topic. How this can be done is examined below.

Third, the convention of narrative order allows recognition of "temporary digressions" in the flow of the narrative. The availability of this category of "digression" within the narrative format allows the interviewer to curtail or legitimize shifts off the main topic as proves useful to his inquiry. Thus, when the patient tries to shift the discussion away from the unfolding narrative, the interviewer can act to define the attempted shift as a digression and reinstitute the interrupted story. In this process he refers back to the happenings that had been mentioned before the digression, citing them one by one in narrative order. He then asks the patient to tell what happened next. For example:

Example 3

I /Interviewer is inquiring about the patient's recent history of seeing a therapist./
That=was when?
P That was right after the custody battle fell through, so that was last winter.
I Kay=
/Shift off narrative order/
P I have a– For some reason there's something abou:t September August
I him
P or September and October and November. Ya know right in that you know not necessarily Christmas time or holiday time
I mmhm
P but– Fall that I always, I donno I always get really really depressed really my husband even knew it.
I mmhm
P You know he knew that (.) I'd start talking about separating or: er: get really depressed you know in the Fall.
I mm
P And he'd say "Well next year we're gunna be prepared for it" Ya know and
I mm

4.0

P It's always been that way. I don't know
/summary, defining shift as a digression and reinstating narrative order/
I .hh But this time you:: after the custody thing – you went to see somebody at Michigan State=It didn't work out.
/continuing in narrative order/
P Right and I–
I and then you found somebody else?
P I waited for a while though.

Conversely, if the interviewer wishes to explore a point of background suggested by something the patient mentions, he can interrupt the narrative to conduct his background inquiry, framing the interruption as a "digression", after which he will reinstitute the main narrative. This process is illustrated in Example 4 and Example 7, below.

Example 4

I Your husband took your medicine away.
P Yeah
I T– Tell me about that.
/narrative starts/
P I had medicine to last me and I was tak'n it proper.
/digression starts/
I uhhuh Wha– what medicine was that?

P Breathine pills and Theolar pills.
I uhhuh and these were from doctor:::
P Arbertine
/summary reasserting narrative/
I Okay you were taking them the way::
P Right
   [
I   he prescribed them
P That's right.
   [
I   and you felt they were helping.
P They were.
I They were helping?
P They were.
/continuing in narrative order/
I Okay, then what happened?

Finally, the narrative format provides the interviewer with a legitimate and relevant next topic which is continually available for discussion. That is, under the narrative format, when a patient is speaking too long and unilluminatingly on an event, or when a patient resists talking further about it, or when the patient stops speaking and the interviewer has no need to inquire further about it, he can proceed to the next happening in the sequence by asking "Okay and then what happened?" The last turn of Example 4 and Example 5 illustrates this use of narrative order to define next topic.

Example 5

I Okay so you were on the— only two pills of Mellaril a night, slightly less than before, but you were doing all right.
P Right.
I Okay, then what happened?

In this way the interviewer can control the pacing of discussion and also establish the next topic.

Thus the narrative format allows the interviewer to maintain an easily understood definition of the situation, while being able at each point in the discussion to control the level of detail on a current topic and to exercise control over the content and level of detail of the next topic, whether it be a continuation of or a digression from the narrative line. Within this basic framework of topic control, the interviewer then regularly pursues detailed information about particular points using techniques concerned with time, magnitudes, and the interviewer's comprehension.

First, the idea of describing a sequence of happenings assumes that the event being considered will have a certain scale or duration in time, but it is indefinite about what that time scale is. Thus when patients are too brief or telescopic in describing a happening of significance, the interviewer can manipulate the ambiguity about the relevant time-scale by shifting the discussion to a description in smaller temporal units. We call this method "slowing down time" because it allows the interviewer to slow down the discussion so that the patient provides more detail. It is one way that the narrative format can be used to expand detail on particular points. For example, a happening described briefly, "So then I went into the bedroom and took the pills", may be investigated by inquiring in sequence about its more microscopic temporal phases, i.e., by asking about the decision to take the pills, their acquisition, the preparation for their ingestion, and the events between their ingestion and the arrival of some help. Also, the general idea of describing a sequence of happenings presupposes that the description will consider relevant *contiguous* happenings one after another. Thus when the interviewer finds that the patient skips ahead and leaves a significant gap in his story, he can make further inquiries to fill the gap about what happened. Filling in gaps is another way of implementing the control which the narrative format allows over next topic. Example 6 is an example of this process:

Example 6

I   Okay there was a scene with your husband where:: he didn't want you to take the pills.
P   Right.

.

.

/Discussion of scene/

.

.

I   What happened to the pills in the course of that?
P   He threw them away and the rest took with him to the hospital.
/filling in gap/
I   hm— how did you end up going to the hospital. I see a fight, but then what led to your going to the hospital?

Both the methods of slowing down time and filling in gaps regularly uncover highly revealing facts about a targeted event. For instance, in the example just cited (Example 6), filling in the gap between throwing away the pills and going to the hospital uncovered a suicide attempt by wrist-slashing which the patient had concealed from a previous interviewer.

To elicit more detailed information from the patient, the interviewer also regularly inquires about specific frequencies and numerical quantities since words like "often", "many", and "few" are usually uninformative and often misleading about order of magnitude. This type of quantitative inquiry can be handled consistently within the narrative format either as an expansion of particular narrated happenings or as a digression from the story line. Usually the interviewer starts out by asking the patient for precise quantities, for example, "How much money did you spend?", "How many times did that happen?", "How many pills did you take?" A patient's evasiveness or inability to answer is usually followed by his asking for an approximation. When the patient claims to be unable to specify a frequency, quantity, or extent, the interviewer may offer rough parameters to prompt an answer: "Was it closer to $2000 or $50 000?", "Was that in the winter or the summer?" In this case the interviewer notes to himself that the patient's response may have been influenced by his suggestion, and he therefore weights it accordingly. Example 7 illustrates the sequence of starting with a specific quantitative inquiry, encountering evasiveness or inability to reply, and offering approximations to prompt an answer. In this example, the inquiry for temporal information was handled as a digression within the narrative line, following techniques already described (i.e., first pursuing and completing the digression, next reasserting the narrative process by summarizing the happenings that were under discussion before the digression, and then continuing with discussion of the next happening in the sequence after the summary).

Example 7

I Okay then what happened?
P And uuh (   ) Well he dropped me because (   ) he would no longer take Medicaid.
  .
  .
  .

/narrative continuing/
P And then I went back to St. John's.
   /Patient describes medication given by new doctors at St. John's./
/digression to determine date/
I Okay when was the change?

2.5

P Quite a while ago
I Okay we started in August
P Yeah
I and: this is October. So that would have been 4 weeks ago, or 6 weeks ago, or longer than that?
P Longer than that.
I Longer than that. Before Labor Day?
P Yeah
/summary, reasserting narrative/
I Okay so you were on the two pills of Mellaril a night, slightly less medicine but you were doing all right.
P Right.
/continuing in narrative order/
I So then what happened?

Often the effort at quantification uncovers surprising new facts which may suggest an interpretation of an event very different from that implicit in the patient's original story.

   In addition to being excessively compressed and abbreviated, having important gaps, and lacking crucial quantitative information, patients' narratives are often confusing because of their contradictory, diffuse, and fragmentary character. To resolve such confusion and to elicit more detail about a happening, the interviewer uses a technique which is based upon a listener's obligation to display understanding (Moerman and Sacks 1974) and a listener's right to initiate repair when understanding is not achieved (Schegloff et al. 1977). This technique consists of displaying his puzzlement. The interviewer defines himself as someone who is trying earnestly to understand the patient's story but is puzzled by certain confusing points and needs the patient's help. Sometimes the interviewer begins with a statement that indicates confusion and then follows with a request for clarification. The last turn of Example 8 illustrates this maneuver:

Example 8

I Tell me about that.
P Well there wasn't much I could do. When I went to the hospital he just took all my pills with him.
I When you went to the hospital
P Yeah
I When was that?
P When I went to umm (   ) here or Jones Hospital.
/expressing puzzlement/
I Okay I'm a little confused. Uh whe– when you went here or Jones Hospital for what?

Sometimes, the interviewer's expression of puzzlement is embedded within a request for clarification:

I But why did they bring you here rather than to the police station?

Often a "puzzled tone of voice" (which includes voice hitches and false starts) and bodily behaviors that express puzzlement are used to further convey the message, "I'm confused; help me understand". Such work to clarify confusion can readily be incorporated into the ongoing interview as an expansion within the unfolding narrative.

As this process unfolds, the search for the information needed to construct an adequate account is not always an easy one for the interviewer or the patient. Puzzlement and earnest request for clarification may not resolve doubts about what happened at any given point. Requests for specific quantitative information may meet with evasion or statements that the patient really doesn't know. Slowing down time may only reveal that the patient has forgotten the actual course of happenings in the interactive scene. Request for more detail about an episode may prompt the patient to wander off evasively on a topic only tangentially relevant. To a greater or lesser extent the interviewer will encounter difficulty or resistance in building the account.

As a general rule, he does not stop his inquiry when he meets initial resistance, but rather persists. As noted above, when a patient is unable to give precise quantitative information in response to a first query, the interviewer persists by asking for an approximation. Similarly, when a patient does not answer an initial request for more detail on an event, the interviewer regularly reformulates the question and asks it again. When a patient denies having access to requested information using a formulation which suggests that he has at least partial access to it, e.g., "I don't remember much about it", or "There isn't much to tell", the interviewer typically says, "Tell me the part that you do remember".

Ultimately the decision about whether to end or persist in pursuing the story of an event involves a complex judgment by the interviewer based on such factors as his assessment of the medical/psychiatric adequacy of the information already obtained, his relationship to the patient, and time constraints. After the interviewer has decided he wants to end the story, he sometimes actively closes off the inquiry by offering an ending summary and initiating a new topic. Sometimes he simply allows what could have been treated as a topical digression to develop into a new topic. Sometimes, if the patient wishes to speak further, he is allowed to do so, but only briefly, with the interviewer responding minimally.

In summary, once the interviewer has identified a significant event in the patient's life, has initiated its exploration at a time and in a manner acceptable to the patient and has listened carefully and critically to the patient's initial narrative response, his inquiry regularly involves a more or less extended process of eliciting clearer and more detailed facts from the patient about the targeted life event. This process of inquiry is organized by a narrative format which the interviewer institutes first by obtaining agreement with the patient about the event's gross time frame (thereby orienting the patient to consider the event as an objective sequence of happenings through time) and by various behaviors which communicate to the patient "We will be discussing the various parts of this sequence in the order in which they occurred". Adopting this narrative format enables the interviewer to maintain a consistent and relatively neutral definition of the situation of inquiry (i.e., we are *describing, not evaluating* a sequence of happenings in your life) while simultaneously being able to control the development of the topic in ways which enable him to elicit needed information from the patient. In order to elicit specific and detailed information within this narrative framework he displays puzzlement, inquires about the frequencies and numerical magnitudes of important points, and, by manipulating the idea of sequential time, slows time and fills in gaps. He persists in this inquiry, despite resistance, until the results obtained, and/or his relationship with the patient, and/or practical constraints indicate it is appropriate to end.

THE RESULTS OF THE INQUIRY: PROCESSING AND ASSESSMENT

As the process of inquiry proceeds, structured by the narrative format, the interviewer gathers a great deal of new information about the targeted event. As information accumulates, the interviewer coordinates the various facts uncovered. Because happenings are elicited sequentially, and because the interviewer inquires about specific dates, most of the facts are naturally coordinated by temporal relations. However, the investigator will sometimes encounter new facts which do not have a clear location within the gestalt of temporal relations, and when he thinks it may be revealing he checks with the patient about their temporal location with respect to the others:

I   Oh, so it was after you cut your wrist that your husband found you and called the police to take you to the hospital?

Also, as the account is being constructed, the investigator will sometimes remember items which the patient had mentioned in an earlier context which seem to fit into the current story. When such items are potentially significant, he inquires about their temporal locations also:

I   Oh, was that when you went to visit your brother?

Intermittently, as the process of inquiry proceeds, the interviewer also formulates his construction of parts of the story and expresses it in summary form for the patient to confirm or correct.

As the complex of temporally coordinated and collaboratively checked facts accumulates, the interviewer is increasingly able to assess the quality of the information offered. His knowledge about temporal relations between the facts allows him to identify significant omissions which he would have been incapable of imagining given only the patient's initial, highly selective, and often distorted narrative. Information about sequencing allows him to assess consistency, since the earlier parts of a process must have an intelligible connection with the later ones. Increase in the detail of description allows the interviewer to see how patient explanations offered earlier accounted selectively for some facts but not others and contained subtle justifications which distorted aspects of the event which were uncomfortable to consider or reveal.

Several kinds of results regularly follow from such a process. As the gestalt of facts in a story expands, becoming more structured and coherent, it becomes harder and harder for a patient who is reluctant to tell about some key feature of a sequence not to mention it, and it becomes harder and harder not to express its felt personal significance. Often as an account is being developed, there comes a point when a patient reveals facts about the genesis of current problems which he or she finds painful, shameful, or threatening, but which contribute significant understanding. Even if such revelations are not made, the rich gestalt of information, whose consistency and reliability can be at least partially assessed, increasingly enables the interviewer to free himself from dependence on the patient's judgment and interpretation of the situation and to arrive at an interpretation of his own. When even this proves impossible, and the interviewer is unable to achieve a clear image of what happened, the process of attempting and failing defines the extent of his ignorance about the problem. In a psychiatric context, the reason the attempt fails is itself always a key datum.

MANAGING THE INTERROGATION FORMAT

In general, the type of process we have described rarely occurs in ordinary conversation. Though justified by the need to make proper medical decisions on the patient's behalf, the interviewer's methodical search for information contains a great many features which have the potential to offend. At the outset, when a topic is plucked out of a patient's developing line of talk to be expanded in detail he had not anticipated, there is the danger that the process will seem to be interruptive. Through repeatedly expressing uncertainty and incomprehension, there is the danger that the interviewer will seem to be accusing the patient of being dishonest, implying, "I don't believe what you've said". By attempting to elicit highly specific details, the interviewer may exceed the limits of the patient's memory or narrative ability, and his inability to provide requested detail may be construed by the patient as a failure or as evidence of his mental incompetence. By probing methodically for what actually happened, the interviewer is likely to touch on happenings whose recollection causes the patient shame, pain, or humiliation. By persisting in seeking certain information in the face of patient resistance and failing to get it, the interviewer may create a situation which appears to define the patient as deliberately resisting his will, thus transforming the definition of their situation into one of conflict.

Thus, though the process of eliciting a story helps achieve the interviewer's basic goal of accumulating the reliable facts needed to make pressing medical decisions, it raises serious interactional dangers of its own since it violates ordinary conventions of politeness and respect for the patient's self. Therefore, another component of the interviewer's style is a series of techniques which he employs to manage the interpersonal dangers which are implicit in this method of inquiry.

First of all, the interviewer is always careful to be courteous. He consciously uses polite forms of address and reference to mitigate the implications of differential power and control. Especially when he persists in inquiring into matters the patient does not want to discuss and would ordinarily not mention, he maintains a polite tone of voice. This tone is respectful and assuaging; it functions to make the process of control less noticeable and less objectionable.

Second, as each story is being developed, the interviewer shows empathic recognition of the distress or anguish which is implicit but not overtly expressed in what the patient is describing. Most patients clearly appreciate an interviewer's recognition of their pain.

Third, the interviewer rarely explicitly confronts, even when the patient is patently evasive, contradictory, or deceptive. Rather, as a motive for his persistence and probing inquiry the interviewer emphasizes his sincere and legitimate desire to understand. Through his behavior he tries to show the patient that he is working hard to understand but is not concerned to judge.

Fourth, the interviewer attempts to avoid defining the patient as incompetent in the work of the interview or resistant to the interviewer's will. Regularly, when the patient stumbles or resists in dealing with an inquiry, the interviewer helps in answering the question, perhaps offering an approximation as an answer. Never is inquiry on a point allowed to end on a note of failure.

Fifth, after every interviewer-initiated inquiry, the interviewer regularly returns to the line of exposition the patient had been engaged in and returns the floor to him so that he can take up where he left off. By connecting with the original intentions of the patient, and by giving the patient the floor to pursue those intentions, the interviewer defines the work of eliciting a story as being a detour or interlude only, after which the patient can complete the expression of his thoughts.

Methods such as these help contain the dangers and mitigate the offenses to ordinary conventions of talking that are implicit in the interview process. Such methods regularly allow the interviewer to avoid overt conflict and bring the process to a satisfactory completion from the technical standpoint of collecting information that is useful, even crucial in making medical decisions on the patient's behalf. These same techniques also make it possible for the interviewer to bring the process to what could be called a satisfactory ritual conclusion, in which respect for the patient's person as well as his medical needs is achieved. In our experience patients who are dependent upon an interviewer's accurate assessment of their situations do not respond unfavorably to being interrogated gently. Rather it is more frequent for them to express feelings of relief when a fuller story has been disclosed and intently heard.

CONCLUSION

This paper has not described many aspects of the interview process, such as the role expectations of psychiatrist and patient, the interviewer's diagnostic knowledge, or his observations on and inquiries about a patient's mental status. Nor, except briefly, has it analyzed the interviewer's specialized way of listening to the patient's talk, a process which has important analogues in other types of professional listening (e.g., Hahn this volume; Spence 1982). Rather, our attention has focused on the publicly observable process of face-to-face interaction in the interview, our purpose being to describe the regular methods of interaction the interviewer uses to pursue his inquiry.

What the interviewer does is to elicit stories from patients about specific events in their lives (especially the sequence of happenings which explain how the patient came into contact with a psychiatrist). The main rule he applies in doing this is that happenings within an event should be described and discussed in the order in which they occurred. Literary and linguistic studies have demonstrated that this rule of narrative order is a basic convention by which individuals construct stories (e.g., Labov and Waletzky 1967; Labov and Fanshel 1977). However, it is not usually recognized that the rule also functions as an important device for organizing social interaction. The way in which topics are organized is a case in point. In improvised verbal interaction such as conversation or psychiatric interviewing, what happens next is not prearranged but decided by the speakers as their talk unfolds (Sacks et al. 1974); at each point, the fate of the current topic is always uncertain. Whatever his intentions might be, the current speaker can never guarantee that his present topic will be pursued by the next speaker; nor, if it is pursued can he be assured of the direction in which it gets developed. Nevertheless an experienced psychiatric interviewer is able to keep a patient's discussion on a single coherently developing topic by using the convention of narrative order. The result of using the convention to organize the unfolding conversational topic is to produce an extended sequence of talk which forms a unified whole, an account of some events progressing from their start to their finish in a patient's life. In related ways, we believe, the principle of narrative order is used to organize topical coherence in many other kinds of collaboratively constructed narratives.

In brief psychiatric evaluation, the task of relating a narrative of personal experience is sufficiently familiar for most patients to be able to perform successfully, even when troubled or distraught. Moreover the process of eliciting a story is such that the interviewer can overcome a patient's possible unwillingness to tell it (due to suspicion, shame, or pain) by defining the process in a non-threatening way as an effort to understand events, not to judge the patient, and by maintaining in all circumstances a respectful, non-antagonistic attitude toward what the patient says.

This process allows the interviewer to encourage a patient to volunteer information and express his personal perceptions. Only by giving a patient freedom to express himself in this way will certain highly relevant types of information come to light. On the other hand, the process of eliciting stories also allows the interviewer control over what a patient says. The interviewer can manage the story-telling process to curtail digressions in a patient's talk; he can also use it to guide a patient's discussion onto points which the patient, being a layman, might not realize are psychiatrically relevant; and most importantly, the process enables the interviewer to direct a patient to talk about unhappy aspects of current troubles which he might otherwise avoid. Thus, the process of eliciting patient stories allows the interviewer to strike a balance between allowing a patient freedom of expression and controlling what a patient says. It enables him to be both non-directive and directive, now encouraging the patient's free expression, now curtailing, guiding, or directing it as he deems necessary in pursuing information relevant to formulating his plan for professional action.

APPENDIX

Special Transcript Conventions [a]	
pauses, in seconds	1.0, 0.5, etc.
micropause (a small "beat" of silence)	(.)
inspiration	.hh
overlapping talk by two or more speakers	[ ]
contiguous words or utterances, without pause or gap	=
elongated sounds	:
truncated or cut off word	—
encloses inaudible or barely audible words	( )

[a] From Sacks et al. (1974).

ACKNOWLEDGEMENTS

Much of the research on which this paper is based was performed in the Michigan State University Interaction Analysis Laboratory. Thanks should go to Drs. Fredrick Erickson, Robert Hahn, and Brigitte Jordan for helpful comments on an earlier draft.

NOTES

1. In ordinary discourse, the terms "event" and "happening" have many meanings, some of which overlap. However, for the purpose of this essay we need to distinguish between the topic of a story, which we will call an "event", and the briefer occurrences which comprise the components of such stories, which we will call "happenings". Though the issue is philosophically and semantically complex, perhaps an example will make our usage clear: how it came about that patient X tried to hang himself can be considered the story of an "event". In the context of that "event", receiving the letter of rejection and purchasing a rope can be considered as "happenings". Which items of patient history are treated as "events" (and expanded by an examination of their constituent "happenings") is negotiated between the interviewer and the patient.

REFERENCES

Garfinkel, Harold
   1967 Studies of the Routine Grounds of Everyday Activities, and Commonsense Knowledge of Social Structures. *In* Harold Garfinkel, Studies in Ethnomethodology. Englewood Cliffs, New Jersey: Prentice-Hall.
Labov, William and David Fanshel
   1977 Therapeutic Discourse: Psychotherapy as Conversation. New York: Academic Press.
Labov, William and Joshua Waletzky
   1967 Narrative Analysis: Oral Versions of Personal Experience. *In* June Helm (ed.), Essays on the Verbal and Visual Arts. Proceedings of the 1966 Annual Spring Meeting of the American Ethnological Society. Seattle: University of Washington Press.
Moerman, Michael and Harvey Sacks
   1974 On Understanding in Conversation. *In* Festschrift for E. Voeglin. The Hague: Mouton.
Sacks, Harvey and Emanuel Schegloff, and Gail Jefferson
   1974 A Simplest Systematics for the Organization of Turn Taking for Conversation. Language 50(4):696–735.
Schegloff, Emanuel, Gail Jefferson, and Harvey Sacks
   1977 The Preference for Self-Correction in the Organization of Repair in Conversation. Language 53(2):361–382.
Schutz, Alfred
   1971 On Multiple Realities. *In* Maurice Natanson (ed.), Collected Papers I: The Problem of Social Reality. The Hague: Martinus Nijhoff.
Spence, Donald P.
   1982 Narrative Truth and Historical Truth: Meaning and Interpretation in Psychoanalysis. New York: W. W. Norton and Co.
Turner, Roy
   1972 Some Formal Properties of Therapy Talk. *In* David Sudnow (ed.), Studies in Social Interaction. New York: The Free Press.

BYRON J. GOOD, HENRY HERRERA, MARY-JO DELVECCHIO GOOD
AND JAMES COOPER

REFLEXIVITY, COUNTERTRANSFERENCE AND CLINICAL ETHNOGRAPHY: A CASE FROM A PSYCHIATRIC CULTURAL CONSULTATION CLINIC

INTRODUCTION

This paper is an exploration of the meaning of "interpretation" as an analytic concept in clinical ethnography. The practical engagement of anthropologists in clinical activities and the "interpretive turn" (Rabinow and Sullivan 1979) of anthropological theorizing during the past decade provide important new grounds for conceptual exchange among anthropologists and psychiatrists. Psychological theory, especially its psychoanalytic school, has long recognized the centrality of interpretation, the importance of studying the relation between public symbols, discourse, and personal meanings, and the theoretical and clinical importance of investigating the "objectivity" of the analyst or observer in clinical encounters. As anthropologists turn new attention to the interpretive process and to the influence of the investigator's own perspective and interests on the encounter with persons of other cultures — the role of "reflexivity" in ethnography (Jules-Rosette 1978c) — and as they begin the ethnographic study of clinical phenomena, issues long contemplated by psychiatrists take on a new relevance. Anthropologists may find theories of transference and countertransference of particular interest. In turn, *clinical ethnography* undertaken from a meaning-centered or interpretive point of view (Good and Good 1980), provides a new opportunity for a critical assessment of certain psychoanalytic theories from an anthropological perspective. This paper is conceived as a contribution to this process.

Hermeneutic, interpretive analysis in anthropology is based on the assumption that social action is analogous to a text (Ricoeur 1979) and that participants in social action and their ethnographic observers both engage in a process analogous to the interpretation and criticism of texts (Rabinow and Sullivan 1979; Agar 1980; Geertz 1973). It is our belief that all clinical practice has a core interpretive or hermeneutic dimension, and that attention to interpretive processes should be central to clinical ethnography. Interpretation is particularly explicit and pervasive in psychiatry. Since Freud's exploration of the "talking cure", interpretation has had an honored place within psychiatric theory and practice. A competent psychotherapist is one who is able to make powerful and timely interpretations, enabling patients to tell their stories and understand themselves with increasing depth and insight. Psychiatric practice thus provides an unusually rich setting for exploring the cultural, symbolic, and discursive elements that constitute the clinical enterprise.

Data for our analysis are drawn from research conducted by the authors in a Psychiatric Cultural Consultation Clinic. This clinic was developed to provide culturally appropriate psychiatric consultation and brief therapy, and to study the

R. A. Hahn and A. D. Gaines (eds.), Physicians of Western Medicine, 193–221.

process of interpretation among clinicians, patients and observers having very diverse cultural and theoretical perspectives. The "case" analyzed in this paper is drawn from our experience in this Clinic.

Focusing attention on the interpretive dimension of psychiatric practice, particularly of a practice designed to highlight contrasting frames of reference, has a dizzying effect. As Agar (1980: 262) notes, "The primary objective of interpretation for an ethnographer is a group of subjects who themselves interpret". Unless care is taken, the enterprise can lose all clarity. In our view, a hermeneutic analysis of clinical phenomena should distinguish three facets of interpretation: (1) the interpretation by patient and clinician of the discourse of the other in terms of their own conceptual models; (2) the interpretation by patient and clinician of a given theoretical or cultural model in terms of their own life histories and personal meaning systems; and (3) the interpretation by the ethnographer of the discourse of patient and clinician. Failure to distinguish between these aspects of interpretation has often resulted in confusion in the literature on hermeneutic analysis in anthropology. Recognition of these distinctions may clarify the relationship of anthropological to psychological theory. Before we proceed to an analysis of our experience in the Cultural Consultation Clinic, a few words about each of these three aspects of interpretation in clinical ethnography are appropriate.

First, recent anthropological theory has conceived clinical discourse as transactions across diverse explanatory models or conceptual systems (e.g., Kleinman 1980). All persons use cultural models, whether scientific or popular, to interpret particular phenomena to construct disease, illness, and other realities. For example, physicians use clinical paradigms to guide their investigation of a patient's condition, beginning with complaints and symptoms, and interpreting them as the result of an underlying pathology (Good and Good 1980:177–181). While the investigation in Biomedicine is increasingly technological, the interpretive processes used by physicians are similar to others studied by social scientists. Physicians use symbolic models in an attempt "to bring to light an underlying coherence or sense" (Taylor 1979:25) that accounts for the patient's complaints and disparate clinical findings, to negotiate a "clinical reality" with physician colleagues, consultants and medical staff (Kleinman 1980), and to communicate or negotiate an understanding of the underlying problem with patients and their families. Analysis thus focuses on the interpretation by clinician and patient of the text or discourse of the other in terms of their own models. Research attends to the differences among clinical or explanatory models (Osmond and Siegler 1974), to the ways in which such models are used in diagnosis and in the construction of illness realities (Kleinman 1980; Good and Good 1980), and to the process of negotiation between client and clinician (Scheff 1968; Katon and Kleinman 1981).

Second, a hermeneutic analysis of clinical phenomena focuses attention on the role of deeply embedded personal texts in the interpretive process. Interpretation is not limited to the cognitive manipulation of clinical models. Many of the symbols, models and images of an individual's therapeutic discourse have unexamined personal meanings and are associated with powerful affects. Clinical or explanatory models that appear to be the same may be linked to quite different contexts of personal significance for different therapists or patients, leading to great differences in the interpretations made with them. One of the finest recent discussions of the relation between public discourse and personal meaning is Obeyesekere's analysis of "the personal meaning of public symbols" — the personal and cultural associations clustering around shared public symbols — and "personal symbols" — "cultural symbols whose primary significance and meaning lie in the personal life and experience of individuals" — of Sinhalese Buddhist ascetics (Obeyesekere 1981). The issue of public and private meaning is equally important in the study of Western medicine. Particular symbols in professional medical discourse have personal meanings quite specific to individual physicians (see M. Good's analysis of the symbol "competence" in medical discourse, in this volume). Not only particular symbols, however, but individuals' whole systems of therapeutic practice are invested with personal meaning and thus are woven into life histories and/or used to resolve personal conflicts in diverse ways (see Day and Davidson 1976). The role of public symbols in carrying personal meanings and affects has, of course, been the subject of extensive psychological theorizing. In particular, theories of transference have been developed to account for the interpretation of the discourse of other persons in terms of one's own hidden personal meanings, the transferring of the intensity of an unconscious idea to a conscious one, and the distortion in the interpretation that results. The psychiatric literature thus has special relevance for analysis of the personal significance of public symbols in therapeutic discourse.

Third, an interpretive clinical ethnography should incorporate an analysis of the encounter of the observer with the "data" and the influence of his/her own experience on the interpretations made. While lip service is often paid to this injunction, only rarely is it made a serious part of the analysis (e.g., see Rabinow 1977; Crapanzano 1980). Critical theory is increasingly calling into question the nature of the "objectivity" of the observer, and making clear the importance of the analysis of the ethnographic encounter with those studied, the role of personal reactions in the evaluation, and the translation of this personal knowledge into theoretical discourse (e.g., Fabian 1971; Jules-Rosette 1978a, 1978b). Very similar issues have been analyzed in the psychoanalytic literature on countertransference. The nature of the objectivity of the analyst, the experience of the analyst in the encounter with the client, and the role of the therapist's reaction to the client in the interpretations made have been central issues in this literature, as they have been in anthropological theorizing on reflexivity. We believe these issues provide fruitful grounds for exchange between symbolic analysis and psychiatric theory. They also represent issues we discovered to be very real in our work together in the case describe below.

Since we will be referring to "countertransference" and the relation of this concept to "reflexivity" throughout the paper, it is necessary to clarify our use of the term. Briefly, an ongoing debate in psychiatry and psychoanalytic thinking concerns the scope of the therapist's reactions to the patient, to which the term "countertransference" should apply. Kernberg (1975) has reviewed two major theoretical positions, which he terms "classical" and "totalistic". In the classical position, as proposed originally by Freud (1910), countertransference is the unconscious reaction of the analyst to the patient's transference; that is, it is the delimited part of the analyst's total reactions to patients that is unconscious, repressed (Little 1960), and evoked by the displacement of the patient's affects, fantasies and behaviors, experienced in early relationships (primarily parental), onto the analyst or therapist (Meissner and Nicholi 1978). With this original meaning, countertransference reactions are viewed as essentially negative, endangering the interpretive process (Little 1951) and thus, by definition, pathological (Langs 1981).

An alternative position, termed "totalistic" by Kernberg, includes within the definition of countertransference the therapist's total emotional reactions to the patient, including both conscious and unconscious reactions, not just those evoked by the transference. The totalistic definition has been criticized for so broadening the concept as to eliminate its usefulness. Chediak (1979), for example, suggests distinguishing a variety of "counter-reactions", but preserving the classical meaning of countertransference. The totalistic definition has also been criticized for its emphasis on the therapist's emotional response to the client, with the implied shift away from technical neutrality (Reich 1960). It supporters have used the redefinition to legitimize a broadened understanding of the relationship that develops in the psychotherapeutic encounter (McLaughlin 1981; Searles 1978). Kernberg (1975: 52) defends the broader definition for its understanding of psychotherapy as an interaction process "in which past and present of both participants, as well as their mutual reactions to their past and present, fuse into a unique emotional position involving both of them".

It is not our intention to enter into the debate about how the term countertransference should be used in the psychoanalytic literature. For the purposes of this chapter, the term will be used in a totalistic sense, because we believe this meaning supports analysis of a more complete range of the interpretive phenomena that are part of the clinical encounter. We came to our analysis of countertransference not primarily from an interest in its theory, but in an effort to understand a clinical encounter in which we were involved. Our subsequent theoretical analysis, however, has led us to believe that transference and countertransference are particularly important subtypes of a more general cultural phenomenon confronting all ethnographers: the groundedness of individuals' interpretations of reality and their encounters with others in multi-layered personal webs of meaning (see Gaines 1982). Symbolic analyses, while focusing on these phenomena, have often failed to attend to the profound affective dimensions of this process, to what Devereux (1967) called the ethnographer's "personal involvement with the material". Our work together in the case we describe below convinced us of the complexity of the frames of meaning we ethnographers bring to our material and the influence of these on our interpretations of the clinical phenomena we observe.

THE CULTURAL CONSULTATION CLINIC

In the fall of 1980 a Cultural Consultation Clinic was established as a subunit of the Consultation-Liaison Service of the Department of Psychiatry at the University of California, Davis.[1] This clinic brought together the four authors of this paper — a psychiatrist (HH), an anthropologist (BG), a sociologist (M-JG) and a clinical psychologist (JC)[2] — and three spiritualist healers (a Mexican-American woman, a Black minister and a Puerto Rican woman), one or more of whom were invited to see each patient with the psychiatrist and social scientists. The Clinic was designed to provide "cultural consultations" for a small number of patients on a trial basis; that is, to conduct culturally appropriate psychiatric consultation and brief therapy and to explore cultural dimensions of the patients' problems. Its goal was to facilitate the work of patients with their own therapists or provide assessments and treatment recommendations to the referring physicians. It was the working assumption of the clinic, based on our confidence in the therapeutic skills of the healers, that they would be particularly valuable consultants in working with many Mexican-American patients, especially those whose first language is Spanish. It was our intention to explore the network of meanings associated with the patients' problems, and to formulate a culturally-relevant psychiatric interpretation.

We consider this paper an experiment in the ethnography of American medical practice because of the unusual nature of the clinic and the definition of the roles of clinician and ethnographer in the clinic. While the psychiatrist and the healers were the primary therapists in the clinic, it was an underlying assumption that the social scientists' interpretations of the patients' conditions were not to be considered merely ethnographic observations, but rather were a central component of the therapeutic work. The ethnographers collaborated in the clinical work, while the psychiatrist, a Chicano, participated as clinician, informant, and ethnographer.

We also consider this paper experimental because of our effort to incorporate into our analysis an exploration of personal issues that emerged in our work together. This focus on reflexivity is not gratuitous, but resulted from our effort to understand a "conflict of interpretation", to borrow a phrase from Paul Ricoeur (1974), that developed among the members of the clinic while we were treating a Mexican-American patient. Our attempts to work through this conflict, while we were preparing to write this paper, forced us to deal with the personal sources of our varied interpretations. At a practical level, this experience convinced us of the complexity of the tacit understandings that influence interpretations and negotiations of clinical realities. At a theoretical level, it suggested that to sustain a hermeneutic analysis of clinical work, we would have to develop an account of countertransference in terms of interpretation theory.

From the outset, at the clinic, it was clear that the consultants brought different epistemological models to the notion of consultation. The social scientists' methodology and skills consisted primarily in the subtleties of interviewing and observations of interactive processes. In contrast, the healers placed less emphasis on formal interviewing and on social and psychodynamic reasoning. They held that their level of understanding derived from intimate knowledge of a spiritual reality, one which by definition was not open to examination by means of verbal discourse.

The communication of formulations among the consultants gave rise to frustrations that required a great deal of mutual respect in order to maintain a constructive atmosphere. In this setting, the multidisciplinary team confronted core problems associated with group and individual affective reactions, formulations of pathology, the communication of those formulations and the exercise of authority. While these have been identified as central tasks of all psychiatric treatment teams (Harty 1979), they became especially salient in a deliberately diverse cultural and clinical atmosphere.

THE CASE

The following case derives from the Cultural Consultation Clinic. It is a case which is central to our understanding of clinical discourse for several reasons. The patient, Mrs. *V*, is a Mexican-American woman with a complicated personal and psychiatric history. Over a number of months our work with her provided an important opportunity to observe and participate in the construction of clinical realities from a number of perspectives. While the two spiritualist healers and the psychiatrist worked with differing models to construct their view of the patient's illness reality, a strong consensus grew early in the treatment that the same basic reality had been discovered from the different perspectives. Late in the treatment, however, a "conflict in interpretation" arose that challenged the certainty of that consensus, and led to our exploration of the interpretive process.

The Healers

The two spiritualist healers who participated in the treatment of the patient were Mrs. Mendez, a Mexican-American spiritualist healer, and Reverend Leonard, a Black minister of a spiritualist church. (Pseudonyms are used throughout to identify the two healers.) Mrs. Mendez, 62 years old, practices healing in the Mexican-American spiritualist tradition described by Macklin (1974) and Trotter and Chavira (1980). She was born in Wyoming of working-class Mexican parents and spent most of her adult life in the Central Valley of California. She was divorced and was remarried to a Mexican-American who is supportive of her work, and has two adult children from her first marriage. She has been active in a variety of important county and state health care agencies, most often as a volunteer appointee, although she was employed as a nurse's aid in a community hospital for six years while in her forties. Mrs. Mendez describes her life as difficult and sad, and she associates the emergence of her healing powers with her life struggles. In her earliest conversation with the sociologist (MJG), she remarked that she was "born with the gift of healing", and that each aspect of her life was like "a new chapter unfolding" her additional capacities for healing.

Mrs. Mendez traces her active involvement as a healer to her search for strength following a serious illness, which she describes as "cancer of the tonsil". She relates how following her illness and subsequent cobalt treatments ". . . my spirit had been broken . . . . I had become . . . this wilted, lonely person . . . . I turned to my Mexican ancestry to study what these people did for themselves in time of distress". Mrs. Mendez made several trips to Mexico and subsequently sought out a Mexican *curandera* who lived in her California town.

The *curandera* "developed" Mrs. Mendez's healing powers through an intensive apprenticeship. Mrs. Mendez heals by giving energy or "spiritual medicine" to clients through her hands and eyes, by ritual cleansing (sweeping the client's body with her hands from top to toe), by utilizing herbal remedies, candles, and incense, and occasionally by extracting malevolent spirits from clients who have been possessed. She accomplishes this by "passing" them through her own body. She also "sees" the cause of clients' illnesses and distress in dreams and visions. The content of these diagnostic dreams were frequently relayed to the researchers in lengthy telephone conversations. Mrs. Mendez has "a protector", "a spirit guide", who heals through her and protects her from the "negativity" and the evil spirits which may possess her clients. Her guide, "a seventeenth century hospital administrator from Mexico", came to her during her development under the apprenticeship of the *curandera*.

Mrs. Mendez sees her unique calling to be the taking of "the message" into professional medical settings. As she noted to the researchers, "When the fluid of the Holy Ghost called me, he said, 'Woman, you are going to be the spiritual dirigible; you will be floating, you will be opening ways; I will give you the spiritual hammer to knock on hard hearts, to open the minds of the professionals' ".

Reverend Leonard is a single, 42-year-old minister of a spiritualist church. He has recently taken the title of "Metaphysician" and conducts healing services several times a week at his non-denominational church. He regularly sees clients at his home in a special consultation room, which is adorned with statues of St. Martin, Jesus and the Virgin Mary. His clientèle is multiethnic: Black, Anglo and Hispanic. The problems for which they seek help range from physical disorders to serious mental illness to affairs of the heart.

Reverend Leonard was "called to 'the work' " in a dramatic and frightening experience of visions at the age of 24, when he was on the streets of Oakland "smoking weed and having a very good time". At first, he said, "I thought I was losing my mind". He came to realize the meaning of the visions, however, and "from that day forth I have been totally involved in 'the work' ". He returned to the Central Valley, transformed his life-style and became a minister. Reverend Leonard acknowledges that his principal gift is that of "prophecy", the ability to "read a person's past, present, and future"; he also claims the ability to see into a person's body, to diagnose disorders, and to heal through the use of herbs, candles, incense, and the channeling of healing energy into the client. He is a skilled counselor who utilizes a pastoral style.

Mrs. Mendez and Reverend Leonard frequently treat clients in collaboration with a Puerto Rican *espiritista*, Mrs. Hernandez, who also participated in the Cultural Consultation Clinic. The three healers, although from different ethnic and healing traditions, both complement and compete with each other as they evolve a common healing language in the process of working with clients.

A Woman With Voices and Headaches

Mrs. *V*, a 42-year-old bilingual Hispanic woman, was referred by her primary therapist, Dr. *K*, for evaluation in the Behavioral Medicine Clinic. Dr. *K* had been treating her for over four years and sought an evaluation surrounding the patient's complaints of persistent head pain and voices, which had not been affected by several medication trials. No neurological basis for her headache could be found. The evaluating psychologist supported previous consultants in concluding that the pain was "functional" and part of a fixed delusion. He recommended she be seen by a folk healer in conjunction with psychotherapy and medication. This recommendation followed an interview in which Mrs. *V* stated that there was a spirit in her. This claim was denied by a priest whom she saw independently, but she persisted in her belief. She was given an appointment in our Cultural Consultation Unit with the hope that a culturally compatible approach to her attribution of illness might prove helpful.

Mrs. *V* presented two main problems: first, she complained of severe chronic headache in the right parietal area, beginning about 12 years previously. Second, she reported hearing voices for the past 8 years.

Our chart review and assessment interviews resulted in a brief chronology of her family, medical, and psychiatric history. It was noted that her chart was unusually thick, with many reports of frustrated treatment attempts. Differential emphasis on particular symptom clusters had led to at least six different primary diagnoses over the years. These focused generally on "histrionic personality" features, a variety of "psychotic" symptoms, and a "unipolar affective disorder".

Mrs. *V* was divorced and unemployed, receiving her income from Social Security disability insurance and Aid for Dependent Children. She lived at home with her 17-year-old son and worked as a volunteer at a community center on an irregular basis.

Mrs. *V* was born and raised in a Mexican city on the U.S. border. She had four sisters and two brothers. Her father managed apartments. Her mother, after the birth of one of the younger children, apparently began to suffer from a severe psychological disorder. The patient was about six years old at this time and recalled sometimes being locked out of her house at night so "the devil would take her". According to Mrs. *V* her mother also heard voices which have continued until the present.

At age 15, Mrs. *V* left home against her parents' wishes to marry a 26-year-old man who had been married twice before and had a three-year-old daughter. By age 17, Mrs. *V* had two sons. Disagreements with the husband over the proper care of Mr. *V*'s daughter, his infidelity, and the patient's "temper tantrums" led to frequent quarrels and physical abuse. At this same age she ingested bleach in a suicidal gesture precipitated by an argument with her husband. She denied suicidal intent. Over the next several years she worked temporarily at a cannery, a bakery, and independent cleaning houses.

At age 27, she had an automobile accident and was hospitalized with multiple somatic complaints, including headache. The medical evaluation revealed no organic basis for her complaints. Thereafter she began to receive "tranquilizers" and "pain pills" from private physicians. When she was 29, she began undergoing psychiatric treatment because of marital problems, depression, and headache. She began to receive antipsychotic and antidepressant medications, which have been continued until the present time in various combinations. She also began receiving psychotherapy, both individual and marital therapy, for about four months. At that point she requested a Spanish-speaking therapist. By coincidence, her new therapist, a man, had the same surname and a first name quite similar to hers.

One year later, after months of deliberation, she separated from her husband and filed for divorce. Three months later, after a year of therapy, the Spanish-speaking therapist took a job in another state and transferred Mrs. *V* to another therapist. She was pregnant by her husband during this period, but miscarried, and she completed the divorce. Over the next 18 months she became more depressed, developed the delusion that the new therapist had hypnotized her, and began to describe "odd things" in her head causing pain, burning, and pulling sensations. In 1972 she revealed that she had fallen in love with the Spanish-speaking therapist and had begun to hear his voice. She had become more socially isolated and withdrawn, claiming that the headache prevented activity.

Several months later she reported a bizarre incident. She had gone to Mexico with a strange man, thinking he might have been the Spanish-speaking therapist. She wanted to know if this stranger would return to marry her. Nine months later, at age 35, she delivered this stranger's child, a healthy male. She gave the baby up for adoption. On the discharge summary, the obstetrician stated, "Except for her hysterical reaction and postpartum psychosis, her postpartum course was unremarkable".

The next year Mrs. *V* was hospitalized involuntarily for about three weeks because of insomnia, depression, deterioration in function, and "strikingly delusional" features, with the central theme of external control over mind and speech, and auditory hallucinations.

After this hospitalization she remained on outpatient treatment, primarily for support and medications. She underwent group therapy for several months, without substantial improvement. For the next several years, until present, she was followed by Dr. *K*.

Mrs. *V* was a very attractive woman, exceptionally well-dressed and groomed. She spoke English well, and her speech was unremarkable. No abnormalities were noted in motor behavior. Although she was initially shy, she had good interpersonal skills and did not appear to be suffering physical pain even though she complained this was severe. She was well-oriented in time and place, but was frequently unsure whether her thoughts were hers or were placed there by others or by a voice. Early personality testing and a recent follow-up indicated her personality functioning to be relatively unchanged over the past ten years. Briefly, her profile suggested a high degree of paranoid ideation, unusual somatic preoccupations, and poorly organized thought processes. Other aspects of formal psychodynamic assessment and mental status will not be reported here, as the purpose of this paper is to describe aspects of interpersonal processes as they developed among the consultants, not to presume the existence of an objective clinical reality.

Session I

After an initial assessment, Mrs. *V*, met with the Cultural Consultation Unit for four sessions. At the first session, the spiritualist healer, Mrs. Mendez, the psychiatrist, and the anthropologist interviewed Mrs. *V*. Mrs. Mendez began by speaking Spanish with Mrs. *V*, and translating to the other consultants. It soon became clear that Mrs. *V* had a good command of English; thereafter interviews took place mainly in English. Initially, the group discussed the nature of Mrs. *V*'s voice. She described how the voice often belonged to people she had met, such as the clinical psychologist. The voice often gave her commands (such as to eat) and, curiously, told her things which made her laugh. Throughout all of our interactions with Mrs. *V*, she would spontaneously burst out laughing. When asked about it, she said, "The voice made me laugh". Upon closer inquiry, we discovered that "the voice" had commented on quirks and foibles of the interviewers or the ironies of the interview situation. Mrs. *V* took no direct responsibility for these very accurate observations; "the voice" had done it.

The spiritualist inquired about Mrs. *V*'s beliefs in spiritual influences. The response was highly ambiguous, including statements that she didn't believe in such powers, that she believed in medicine and psychiatry. Her perception of psychiatric methods, however, interpreted to her through her voice, included a notion of doctors trying to stimulate her mind which had become weak. She thought she could be influenced by others, including doctors, but she differentiated this from outright possession by a spirit. Regarding the voice, she said she sometimes learned from it, but was often frightened of it as well. She became confused in discussing the source of her thoughts.

The psychiatrist soon commented that Mrs. *V* seemed to feel ashamed to talk about what the voice said. This quickly led to an abandonment of the voice and to recollections of early painful memories of her parents fighting and of sexual incidents with her father. Both Mrs. Mendez and the psychiatrist experienced a shared intuitive perception about Mrs. *V*. Their empathic experience suggested to them that she had been sexually abused by her father and perhaps by other men. Both interviewers sensed a level of trust from Mrs. *V* which encouraged a rapid approach to this central issue. The psychiatrist asked Mrs. *V* about this possibility.

She disclosed that her father had attempted to have sex with her on at least a few occasions when she was 10 years old. Mrs. *V* denied actual intercourse but could not be explicit in recounting the actual events that took place. She described an incident when her mother, abhorring sexual intercourse, placed Mrs. *V* in bed between her and her father and told him to "do it with her". She indicated that her mother felt Mrs. *V* was "too religious" as a girl and that offering her to her father constituted a form of punishment from God. She said, "God and the devil were proving who was stronger. The voice says God and the devil don't want me. God says he doesn't want me because I do things he doesn't like". Again she was unable to explain further, and was quite embarrassed. In eleven years of treatment, Mrs. *V* said she had never previously described these incidents. She had apparently hinted at this problem two months previously to Dr. *K*, but according to his note he had discounted her report.

At the end of this first brief session, the spiritualist healer concluded that Mrs. *V* was possessed by a spirit. Both she and the psychiatrist felt that they had discovered the same historical issues, and that psychosexual problems were central aspects of her present illness. There was initially a good deal of enthusiasm and accommodation of each other's etiological views. It became clear in subsequent sessions that the interpretive processes of the consultants were differentially shaped by personally meaningful reconstructions of aspects of the clinical material which each held to be the most salient. This led to critical differences in views regarding the role of the patient in her illness, and the constitution of the therapeutic process.

Six days after this session, Mrs. *V* voluntarily entered the psychiatric inpatient service, with increased discomfort due to depression and persistent hearing of voices. She was discharged two days later after a change of medication had led to an improvement in her condition.

Session II

The next session took place three weeks later. Dr. *K*, the healers, Mrs. Mendez, and Reverend Leonard, the psychiatrist and the anthropologist interviewed Mrs. *V*. The sociologist observed the meeting through a one-way mirror. This session began with a discussion among the members of the Cultural Consultation Unit before bringing in Mrs. *V*. During the discussion, Dr. *K* expressed doubt about the validity of Mrs. *V*'s report of molestation. Mrs. Mendez emphasized her viewpoint that Mrs. *V* had "picked up a strange entity" with men, and implied she had done something immoral with men, and needed to "get it out".

Reverend Leonard said he saw different "spirits" affecting Mrs. *V*, including one which affected her brain, causing headaches, and other entities which he characterized as being "like a war" going on inside her. He described physical sensations he felt she had, and said that she could not report what was happening to her because of her confusion. He made these statements before ever meeting the patient, saying he knew these things through Dr. *K*'s presence in the room. The psychiatrist and Reverend Leonard shared a sense that Mrs. *V* suffered from great internal conflict, and the psychiatrist further framed this as a desire for the companionship and the company of men along with a great fear of them.

When Mrs. *V* came in, Mrs. Mendez and Reverend Leonard received permission from her and began a healing titual. The healing consisted of Mrs. Mendez channelling healing energy into Mrs. *V*. She stood behind the patient, laid her hands on the patient's head and shoulders, and stroked her in sweeping motions, all the while saying prayers. At one point she went into a trance, and a spirit spoke through her, mimicking Mrs. *V* when she broke into laughter, reincorporating the laughter into the ritual context. Reverend Leonard stood in front of Mrs. *V*, directing healing energy into her, and stood by protectively when the spirit entered Mrs. Mendez. Mrs. *V* interrupted the ritual several times with laughter and, finally, the healers discontinued their efforts.

Throughout the remainder of this two-hour session, the healers and psychiatrist addressed the several functions which the "voice" performed for her. Through the healings and discussions around this and further historical material, each consultant arrived at an interpretation of Mrs. *V*'s illness which included an etiological hypothesis, a characterization of her present illness, a model for therapy, and aspects of resistance to therapy.

The interviewers all concurred on the salience of the issues of sexuality, the need for intimacy, and the patient's experience of shame and guilt. They raised the issue of her feelings about her father's sexual abuse and her husband's infidelity and physical abuse. They discussed her mistrust of other men she had met. They gave her "permission" to have these feelings and, at the same time, to continue to use "the voice" as necessary to protect her from the intense emotions associated with these experiences. With this sanction, Mrs. *V* began to acknowledge some of her own feelings while continuing to attribute most of her troubles to "the voice" and her pain. Each interviewer approached these issues with a different interpretive framework.

Mrs. Mendez suggested several times that Mrs. *V* had led a "corrupted life" and had "picked up a lot of entities" on the streets. She never confronted the patient with this impression, however, and saw herself as working through direct spiritual healing as opposed to verbal therapy. She respected the voice as a manifestation of spirit which caused suffering, and she related this directly to religious themes. She said she knew Mrs. *V* had withheld information about sexual activity before marriage and possibly after. Her knowledge was attributed to her "reading" during the healing ritual and subsequent trance state. It was noted that after the trance and a translation and clarification with the psychiatrist, Mrs. *V* appeared to talk more openly about actual life events.

Mrs. Mendez viewed the patient's suffering in terms of her leaving God and the Catholic Church. In a discussion after the session she said: "In the first place there was a current of the parents' problems coming through. She is making it grow, all this fantasy, imagining that this man loves her. She cannot be alone . . . . She has no faith, she doesn't pray, she doesn't believe . . . . She always believes in the admiration of men, that's all, that's her God." Mrs. Mendez was impatient with the efforts of Reverend Leonard and the psychiatrist to explore the patient's feelings of shame and moral conflict. Her goal for therapy was to "open her up more", which could be accomplished through direct spiritual means and by Mrs. V's explicit acknowledgment of her history of sexual activities. Her ultimate goal was to restore the patient to the Catholic Church: "I want her to accept her God-given right, open her heart to God; she said she is Catholic." Mrs. Mendez appeared to regard as resistance the continued efforts of the patient to divert attention to her physical pain. Mrs. Mendez noted several times during the session the inconsistency between the patient's complaints of pain and her actual appearance and mood.

Reverend Leonard understood the origins of Mrs. V's illness as a conflict between her natural feelings and a moral-religious prohibition against these feelings. He said to the group: "Her mother was a religious woman. She was very dogmatic. You rejected it but it stayed there anyway . . . . The moral was implanted a long time ago, age 3. It's gotten to the point that the moral is larger than herself". In a long hypnotic recitation he explained to Mrs. V how her "moral" and "human" parts are at odds with each other. He also believed she had seen her mother with another man, but could not accept this because she was a religious person. In a later discussion he said, "she wants to confess to herself that she's after a man, but the moral part doesn't accept that". He continued to make metaphorical use of his sense of her as accepting and rejecting at the same time. He experienced this several ways, saying that "she hears but doesn't hear", and that her pain was "there but not there". He described her resistance to the healing process: "She's the receiver and the sender as well. It resists being worked on. My hand burns from it. It stops and doesn't move."

Throughout all of the sessions, Reverend Leonard alternated between two modes of interpretation. One was an explanation of physical aspects of energy flow, tension, and blockage which he experienced during healing rituals and by directly "seeing" internal processes. The other was an interpretation based on internal conflicts. Interestingly, he appeared to utilize both physical and psychological metaphors as different manifestations of the same fundamental contradiction he experienced in Mrs. V. At a well-timed moment he commented on his own perception of this to the patient, "You don't know whether you are the voice or yourself!" He had previously accepted the validity of the voice as part of herself, and this comment was met first with group laughter and later by a moving and lucid statement by the patient about her disappointments in intimacy with men, her hopes to remarry, and her inability to cry.

Reverend Leonard felt that she would improve if she could accept her desire for intimacy with a man, with a de-emphasis on moral prohibitions. His method was both indirect and powerful. He showed the patient that he accepted the different representations of her conflict while presenting long monologues, punctuated with suggestion and subtle reframing of her situation. At one point when Mrs. V complained about men always wanting sex but without marriage, he said, "You're having the same problem as everybody else, you're not any different".

The psychiatrist focused on the shame and guilt associated with sexual abuse and parental instability as the main etiological contributions to her illness. He was more explicit than the other interviewers in identifying "the voice" as a way for her to avoid taking direct responsibility for her thoughts, feelings and behavior. He communicated that he understood her need for the voice, but periodically confronted her on her attribution of life's difficulties to its presence. During the session he commented to one of the spirtualist healers, and therefore indirectly to the patient, his feelings on this,

I think that if she gave up the voice she would have to accept that she wanted to leave her husband. She would have to accept that he was bad to her, she would have to accept being angry with him, with being angry at the social worker . . . with the guy who got her pregnant. She would have to deal with giving up her child, and with not being able to find a satisfying life since then.

The psychiatrist felt that Mrs. *V*'s resistance to therapy was evident in an understandable and generalized inability to trust others. He further commented that she appeared to be punishing herself or to be acting as if she needed punishment for unacceptable, but unspecified early acts. He later said that Mrs. *V* related to men with seductiveness but was unaware of this, and when men responded with interest in her, she repulsed them and used the experience to confirm her expectations regarding the sexual motives of men. He saw her as splitting off behavior from morals, reflecting an inability to integrate these two contradictory sides of her mother. Her inappropriate laughter and use of "the voice" were taken as evidence of this split.

The session concluded with a different approach to "the voice". At one point Mrs. *V* began to laugh and reported that "the voice" made her laugh by pointing out the causal posture of the psychiatrist in his chair. The psychiatrist then began to laugh, slightly embarrassed but acknowledging the reality of "the voice's" observation. Indeed, he sat with an exaggerated slouch. By acknowledging this reality, he validated the observation and allowed Mrs. *V* to see it herself. Vigorous laughter suddenly spread throughout the whole group, and Reverend Leonard and the psychiatrist commented that possibly "the voice" had left Mrs. *V* and gone to all the others. These comments provoked further laughter and a kind of unguarded appreciation of simple human experience free from fear.

Within four weeks of this session, Mrs. *V* stopped hearing "the voice". At the same time, Dr. *K* had made a change in medications, substituting one antipsychotic for another. Obviously, we can only report the sequence of events without making any kind of guesses about the relative contribution to the remission of symptoms. We can note that Mrs. *V* had received both antipsychotic medications in the past with no discernible change in symptoms. Except for a brief return of "the voice" when Dr. *K* terminated with her and she began to work with the psychologist as her new therapist, Mrs. *V* remained free of "the voice" for at least 16 months following this session.

Session III

The third session took place four months after the second. During this session, Mrs. Mendez, Reverend Leonard, the anthropologist, the sociologist, and the psychiatrist interviewed Mrs. *V*. The interview covered much of the same material as the previous one, i.e., taking responsibility for her life experience, associated emotions, and patterns of interpersonal interaction. Mrs. *V* was fairly cooperative throughout the interview and, in fact, became much more directly self-disclosing and emotionally expressive.

During the healing ritual, Mrs. *V* experienced temporary relief of pain when Reverend Leonard applied pressure to the source of her head pain. She also reported feeling slightly better after a healing session with Mrs. Mendez. She was hearing "the voice" for a short time during this session, which the psychiatrist noted as coinciding with discussion of her termination of therapy with Dr. *K*. When engaged with affectively arousing material, however, she did not complain of voices or headache. This appeared to be a radical change in her defensive style.

Mrs. *V* cried during this session, expressing confusion over her inability to trust others and a fear of death which she felt might occur through medical treatment of her pain. When asked who in her life loved her, she replied, "There is not such a thing in this world that a man could love a woman, I guess". A tearful exchange followed next in which the psychiatrist offered his view of Mrs. *V*'s illness to her and the other consultants. He emphasized her strong desire to be loved and cared for and the healthy nature of this desire. He elaborated on her history of being hurt in relationships, saying that her pain may have been from muscle tension physically, but that it represented a fear to let go. He saw the pain as a protection against an overwhelming sense of loss.

Reverend Leonard's explanatory model coincided closely with that of the psychiatrist. He described her voice as a companion helping her with stress. He said she retained a certain pride and elegance which is the moral part she is unable to turn loose. He likened her punishing sense of morality to a wall which needed to come down, and he created an image of a wall which she had built but which closed her off from her human need to communicate with others. Mrs. *V*, sobbing, acknowledged that her life had indeed felt cut off since her divorce.

The remainder of the session was concerned with practical suggestions for Mrs. *V* in social situations with men. She complained about expectations of sex when going out with a man. Mrs. Mendez implied that these suggestions for setting limits were somewhat naive when dealing with a Mexican man. She did not elaborate.

Much in contrast to the previous session, where the interviewers attempted to accommodate each other's perceptions, discrepancies between the different interpretive models became strikingly apparent in the discussion after the interview. Mrs. Mendez, Reverend Leonard, and the psychiatrist all felt quite positive at the conclusion of the interview. The sociologist had become increasingly uncomfortable with the judgmental quality of Mrs. Mendez's attitude toward the patient which she perceived as less than therapeutic. She also saw the psychiatrist as accepting the moral content of Mrs. Mendez's explanatory model of the source of the patient's distress and voice. In the post-interview discussion, she expressed these concerns, with anger, initially and directly to the psychiatrist, and indirectly to Mrs. Mendez. Both the psychiatrist and the healer felt attacked and responded quite defensively.

Suddenly the group plunged into an emotional whirlpool which led to an abrupt termination of the meeting. Gradually, over several days, as feelings subsided, the participants began to approach each other in a spirit of serious cooperative inquiry. That process has led to the present paper's observations.

Session IV

One month following the previous session, Mrs. *V* was interviewed by the psychiatrist, the anthropologist, and Reverend Leonard. Mrs. *V* initially talked about her pain and about her disability claim. She occasionally heard the voice but refused to say what the content of this was. The psychiatrist, through a series of gestures and suggestions, tried to show the patient that she was quite capable of detecting when someone was influencing her. She acknowledged this somewhat, but became more demanding about what could be done for her. She expressed continued uncertainty about Reverend Leonard, who was standing behind her briefly during a healing session. She explained her difficulty in knowing when men were tricking her, and she talked about her painful early years in marriage. The psychiatrist felt that her uncertainty about receiving continued psychiatric treatment was reflected in her resistance in this session. Also, this was to be the final session for Mrs. *V* in this group. This resistance was felt directly by Reverend Leonard as he tried to work on her pain spiritually: "... the voice is like a wall, a fence ... not allowing energy into her. There's an energy flow between people and she kicks it back to them. And she goes out and she wonders why people don't come back ... it's because she throws back to them the very same thing that she thinks they are sending to her".

Her sadness and disappointment at not feeling confident about her ability to further improve was acknowledged at the end of the session. She had managed to do volunteer work on a regular basis, and she thereby significantly increased her social contact. More importantly, she had begun to accept some of her anger and pain as related to real events in her life. She was seen once more in this clinic two weeks later, in order to talk about a referral for therapy to the psychologist who participated in the clinic activities. The psychiatrist also reviewed her treatment, which provided little new information and will not be reported here. The psychologist followed her for a period during Dr. *K*'s absence.

At the time of the writing of this paper, Mrs. *V* had been able to arrange continued treatment with Dr. *K*, her original therapist. She continues to be disturbed by headaches, but has been essentially free of hearing voices. Her major concern is the possibility of her son leaving home, and the practical problems of living more independently.

DISCUSSION

Early in this case, our work led us to believe that the three therapists, while using quite different clinical models and approaches, had elicited or discovered the same reality underlying Mrs. *V*'s suffering: previously unrevealed sexual abuse in child-hood, unresolved feelings about her husband and the divorce, the giving up of a child for adoption, a sexualized relationship with a previous therapist, all of which led to severe conflicts about her sexuality, problems of attribution, a defensive splitting off of a part of herself, and a focusing on pains in the head and the magical power of physicians to remove them. While at this level of generality there was agreement, the "conflict of interpretations" following Session III forced us to take more seriously the differences in interpretations that existed, and to explore the sources of those differences.

At the first level, that of explicit clinical models, the sharpest differences among clinicians were between the psychiatrist and the two healers. The psychiatrist worked within the framework of dynamic psychotherapy, and sought the sources of the patient's pain both in early childhood experiences and in her defensive responses to later life traumas. The healers, on the other hand, worked within a common spiritualist tradition, although they disagreed about the specific sources of Mrs. *V*'s problems. Mrs. Mendez focused on the voice as the primary problem, and identified it as an "entity" that Mrs. *V* had "picked up" while involved with unspecified men. Reverend Leonard focused more concretely on physical aspects of the head pain, described in terms of scarring that affected the energy flow. He further elaborated this as a metaphor for her problems in relating to other people. He interpreted the voice not as an entity but as part of her self, a part that both "tells you the truth" and "entertains you" in times of loneliness.

Mrs. *V*'s own explanatory model did not include the existence of spirits. She believed her problems resulted from a physical disorder in her head, which she hoped some physician could take away, and from the voice, whose origin she could not explain. She feared she had mental problems, and felt her symptoms severely affected her social functioning. Through the therapy, she increasingly came to relate her symptoms to trauma in her life; she came to redefine the voice as thoughts.

While the formal aspects of the spiritualist and psychiatric models differed, with the healers constructing reality in terms of entities or spirits and energy fields, these did not prove to be the most significant differences for the interpretations made by the three clinicians. While Mrs. Mendez was convinced that Mrs. *V* was possessed by a very real "entity", she focused her attention on the "corrupted life" she was convinced Mrs. *V* had led. Following the first session, all the clinicians agreed that Mrs. *V* had suffered sexual abuse as a child and that these experiences should be explored in future sessions. By the second session, however, Mrs. Mendez had become convinced that the patient had been "sold on the street" as a youth, that she had continued to lead a promiscuous life, especially since her divorce, and that her voice was an entity that she had picked up while she was "running around with men". Mrs. Mendez's goal for therapy was to elicit a confessional recital from the patient of her immoral activities, and to encourage her to change her life. She did not state this to the patient, however, and it was noteworthy that she implied that the psychiatrist and/or Reverend Leonard should confront the patient. She usually remained silent, and her work consisted mainly of conducting healing rituals and asking a few questions.

While the rationale was quite different for the psychiatrist, the over-arching structure of his therapeutic paradigm and strategy had important parallels to that of Mrs. Mendez. He felt that the patient had powerful conflicts over her own sexuality. He believed these conflicts led her to relate to men in ways that validated her fears that men only treated her as a sexual object. He postulated that these conflicts originated in early childhood experiences, and that a reconstruction and rehearsal of these experiences was one of the necessary elements in her therapy. He had a strong intuition that Mrs. Mendez's belief that the patient had once been sold on the streets would prove historically accurate, although that was not essential to his understanding of her conflicts.

Reverend Leonard had a distinctly different formulation of the patient's illness. Contrary to Mrs. Mendez, he believed that the voice was part of herself. In this he was joined by the psychiatrist, and together they attempted to reformulate Mrs. *V*'s attribution of the source of the voice, that is, to help her acknowledge that the voice was a part of herself. Second, he believed that Mrs. *V*'s conflicts over her sexuality arose not so much from her sexual exploitation in her childhood and youth as from her mother's condemnation of her sexuality as "immoral". In his opinion, the major therapeutic tasks were to help her find relief from this internalized maternal moral punishment and to increase her interaction in the social world.

Mrs. Mendez's strong moral condemnation of the patient's sexual promiscuity aroused the most powerful responses of the other members of the clinic. Specifically, the "conflict of interpretations" focused on whether Mrs. *V* had actually been "sold on the street" in her youth. In our attempt to evaluate the validity of this claim and to understand the roots of the interpretations made by the three clinicians, the "observers" (including the psychiatrist) were forced to examine the personal grounds of their own interpretations. Exploration of the conflict began to reveal to us the multiple levels of meaning and the complexity of the subjective frameworks brought to the case by all participants. The format for exploring these issues was a series of long, tape-recorded discussions among the psychiatrist, anthropologist, sociologist, and psychologist, and separate discussions with the healers about their understanding of the case and the differences in interpretation.

First, each person brought a particular set of personal and cultural meanings to the issue of the patient's hypothesized sexual promiscuity and Mrs. Mendez's moral stance. The psychologist recalled that Mrs. Mendez's belief that Mrs. *V* should confess her sexual activities stimulated issues raised for him in both early exposure to the Catholic Church and in his therapeutic work with an excommunicated Mormon. He felt Mrs. Mendez's model accurately saw the patient as suffering tremendous guilt, but he reacted against the use of guilt to restore moral prohibition which he could not accept at a personal level. He found confession to be a restrictive solution that did not respect the patient's personal conflicts over moral issues. His reaction was deepened through independent, research-oriented interviews with Mrs. *V*, in which she detailed her sense of unhappiness with her religious background. At one point she stated that she wished she could return to the Catholic Church, but literally could not comprehend the meaning of religious belief in view of her overwhelmingly negative life experiences. He strongly identified with her confusion over this issue, and therefore saw Mrs. Mendez's stance as a missed opportunity for siding with the adaptive forces within the patient. His emotional reaction was quite mixed also, for in other respects he found Mrs. Mendez to be a powerful, compassionate presence within the sessions.

The anthropologist responded more strongly to Mrs. Mendez's fundamentalism. Having been reared as a fundamentalist Protestant, Mrs. Mendez's insistence on the propositional truth of her claims and her unwillingness to accept a stance that would relativize those statements aroused for him unresolved conflicts related to his own religious heritage and the moral stance of his own mother. He believed that sexual promiscuity was a metaphor that allowed exploration of the patient's conflicting feelings about her own sexuality. Although he felt Mrs. Mendez was making historically inaccurate judgments and assuming an inappropriate moral stance, he found direct confrontation with her unthinkable. It was thus particularly conflictive when the sociologist, his wife, angrily confronted the psychiatrist and Mrs. Mendez about what she felt were judgmental aspects of their model. The sociologist felt that Mrs. Mendez had formulated her conclusions about Mrs. *V*'s promiscuity partly in reaction to the patient's resistance to Mrs. Mendez's treatment and interpretation, and by means of "cultural stereo-typing"; i.e., Mrs. Mendez assumed the patient fit a negative cultural type. The sociologist felt particularly strongly that the patient's own claims regarding her early sexual experiences were being disconfirmed, and that she was being regarded as an immoral participant rather than as a victim. The sociologist's perceptions were based not only on clinic sessions but also on lengthy telephone conversations with Mrs. Mendez. In one conversation, Mrs. Mendez remarked that she felt the patient

... had some kind of Satanic entity in her. She was raised in a religious environment but turned from the Church .... She wanted to be willful. She used her nice face, her youth to conquer men in Mexico. Let us not forget cultural awareness; not every woman goes on the street. Her father ... gave her the training so she'd know she could do it for money. Her mother was on the good, submissive side; her father was a little devil ... the lady was a drinker, a bar woman ... her gestures are from a bar person, of conversing and drinking with men ... she spent her youth doing that kind of work. (1980, December 31, telephone conversation)

Although the sociologist recognized the patient's struggles with her sexuality and her early traumatic experiences, she felt there were no data, other than Mrs. Mendez's intuition, to support the claim that the patient had been a prostitute. During subsequent intensive discussions of the case, the sociologist recalled experiencing intense anger as a young single woman in the Middle East when she had been wrongly accused of promiscuity. She acknowledged that her feelings regarding the treatment of Mrs. *V* were rooted in part in this earlier experience and in part in a strong aversion to the psychiatrist's and healer's wielding of power and control through the idiom of sexuality. Although the sociologist realized that Mrs. Mendez's evaluation of the patient was quite appropriate within the context of her cultural milieu, she began to question the therapeutic validity of Mrs. Mendez's interpretations.

The psychiatrist continued to have a strong intuition that the patient had actually been victimized as a prostitute in her youth. In part he recognized the association between this conviction and his investment in finding that the healers have powers of intuition born of remarkable acuity in nonverbal communications. He felt his own cultural heritage provided him with a basis for intuiting the structure of the patient's experience and for making reasonable guesses about her history.

While we do not have adequate life history material to fully understand the personal grounds of the healers' interpretations, it appears their life experiences were significant in structuring the relationship each formed with the patient. For example, Reverend Leonard told the researchers that he believed Mrs. Mendez's own personal history and family life, her religious upbringing, and her cultural values influenced her moral stance. "I told her later", he said to us, "what we need to do is to get rid of the mother, to kill the mother. Instead you have become the mother", While Mrs. Mendez clearly took on the role of a morally punishing mother, Reverend Leonard was able to play the role of a supportive male figure, showing that this person need not be sexually threatening. He was therefore able to develop a strong therapeutic relationship with the patient.

In reviewing videotapes, Mrs. Mendez appeared to be reacting to a sense that the patient had successfully seduced the male interviewers into a position of supporting her "natural" sexual drive, perhaps as a validation of her covert wish to be pursued and admired by men. In giving suggestions for her interactions with men in social situations, the male therapists could therefore have been seen by Mrs. Mendez as acting out the very conflict with men that each had previously cited as evidence of the patient's pathology. This hypothesis is speculative since Mrs. Mendez could not articulate her reaction. It is offered in order to provide an alternative view of a clinical vignette, one which was generally evocative of an image of a morally punitive maternal figure, but one which contained a request for the group to attend to a potentially critical manipulation of the therapists by the patient. The group and individual affective reactions prevented a useful discussion of this subject for a time.

While our personal responses to the perception of promiscuity in the patient played a significant role in our conflicting interpretations, our discussions also revealed that other dimensions of our relationships to the healers and to each other provided important grounds for our interpretations. From the very beginning, bringing the healers into the Cultural Consultation Clinic as therapists produced the potential for conflict between the social scientists and the psychiatrist. The anthropologist and the sociologist had worked with the healers for several years before they introduced them to the psychiatrist. The anthropologist in particular responded with ambivalence to the psychiatrist's decision to bring the healers into the clinic. While it would provide the opportunity for a very special form of anthropological collaboration and research, it might jeopardize his privileged relationship with important informants.

The potential for conflict was heightened by changes that developed in the relationships between the healers and each of the researchers. These relationships were negotiated most explicitly in "readings" done by the healers. When Mrs. Mendez first met the psychiatrist, just prior to opening the clinic, she saw around him a "blue light", indicating his healing powers. In readings done during the course of the clinic, Mrs. Mendez and Mrs. Hernandez, the Puerto Rican *espiritista*, represented him as having a special healing gift, as being warm and caring, and as having personal sadness resulting from actions by significant persons in his life. These readings were in sharp contrast to those they gave to the three social scientists.

Mrs. Hernandez gave the anthropologist a reading which characterized him as having a "docile spirit"[3] and as having suffered genital torture and great physical torment in a previous life. Her reading of the sociologist represented her as strong and difficult to read and as unfulfilled because she had not borne children. These readings were interpreted to mean that Mrs. Hernandez intuited that they failed to live up to a Hispanic cultural ideal of male-female and husband-wife relationships. Neither Mrs. Hernandez nor Mrs. Mendez characterized either social scientist as having healing powers. In contrast with these readings, the sociologist remembered feeling as if the two spiritualists had engaged in a "love feast" with the psychiatrist during their reading of him. She later recalled feelings of annoyance at the special relationship between the psychiatrist and healers which these readings indicated.

In addition, the anthropologist and sociologist felt that once they introduced the healers into this clinical setting, they themselves were considered peripheral. For example, Mrs. Hernandez suggested in a reading that her role should be to establish a foundation to receive grants to support and disseminate the spiritualists' work. Thus, while the anthropologist and sociologist continued to work closely with the healers, bringing the latter into the clinic with the psychiatrist altered relationships between all participants in ways that were conflicting.

The psychologist, who came to know the healers when he joined the clinic staff, primarily as a researcher, had a similar experience. He remembered a reading by Mrs. Hernandez characterizing him as a researcher whose clinical intuition was undermined by too much intellectual reasoning. (The psychologist ran the video camera.) He felt that the contrast between the readings of the social scientists and the psychiatrist reflected a splitting which attributed significant deficiencies to those seen in the role of observer. Positive healing qualities could then be retained only in the psychiatrist and in the relationship between the psychiatrist and the healers.

The three social scientists experienced the differential respect shown to the psychiatrist as mirroring other experiences. For the anthropologist and sociologist, this relationship reflected the status differential between the physician and non-physician faculties within the medical school. The social scientists were often addressed by their first names by the healers, the psychiatrist was addressed as "Doctor". This differential form of address aroused the strong sense of frustration that accompanies the routine experiences of personal disconfirmation of non-physicians in a medical school. Within the clinic, this issue also surfaced as a conflict over the role of the social scientists. There was unresolved ambiguity over their dual roles as observing ethnographers and participating co-therapists, and this ambiguity reflected the more general status issues.

The issue of ethnic identity provided another important personal meaning frame for the interpretations in the multiple relationships. For the psychiatrist, a native California Chicano, the experience of working with the healers was emotionally complex. When he was recognized by Mrs. Mendez as having a "blue light", he had recently returned from a trip to Mexico where he had accompanied two anthropologists on a visit to a powerful village healer. This visit raised important issues of personal and ethnic identity. Working with a powerful Mexican *curandera* (Mrs. Mendez) aroused for him associations with the mysterious Mexican folk healing tradition and its special powers. On the other hand, working with popular healers in a professional setting aroused anxieties about potential ethnic stereotyping and discrimination by his physician colleagues.

The issue of ethnic identity was particularly important in the dynamics of the clinical case. It was a basic working hypothesis that the healers would have special abilities to work with Chicano patients because of their "empathy", that is, their skill in non-verbal communication with Chicano patients and their implicit knowledge of the meaning structure of popular Mexican-American culture. However, this identity also provided Mrs. Mendez and the psychiatrist with a common, privileged vantage point that made it difficult for the social scientists to disagree with their clinical formulation. Thus, since the social scientists were non-Hispanic, the ethnic boundary coincided with other differences — between healer and non-healer, clinician and observer — that were markers of power and status in the clinic.

The question of cultural contributions to countertransference has not been well-developed in the literature (Spiegel 1976). To restate, the authors worked from the assumption that ethnic similarity between the patient and some of the consultants would provide crucial information not available to the other consultants. Herrera and Frank (1976) develop this argument in terms of reflexive behavior and cultural stereotyping. While this assumption was validated in the case in our clinic, we do not believe it extends to an *a priori* validation of interpretations arising from cultural similarity. Culturally based impediments to therapy must also be acknowledged.

In order to develop this discussion, the core clinical function of empathy must be examined. Across theoretical orientations the concept of empathic understanding suggests an ability experientially and emotionally to grasp the quality of the patient's experience (Bachrach 1976). Through empathic understanding, the therapist helps to clarify the emotional struggles and self-perceptions of the patient. This has been most usefully described in the psychoanalytic literature as being achieved through a series of "transient trial identifications" with the patient (Fliess 1942).

In such identifications the therapist takes in (introjects) central aspects of the patient's identifications (objects). Herein lie both the strength and the danger of this process. In theory, the empathic identification is not sufficient to obscure the portion of detached, observing ego which the analyst uses in interpretation and therapeutic facilitation (Baum 1973).

The hazards of these trial identifications have been reviewed by Reich (1960), Fliess (1953), Chediak (1979) and others, who stress the revival of strong affective material stimulated in the regressive identification. This can result in a failure to usefully detach oneself from the intrapsychic conflicts aroused, to such a degree that the transference needs of the analyst are acted out regressively (Baum 1973). Alternatively, the analyst may fail to relinquish the identification due to the narcissistic gratification it provides (Kernberg 1975).

Racker (1957) discusses a particular danger when the therapist identifies with the original transference objects of the patient. He labels this "complementary identification". Kernberg (1975: 59) provides an example of this phenomenon:

For instance, the analyst may identify with a superego function connected with a stern, prohibitive father image, feeling critical and tempted to control the patient in some particular way, while the patient may be experiencing fear, submission, or rebelliousness connected with his relationship to his father.

To bring this discussion back to the present clinical material, it is possible that the reaction of Mrs. Mendez was an example of such an identification, in this case with an internalized image of a morally punitive mother. As the sociologist remarked, this reaction may have been the only one available to Mrs. Mendez for a variety of reasons. First, the content of her interpretation of pathology and her curative suggestions derive in part from her cultural and religious heritage. Second, the intensity of her affective response is likely to be related to her methodology. She uses not only empathic understanding as it is commonly understood, but a deliberate attempt to merge with the patient in the form of a trance. The profound impact of this quest is evident in her extensive ritual cleansing which follows these experiences.

This example is discussed to suggest that the issue of ethnic similarity does indeed profoundly affect the quality and intensity of empathy in the clinical interaction. Vividly shared cultural archetypal images may thus be evoked in the negotiation of "clinical reality" which are not shared by ethnically dissimilar dyads. Complementary identification is, of course, a danger for all therapists if it is acted out and not recognized and interpreted. Ethnic similarity may provide a particularly fertile ground for both the positive aspects of empathic understanding and communication, and the negative prospect of a repetition of earlier pathology. Gottesfeld (1978) provides a rare description of how "ethnic collusion" impeded her interpretation of a case and became manifest in her countertransference reactions.

Our point in describing these complexes of meaning within which our work was embedded is to show their importance for the interpretations we as observers made of the work of the clinic. Not only was the work of the clinicians with the patient a series of negotiations between quite different models, and not only were these models grounded in personal frames of meaning; the interpretations of the clinical discourse by the observers were embedded in a complex set of personal and professional relationships and webs of personal significance that influenced their investment in the validity of various approaches to understanding the patient.

Finally, we should note that while this paper is not intended as an analysis of the therapeutic efficacy of our approach to treating Mrs. *V*, careful review of the videotapes has convinced us that the patient did excellent work in this unorthodox clinical setting. In a few intensive sessions she was able to grapple with issues not previously addressed in years of treatment; she was able to relinquish attribution of her thoughts to the "voice", and her appearance, demeanor and social functioning improved over the seven months. While there can be no final interpretation, the therapy clearly enabled the patient to work with very real issues in her life.

CONCLUSION

In this paper we have used an intensive analysis of a single case to provide a view of the complex layers of meaning involved in psychiatric practice. While multiple practitioners and alternative healers are not common to most psychiatric practice, the fundamental task of interpreting across diverse meaning frames is universal. We believe that a hermeneutic model provides a guide to exploring the dialectic of interpretation that constitutes clinical discourse. While algorithmic decision-making has a part in determining psychotropic medication and the disposition of emergency cases, the process commonly associated with the hermeneutic circle is more salient in psychiatric practice. The clinician begins with a text-like fragment, then seeks contexts in the life history of the patient that will allow a coherent interpretation of that text. This in turn facilitates self-understanding that stimulates renewed disclosure of personal texts by the patient. While the extent of this process is unique to psychiatry, this form of interpretive discourse is common to all clinical work and deserves serious study.

The Cultural Consultation Clinic provided us with the opportunity to contrast the construction of illness realities by therapists using spiritualist and psychiatric clinical models (see Gaines, this volume). These models differ significantly in their identification of etiological agents and processes (invading spirits and distorted energy patterns in the spiritualist tradition, and childhood and adolescent trauma resulting in disturbed object relations and pathological thought and attribution processes in psychiatric terms). Models of treatment (spiritual healing versus psychotherapy) and interpretations of the patient's resistance also vary in these two clinical paradigms. The spiritualist and psychotherapeutic discourses provide the clinician with tools for constructing quite different interpretations of reality.

In this case study, perhaps most striking were the similarities and differences of interpretations by the three primary clinicians that *did not* follow from the differences in their healing traditions. On the one hand, all three therapists encountered the same patient, developed a close, empathic relationship with her, and intuited moments of great pain in her life that resulted in impairments in social and psychological functioning. All therapists helped the patient provide a deeper and fuller recounting of her life story. The same historical issues and psychosexual problems were identified as central aspects of her present illness. On the other hand, the three clinicians developed interpretations of the patient's condition that had very significant differences.

Especially noteworthy was the fact that Reverend Leonard and Mrs. Mendez, while operating within very similar therapeutic traditions, developed quite different understandings of Mrs. V's pathology. While we have limited data for interpreting this, countertransference issues were clearly important in the relationship that each healer developed with the patient. The interpretations of each healer were grounded in these relationships. Classical issues of countertransference and counter-identification — for example, the patient's projections from her relationship with her mother onto Mrs. Mendez, and Mrs. Mendez's response in ways rooted in her own life history — played an important role in the way the two healers drew upon the range of potentialities in their spiritualist tradition to develop a specific interpretation of the patient's condition. In addition to the issues usually discussed in the psychiatric literature, ethnic identification, culture-specific perceptions of family and sex-role relationships, and culturally patterned metaphors and networks of symbols and associations played an important role in the countertransference reactions of all three clinicians.

The conflict that developed about treatment, our analysis of the case and our subsequent efforts to understand the sources of that conflict revealed that countertransference reactions were significant not only in the therapist-client relationships but in the ethnographer-therapist-client relationships as well. The ethnographers, along with the therapists, went through a process described in structurally similar terms in the literature on reflexivity and countertransference. They first encountered the "other", entering into a communicative relationship, using "trial identifications" or empathy to intuit the perspective of the other, and developing mutually validated (though at times conflicting) intersubjective realities. Second, they subjected their experiences to evaluation and analysis, returning to test hypotheses by articulating their interpretations and seeking responses. Third, they made an effort to develop a coherent interpretation and translate their experience into the language of their theoretical discourse (spiritualist, psychotherapeutic, anthropological). At each step, their experiences and interpretations were grounded in their own personal meaning system as well as their theoretical traditions. We suggested in the Introduction that as each participant brings multi-layered and personally grounded webs of meaning to the clinical encounter, so the ethnographer brings implicit personal understandings to the attempt to construct a coherent interpretation. Our own exploration of the conflict of interpretations described above led us to an increased respect for the complexity and power of such personal frames of significance.

While psychiatric theory and interpretation theory in anthropology share important insights, significant differences remain, particularly at the level of epistemology. Much of the history of theorizing about transference and countertransference is based on an assertion of an objective "external reality" available to the self-conscious analyst or observer, and distinct from the distortions of "psychic reality". In this paradigm, countertransference is viewed as a deviation from "objective" interpretation based in (an absolute) reality.[4] Interpretation theory assumes the relativity of the realities constructed through universal interpretive processes, not a universal objective vantage point from which interpretation is made. Self-analysis cannot produce an objectivity that is free of value and cultural perspective; nor can it allow unmediated confrontation with a reality that is external to language and discourse. Since the 1960s, psychiatric theorizing has paralleled anthropological discussions in challenging this view of the role of the observer/analyst. McLaughlin argues against a view of the analyst as occupying a "secured and superior reality-view" and in favor of a recognition of the analytic process as "as evolving, mutual authentication of the psychic realities of the two parties in the analytic search" (1981:658). This perspective provides grounds for further theoretical exchange. Anthropological research findings should challenge psychiatric theorists to recognize the broader set of phenomena (interpretations across diverse systems of public and personal meanings) of which transference and countertransference are particularly important subtypes. Anthropological theory is challenged, in turn, to account for transference and countertransference within a hermeneutic analysis of the interpretive process. The clinical ethnographer in particular is reminded that clinical realities are negotiated by clinician, patient and observer not merely in terms of cognitive models, but in terms of cultural frames that are deeply invested with personal, psychosexual and affective meanings.

Finally, we are left with the strong impression that the work of the healers is neither unique nor exotic, but a specific form of therapeutic practice carrying out "core clinical functions" (Kleinman 1980:71–83). Both professional and folk psychiatric therapists use empathy and intuition as means of understanding. It *does* make a difference what clinical models are employed; but whatever the interpretive device, the therapists (as observing ego or spirit guide) each confront the reality of the client's pathology and resistance. Efforts are made to interpret and work through the resistance and to increase the client's flexibility. Ultimately, interpretation occurs in the encounter with the reality of the other, resulting, for therapist or ethnographer, in a renewed comprehension of the self.

NOTES

1. Special thanks to Dr. Nawaz Kaleel for his generous assistance in our work in the Clinic.
2. During the period covered by this report, Dr. Herrera was chief of the Consultation-Liaison Service. He is a California-born Chicano. Dr. Byron Good and Dr. Mary-Jo Good, who are husband and wife, were each members of the Department of Psychiatry. James Cooper was a doctoral student in the Clinical Psychology Graduate Program.
3. The characterization of "docile spirit" was used consistently for Anglo men "read" by Mrs. Hernandez.
4. See McLaughlin (1981) for a critical discussion of the history of this position.

REFERENCES

Agar, Michael
    1980 Hermeneutics in Anthropology: A Review Essay. Ethos 8:173–203.

Bachrach, Henry
    1976 Empathy: We Know What We Mean But What Do We Measure? Archives of General
          Psychiatry 33:35—38.
Baum, O.
    1973 Further Thoughts on Countertransference. Psychoanalytic Review 60:127—139.
Chediak, Charles
    1979 Counter-Reactions and Countertransference. International Journal of Psychoanalysis
          60:117—129.
Crapanzano, Vincent
    1980 Tuhami: Portrait of a Moroccan. Chicago: University of Chicago Press.
Day, Richard and Ronald H. Davidson
    1981 Magic and Healing: An Ethnopsychoanalytic Examination. In Werner Muensterberger,
          Aaron H. Esman, and L. Bryce Boyer (eds.), The Psychoanalytic Study of Society,
          Volume 7. New Haven: Yale University Press.
Devereux, George
    1967 From Anxiety to Method in the Behavioral Sciences. The Hague: Mouton.
Fabian, Johannes
    1971 Language, History and Anthropology. Philosophy of the Social Sciences 1:19—47.
Fliess, Robert
    1942 The Metapsychology of the Analyst. Psychoanalytic Quarterly 11:211—227.
    1953 Countertransference and Counteridentification. Journal of the American Psycho-
          analytic Association 1:268—284.
Freud, Sigmund
    1900 The Interpretation of Dreams. Standard Edition 4 and 5. London: Hogarth Press.
    1910 The Future Prospects of Psycho-Analytic Therapy. Standard Edition 11. London:
          Hogarth Press.
Gaines, Atwood D.
    1982 Cultural Definitions, Behavior and the Person in American Psychiatry. In A. J.
          Marsella and G. M. White (eds.), Cultural Conceptions of Mental Health and Therapy.
          Dordrecht, Holland: D. Reidel Publ. Co.
Geertz, Clifford
    1973 The Interpretation of Cultures. New York: Basic Books.
Good, Byron J. and Mary-Jo DelVecchio Good
    1980 The Meaning of Symptoms: A Cultural Hermeneutic Model for Clinical Practice. In
          Leon Eisenberg and Arthur Kleinman (eds.), The Relevance of Social Science for
          Medicine. Dordrecht, Holland: D. Reidel Publ. Co.
Gottesfeld, Mary
    1978 Countertransference and Ethnic Similarity. Bulletin of the Menninger Clinic 42(1):
          63—67.
Greenson, Ralph
    1976 The Technique and Practice of Psychoanalysis. Vol. I. New York: International
          Universities Press.
Harty, Michael K.
    1979 Countertransference Patterns in the Psychiatric Treatment Team. Bulletin of the
          Menninger Clinic 43(2):105—122.
Herrera, Henry and Jerome Frank
    1976 On Helping the Underprivileged — Some Pitfalls. Paper presented at the American
          Orthopsychiatric Association Meeting. Atlanta, March, 1976.
Jules-Rosette, Benetta
    1978a The Politics of Paradigms: Contrasting Theories of Consciousness and Society.
          Human Studies 1:92—110.
    1978b The Veil of Objectivity: Prophecy, Divination, and Social Inquiry. American An-
          thropologist 80:549—570.

1978c Toward a Theory of Ethnography: The Use of Contrasting Interpretive Paradigms in Field Research. Sociological Symposium 24(2):81–98.

Katon, Wayne and Arthur Kleinman
1981 Doctor-Patient Negotiation and Other Social Science Strategies in Patient Care. *In* Leon Eisenberg and Arthur Kleinman (eds.), The Relevance of Social Science for Medicine. Dordrecht, Holland: D. Reidel Publ. Co.

Kernberg, O.
1975 Borderline Conditions and Pathological Narcissism. New York: Jason Aronson.

Kleinman, Arthur
1980 Patients and Healers in the Context of Culture. Berkeley: University of California Press.

Langs, Robert
1981 Resistances and Interventions: The Nature of Therapeutic Work. New York: Jason Aronson.

Little, Margaret
1951 Countertransference and the Patient's Response to It. International Journal of Psychoanalysis 32:32–40.
1960 Counter-Transference. British Journal of Medical Psychology 33(29):29–31.

Macklin, June
1974 Belief, Ritual and Healing: New England Spiritualism and Mexican-American Spiritism Compared. *In* Irving I. Zaretsky and Mark P. Leone (eds.), Religious Movements in Contemporary America. Princeton, New Jersey: Princeton University Press.

Meissner, William and Armand Nicholi
1978 The Psychotherapies: Individual, Family and Group. *In* Nicholi, A. (ed.), The Harvard Guide to Modern Psychiatry. Belknap Press: Cambridge.

McLaughlin, James T.
1981 Transference, Psychic Reality, and Countertransference. Psychoanalytic Quarterly L:639–664.

Obeyesekere, Gananath
1981 Medusa's Hair: An Essay on Personal Symbols and Religious Experience. University of Chicago Press: Chicago.

Osmond, Humphry and Miriam Siegler
1974 Models of Madness, Models of Medicine. New York: Macmillan Publishing Co.

Rabinow, Paul
1977 Reflections on Fieldwork in Morocco. Berkeley: University of California Press.

Rabinow, Paul and William M. Sullivan
1979 The Interpretive Turn: Emergence of an Approach. *In* Paul Rabinow and William M. Sullivan (eds.), Interpretive Social Science: A Reader. Berkeley: University of California Press.

Racker, H.
1957 The Meaning and Uses of Countertransference. Psychoanalytic Quarterly 26:303–357.

Reich, Annie
1960 Further Remarks on Counter-Transference. International Journal of Psychoanalysis 41:389–395.

Ricoeur, Paul
1974 The Conflict of Interpretations: Essays in Hermeneutics. Evanston: Northwestern University Press.
1979 The Model of the Text: Meaningful Action Considered as Text. *In* Paul Rabinow and William M. Sullivan (eds.), Interpretive Social Science: A Reader. Berkeley: University of California Press.

Scheff, Thomas
1968 Negotiating Reality: Notes on Power in the Assessment of Responsibility. Social Problems 16:3–17.

Searles, Harold F.
  1978 Concerning Transference and Countertransference. International Journal of Psycho-
        analytic Psychotherapy 7:165–188.
Speigel, J. P.
  1976 Cultural Aspects of Transference and Countertransference Revisited. Journal of the
        American Academy of Psychoanalysis 4:447–467.
Taylor, Charles
  1979 Interpretation and the Science of Man. *In* Paul Rabinow and William M. Sullivan
        (eds.), Interpretive Social Science: A Reader. Berkeley: University of California
        Press.
Trotter, Robert T. and Juan Antonia Chavira
  1980 Curanderismo: An Emic Theoretical Perspective of Mexican-American Folk Medicine.
        Medical Anthropology 4:423–487.

ATWOOD D. GAINES

THE ONCE- AND THE TWICE-BORN: SELF AND PRACTICE AMONG PSYCHIATRISTS AND CHRISTIAN PSYCHIATRISTS *

INTRODUCTION

This chapter analyzes certain key beliefs, assumptions, conceptions, and clinical practices based upon them, of American psychiatrists. It focuses on two categories of American professional ethnopsychiatrists. The members of the first category are generally referred to as "Christian psychiatrists" by these practitioners themselves and by others; the second category of professionals is commonly labeled simply "psychiatrists" by self and others but often "secular psychiatrists" by some members of the first category.

As will be seen, one of the tasks of this analysis of belief and practice among these professionals involves some sorting out of the terms of reference and a consideration of the autonomous, independent reality of these two 'groups' of practitioners. One goal of this paper is to point out some theoretical implications of a comparison of psychiatric and Christian psychiatric belief and practice in America. This exploration has relevance for both anthropological theory and research and for psychiatric practice. To accomplish this task, the paper will focus on the following elements of psychiatric belief and practice: the cultural construction of some "core clinical functions" (see Kleinman 1980b) including help-seeking, the cultural construction of illness and clinical realities, the hermeneutic nature of clinical encounters, including the issue of transference, and the appropriateness of therapeutic modalities. Two issues receive emphasis in this paper, the significance of unconscious cultural constructs (e.g., the concept of person) in medical contexts and in health and sickness related behaviors, and the symbolic construction and reality of professional and, by implication, lay 'groups' of healers corporateness.

In the course of the paper, I shall construct and then deconstruct the distinctive Christian and 'secular' psychiatric 'group' realities. Since I suggest that the reality of groups is psychological (or better, psychocultural), I mark the name of such collectivities in quotes or refer to them as "categories".

THE ONCE- AND THE TWICE-BORN

Recently, Christian psychiatrists were introduced into the growing anthropological literature on Western biomedical specialists (Gaines 1982c). I here summarize briefly key characteristics of this 'group' and introduce new ethnographic material all in order to facilitate the comparison of Christian and 'secular' psychiatrists, the latter being the subject of some earlier works (see Gaines 1979, 1982a, 1982b).

The data for the present paper derive from several sources. In 1977, I spent some months studying psychiatric residents' psychodiagnostic practices in emergency

223

R. A. Hahn and A. D. Gaines (eds.), Physicians of Western Medicine, 223–243.
© 1985 *by D. Reidel Publishing Company.*

room contexts in a West Coast city. This was followed by thirteen months of participant observation spent studying 'secular' psychiatry in Hawaii (1978–79). And, from 1982 through 1983, I did research on Christian psychiatrists, primarily through the use of semi-structured, serial interviews, at Mason Medical Center (a 'nom de centre') in America's 'Bible Belt'.

My first task should be to explain what my informants and I intend by the use of the term "Christian psychiatrists". The reader will note that the term "Christian psychiatry" is not employed. I refrain from using this term because research indicates that it does not correspond to any extant, corporate body within psychiatry (see Gaines 1982c).

My research indicates that an individual did attempt to create a unified, coherent body of Christian psychiatrists, a 'Christian psychiatry'. However, the attempt failed and a distinct, relatively homogeneous group did not emerge. (It should be noted that some observers and participants in the religious scene who have an interest in promoting religion sometimes use the term 'Christian Psychiatry' (and even 'Christian law', e.g., Christians practicing law) as a means of showing that the new religious thought in America is quite widespread even among professionals and other high status groups.)

A Christian psychiatrist respresents the coincidence of at least two distinguishable identities, as is implied by the appellation. In suggesting that the identity of a Christian psychiatrist is at least a dual one, note that for the sake of simplicity of presentation I leave aside the several other components of the total identity of these or any other individuals such as age, gender, marital status, ethnicity, nationality and the like (see Devereux 1982 on the nature of personal identity as a unique combination of a number of identities).

To be called a "Christian", in the sense of the term which my informants intend, indicates to them and to others of their subculture that the individual has developed an on-going, personal relationship with "the Savior". This relationship is generally believed to have developed during a specific episode or event in which the individual "realized the power of God", or that "Jesus truly loved" him or her or that "it was time to let Jesus into" his/her life. However it occurs, an individual has an experience which is interpreted as a personal experience of "the Savior" and as such constitutes a "second birth". Thus, the individual is said to be "born again". The experience is of sufficient emotional significance to the individual that she or he will later frequently relate it to others in a process called "testifying". (One usually testifies to another believer, and so it is that one will both testify and bear witness to others' testimony.)

Members of the traditions who adhere to these beliefs may be called Evangelical and/or Fundamentalist Christians. Some people, including one of my informants, prefer to describe the transformative experience as becoming "alive in Christ". He believes that the phrase "born again" has become "too commercialized", and so he refers to himself as "alive in Christ", not "born again". He means by this that Christ, and the other two constituents of the Holy Trinity, are alive, dwelling within the individual; he also believes that the person is animated, enlivened by that in-dwelling presence. In his view and that of his co-believers, a person is both physical and spiritual, sacred and profane.

The first portion of the dual identity, as Christian and psychiatrist, involves a religious transformation and is a set of experiences and beliefs ostensibly not found associated with the second half of the identity, considered below.

Psychiatry is a speciality of Western Biomedicine which deals with a number of problems considered in the West to comprise a single domain called "mental disorders (or illness)". To a lesser extent, this medical speciality is also concerned with questions of what is called "mental health". The field of action of this specialty is wide and includes the diagnosis, management, research on and treatment of a host of often ill-defined "diseases" of the "brain", conceived as a physical entity, and the immaterial "mind", seen as the seat of emotion, perception and cognition. The field also treats of behavioral disorders of the young and of adults and the elderly (American Psychiatric Association 1980).

Psychiatric disorders may be present in the absence of abnormalities of brain and, conversely, abnormalities of brain are not necessarily manifested as abnormalities of mind. The specialty thus treats disorders said to be psychogenic (purely problems of mind), organic (problems of brain structure or processes), developmental (either problems of mind or brain seen developmentally), characterological (usually problems of mind but referring to distortions, disorders, malformations, etc. of the 'personality', which itself is the total psychological organization or being of a person), toxicological (acute or chronic problems of mind or of brain resulting from ingestion of noxious substances), and also, apparent social problems ("conduct disorders") which cannot be easily attributed to problems in either brain *or* mind (American Psychiatric Association 1980).

Within the specialty, there exist a number of subspecialties including child, consultation-liaison, geriatric, forensic, social, community and "cultural" psychiatry Kleinman (1980a). A practitioner in one or more of these subspecialties is a psychiatrist, though the approach to problems which a given psychiatrist will take may vary widely from his or her colleagues within any given subspecialty (Gaines 1979; Johnson, this volume).

This portion of the dual identity is, like the first, anchored in a set of experiences, called "medical education", and "psychiatric residency", and in the certification of such experiences and knowledge acquisition. Research suggests that preresidency medical education and residency itself only minimally affect training psychiatrists' conceptions of the etiology of mental illnesses (Gaines 1979; Light 1976), though such experiences seem powerful in terms of role behavior. Rather, professional training provides a means for *refining preexisting* notions of mental illness. For this reason, research indicates the similarity of folk and professional beliefs in particular cultures (Townsend 1978; Kleinman 1980b). It is suggested here that previous cultural experience has established cultural conceptions of mental disorders which remain relatively stable through medical education (see Gaines 1979).

The co-occurrence of two sets of experience, one which transforms the individual in terms of his relation to a perceived divinity, and the other a lengthy, secular educational experience in accredited institutions, *may* produce a Christian psychiatrist. Individuals known as Christian psychiatrists also may have had some rather lengthy educational experiences in seminary or bible college. In fact, all of my Christian psychiatrist informants have done missionary work for periods of up to a year or more, usually in other countries. Ironically, these experiences give to some of these psychiatrists an interest in and affection for anthropology.

Christian psychiatrists hold views in common which (more apparently than actually) distinguish them individually and collectively from other psychiatrists. First, they all believe in "salvation" through being born again. They believe that they, as individuals and collectivities, professional, familial and congregational, have an on-going, personal relationship with Jesus Christ, the Savior and they are thereby "saved".

They further believe that Jesus, God and the Holy Spirit are, like the Nuer's notion of *kwoth*, refractions of a single divinity. They also believe that there is a connection between the world of their God and that of humans. The connection is at least twofold: God may act in the lives of people, and, indeed, dwell within them, and people may communicate with God (or Jesus) through prayer.

Prayer may involve communication with divinity through thoughts or through speech. Prayer activity may be conducted in solitude or in groups, wherein individuals may be praying for the same or different desires or goals. Related to the belief in communication with divinity is the notion that divinity may speak to the individual. This speech act often seems to be regarded as divine placement of words or thoughts into the mind of the individual. Communications thus may flow in two directions, each side 'hearing' the other and potentially being affected by such communications.

Based upon these beliefs, it is understandable that my informants believe that prayer is a potentially efficacious therapeutic tool. They do not, however, agree on the extent to which prayer should or could be used; nor do they agree on the appropriateness of specific contexts of prayer, 'with' or 'for' their patients.

Christian psychiatrists also believe that Scripture is the ultimate authority. In all matters, Scripture serves as the final, unequivocal word. However, my informants are Evangelical Christians, and hence should be distinguished from Fundamentalist Christians. That is, while all of my Evangelical informants (who in fact belong to several different denominations, including Baptist, Church of God and Southern Presbyterian) share the view that Scripture is the final authority, none would accept literal interpretations of Scripture. Their nonliteral interpretations distinguish them from Fundamentalists, though the two groups do in fact share many theological beliefs. Evangelicals do not seem to establish unitary doctrines or to exact conformity to particular theological conceptions. Hence, there are differences of opinion within the 'group' and there seems little effort to exact unanimity on particular issues. A final commonality of those called Christian psychiatrists is the belief that such individuals should manifest "Christian love" toward all other people, whether they are believers or not, whether patients, friends or acquaintances.

Christian psychiatrists seem to contrast with other psychiatrists in several ways. Christian psychiatrists often use a term for themselves which, taken literally, does not distinguish them from a host of others. That is, there are many psychiatrists with few, if any, of the beliefs noted above, who nonetheless describe themselves as "Christians". Several people I interviewed, some of whom were not psychiatrists and some of whom were, stated that they "resented" what they saw as a "restricted" use of the term "Christian". Some lay persons felt that the designation "Christian" is inappropriate for people such as my informants. For example, Catholics regard themselves as Christians and dislike the cooption of the term by Protestant Fundamentalists and Evangelicals.

My informants are not the only Evangelicals or Fundamentalists who are psychiatrists. That is, not all individuals with a personal relationship with God who are psychiatrists call themselves or are known as Christian psychiatrists, though they certainly are known as Christians. Many Christians, in fact, do not even regard my Evangelical informants as "proper" Christians, but as rather "strange birds" who give a bad name to the larger flock, which includes Catholics, Lutherans, Calvinists and others.

There is still another level to consider. The label implies for some that Christian psychiatrists are the only psychiatric professionals who have a regard for or interest in specifically Christian values in their practice in particular, or for spiritual issues in general. Other informants have stated that while they are not the same sort of Christians as my informants, they too are concerned with and take account of spiritual values and beliefs in their clinical practice, and sometimes in their private lives.

Several informants who are atheists have stated that they feel the appellation makes it appear that they, as labeled "secular" psychiatrists, are unconcerned with spiritual issues when, in fact, they often concerned themselves with these issues in their clinical work.

We may now look at secular psychiatry to ascertain just how distinctive is the faith of the Christian psychiatrists. We will see that religious beliefs are in fact quite widespread among psychiatrists other than those who define or conduct their work in religious terms. In a recent survey conducted by the American Psychiatric Association (1975), a subsample of 900 randomly selected individuals was asked to state theological viewpoints in terms of three choices, "theistic", "agnostic", and "atheistic". (The total sample was 14,843).

Fully 86% of the respondents gave clear answers, and 70.3% of this group stated they were "theistic" (APA 1975:19). Eleven percent stated that they had at least some theological training. Of this figure, half had sufficient training, three years, to complete their seminary education (APA 1975:18). Some 75.3% of providers attended church or temple at least occasionally, and only 9.2% "never" attended a place of worship (APA 1975:21). Christian psychiatrists are thus not alone in their belief in divinity among those in this professional cadre. These data provide our first look at what is perhaps less of a singular, distinct group than might have been anticipated by the reader newly acquainted with Christian psychiatrists.

Next, I want to consider some aspects of Kleinman's formulation of "core clinical functions" of "all health care systems" (Kleinman 1980b:71). There are five functions as he outlined them:

- The cultural construction of illness as psychosocial experience.
- The establishment of general criteria to guide the health care seeking process and to evaluate treatment approaches that exist prior to and independent of individual episodes of sickness.
- The management of particular illness episodes through communicative operations such as labeling and explaining.
- Healing activities *per se*, which include all types of therapeutic interventions, from drugs and surgery to psychotherapy, supportive care, and healing rituals.
- The management of therapeutic outcomes, including cure, treatment failure, recurrence, chronic illness, impairment and death [Kleinman 1980b:71–72].

HELP-SEEKING AND CLINICAL REALITY

I shall consider first the means of help-seeking which lead individuals to psychiatrists and to Christian psychiatrists. Looking at some commonalities and dissimilarities may be enlightening as concerns several core clinical functions of the local health care system. First, it should be mentioned that there are rich traditions in both Christian and secular medicine. And Christian psychiatrists are by no means the only Christian (in the 'born again' sense) medical professionals practicing in the area where this study was undertaken. In addition, there are numbers of folk healers including "power doctors", root doctors, spiritual healers and readers, clergypersons of different denominations who provide help for various problems and, of course, herbalists. I have also encountered a lovely old woman who receives payment in goods from others for her abilities in producing efficacious prayers for them. Finally, the popular, family-based level of health care is alive and well even in this area sometimes called the "City of Medicine".

Help-Seeking

In an earlier study, I looked at how psychiatric patients found their way into the psychiatric emergency room and hence into the psychiatric system (Gaines 1979). This work confirmed that of earlier researchers by pointing out that the diagnostic process which leads to the psychiatric system is a lay diagnostic process wherein friends, relatives, workmates, neighbors or even the future patient him or herself makes the initial judgment that the problem at hand is psychological or mental and not "physical" (Mechanic 1962), according to the bifurcate division of disorders in the indigenous ethnomedical system.

In brief, Christian and secular psychiatrists obtain their patients in many of the same ways, through referrals from lay persons, other physicians, and from emergency rooms and wards if they are "attending" at one of the local hospitals. Increasingly, however, Christian psychiatrists are receiving referrals from other Christian physicians and Christian lay persons. I have a number of cases, for example, in which Christian surgeons make referrals to Christian psychiatrists when some post-operative emotional problem, usually depression, evidences itself. There seems to be developing quite a bit of this "in-house", or "in-faith" referring (and consulting).

There are cases also of secular psychiatrists referring patients to Christian psychiatrist. This seems to occur when a patient's clinical presentation includes a considerable amount of religious ideation.

Clinical Reality

Here we can note that religious orientation, or lack thereof, may be added to the list of factors affecting help-seeking, at least in America's "Bible Belt". But we should also be aware that the definition of problems, the illnesses, will likewise be cultural, i.e., "meaningful" in cultural terms (Good 1977). Christians may seek aid for illnesses which seem distinct from those found in the dominant culture. I will consider two such problems, the first of which is divorce. Divorce is seen as a problem requiring both spiritual and Christian psychiatric assistance. In the Christian tradition we are focusing on, divorce is both an illness and a disease, the latter in the sense that it is a problem seen as a clinical entity by the professional healers of the health care system.

Because of the strong male bias of the tradition, which is consistent with the Mediterranean culture area from which it comes, the desires of a woman seeking divorce may lead her to be treated by a Christian psychiatrist (though many Christian psychiatrists would not accept such a "case"). To understand the construction of divorce as both illness and disease (in using this distinction, I assume these two realities are independent of one another, not mirror images), we must recognize the sacred nature of this institution among my informants. Marriage is taken with enormous seriousness and the maintenance of the union is of utmost importance to them.

In one case, a woman of about thirty-five years of age was admitted to Mason Medical Center for emotional and behavioral problems with which her family and friends could not cope. She had decided to leave her husband of fifteen years. One might think that she had good reason to leave him; he had a drinking problem, had had affairs with other women, and he physically abused the patient. However, it was reported to me by a psychiatric nurse that the case was referred to a very well-known Christian psychiatrist on the staff of Mason Medical. This psychiatrist recommended that the woman return to her husband, and that such was her "Christian duty". She "should ask God" for the ability to understand her husband and to allow her to have "Christian patience and endurance". In a sense he suggested she would be a better Christian and a better person if she returned to her husband, without making any changes in her situation. This kind of recommendation is not uncommon. A psychiatrist on the staff of Mason who is psychoanalytically trained, in a discussion about this sort of case, examples of which were known to him, felt strongly that such recommendations were wrong; they served only to "confirm and validate the sadistic tendencies of the husbands" in question (and the masochism of some women).

There is another sort of case which may end up under the care of a Christian psychiatrist. These are "cases" of homosexuality. Interestingly, these cases, and those of divorce above, are referred not only by other professionals, but often by members of the congregations or fellowship groups of the Christian psychiatrists. This is a source of referrals which other psychiatrists would be less likely to have. Homosexuality is considered a sin, an "abomination", to Evangelicals and Fundamentalists alike. One of my informants has had great "success treating homosexuality". His major tools are prayer and conversion, the leading of the patient to God. If a person undergoes the 'born again' experience, he or she often may cease the practice of homosexuality (Gaines 1982c). It is thus seen as both an illness (or sin) and a disease which a Christian psychiatrist may be very effective in "treating".

CONCEPTIONS OF PERSON

This section explores notions of person which distinguish the two sorts of psychiatrists and which seem to be responsible for discernible differential interpretations and subsequent actions in the clinical sphere. Later we shall look at aspects of psychiatric practice among both the Christian and "secular" psychiatrists. In that regard, the focus will be on the logic of praxis in psychiatry for these two categories of psychiatrists, and also their respective notions of therapeutic efficacy. Several cases will illustrate the belief of Christian psychiatrists that a "Christian perpective" made a difference in the clinical outcome. We shall see the essentially hermeneutic nature of clinical interactions grounded in cultural assumptions and conceptions which preexist, but which may be refined in and brought to bear on, particular interactional encounters. A key cultural conception appearing in clinical contexts is that of person.

Early in the 1950s, and again recently, researchers have focused their attention on cultural conceptions of the person (Lee 1959; Hallowell 1955; Shweder and Bourne 1982; Geertz 1973; Gaines 1982a; Conner 1982). It is now seems beyond doubt that different cultures hold differing conceptions of the person, and that these conceptions vary radically across cultures in ways which are not related to economic or educational variations (Shweder and Bourne 1982).

I will mention briefly here and explore later a suggestion for a means of giving context to, and providing insight into, patients' conceptualizations of their illness problems. Kleinman et al. (1978) and Kleinman (1980b) have found that patients have cognitive models of their illness episodes; they refer to these models as 'Explanatory Models' (EMs). They recognize that not only do patients have EMs, but so do healers. What I will suggest here is that EMs are in part reflections of larger cultural conceptions; in particular, conceptions of the person. I suggest that the key conception of person *organizes* cultural knowledge which gives rise to the EM of patient and healer. That is, a non-medically focused notion, that of person, lies behind and organizes patients' and healers' thinking about sickness episodes. Put another way, we may say that a cultural or folk theory underlies and gives shape to cultural knowledge and direction to cultural thinking about sickness. I shall return to this point below.

It was Geertz (1977) who may be said to have rekindled, among many other topics, our interest in cross-cultural conceptions of person. He gives us some insights into our own, Western, conception of self in the course of his examination of Balinese, Moroccan and Javanese concepts of person and self. Geertz describes the Western self as:

a *bounded, unique*, more or less *integrated* motivational and cognitive *universe*, a dynamic *center* of awareness, emotion, judgment, and action organized into a *distinctive whole* and *set contrastively both against other such wholes* and *against a social and natural background* ... (1977:9). (Emphases added.)

Geertz assumes a unitary notion in the West though his own work on the pervasiveness of religious orientations (1973) would suggest a division in the West into at least several traditions.

I suggest there are two major cultural traditions in the West, the Protestant European and the Mediterranean Traditions,[1] each with it distinctive conception of person and self (Gaines 1982a). I suggest that Geertz' description of person refers to the Protestant European conception which I have termed "referential". This is the concept of person which is to be found in the dominant ideology, including that of medicine and psychiatry, in America. I want to emphasize some of the features of this conception.

The person is a bounded, physical entity; personhood is coterminous with the extent of the physical body, the domain of the core of medicine, internal medicine (Hahn 1982, and this volume). The person, furthermore, is seen as unique, though a combination of 'typical' features. The person is a center of awareness, judgment and action whose organizational integrity stems from inner affective and cognitive, i.e., psychological, resources and strengths. The self is seen as whole, complete unto itself, and it is thought to exist in an environment consisting of other such unique, distinct, separate "individuals" — a word which conveys the notion of bounded uniqueness and autonomy.

Disorder conceived of in a worldview containing such a notion of person logically must locate the problem *within* an "individual", that is, within the physical confines of a person so conceived. So too must therapy be directed toward the individual and healing activities focused on the body and mind (as constituents) of the individual person. A concrete, constant person exists which is referred to in discourse.

In contrast, the conception of person which can be elucidated from expressed thought and action of our Christian psychiatrist informants provides a rather different view of personhood. The Christian person is in fact quite similar to that outlined for the Mediterranean Tradition, the "indexical" person (Gaines 1982a). This should not be surprising as both are, as Arensberg once called them, "people of the Book" (also see Davis 1975). First of all, the Christian self and the reflection of the self seen in others, the person, is a spiritual self. That is, the self is not solely, or even primarily, a physical entity — a unique, corporeal object. The boundary (if indeed there is a boundary in the same sense, the notion of boundary perhaps being a function of *a particular* view of person in the first instance) is drawn around, or is permeated by extra-corporeal elements. Specifically, the self *includes* spirits (see also Hallowell 1955; Conner 1982), in this case the several elements of and the totality of the Trinity. Discourse about it indexes *only* a given encounter and thus may change over time.

The in- and extra-dwelling spirits observe, involve themselves in peoples' lives, listen to them, hold expectations, even tempt them. For the latter, we should note that there are "evil" as well as good spirits. Not the least of these evil spirits is the devil. It is believed that the devil can move people to act and is thought to be capable of residing within an individual or remaining outside of him or her and from that vantage point directing the actions of the person.

Likewise, good spirits are believed to be in-dwelling as well as external. As Saint Paul said, "I live; yet not I; but Christ liveth in me". The spirit dwells within the believer from the moment of his or her second birth. The in-dwelling spirit is seen as animating the person and "leading" the person in his or her life.

The presence of a unified, in-dwelling overseer and sovereign implies several things of importance to us here. First, the uniqueness of a person is in some sense diminished, for all believers share an in-dwelling and animating spirit. Second, the sharing of a spiritual dimension makes an individual a part of a total Christian community and family. And it is the family that is considered a sacred social unit, not the individual (or his or her rights, or wants or needs). According to this view, what animates an individual, what is good and positive about a person, are things not unique to a given person; they are elements shared by all believers. The focus of thought is not on that which is unique about a person, but that which is held in common. The individual is a refraction of the Christian community and family and, as such, the self is *not the center* of awareness as in the case of the referential conception of person. Nor is the person or self seen as complete. On the contrary, a person without the spirit is by definition *incomplete*.

Further, the person is *not the source* of action, whether good or bad, since the person is animated by spiritual entities. Clearly the person is not conceived of as autonomous, but rather is a sort of shell filled and moved by superior spiritual forces and entities.

All this makes for a person who is "socio-centric" rather than "ego-centric" (see Shweder and Bourne 1982). It can be seen that the person is *both self and other* in this tradition, just as Lacan has claimed in his formulations in French psychoanalysis (Turkle 1978). And, importantly, White and Marsella have recently pointed out that when behavior is seen to emanate from an individual, seen as bounded (a corporeal self), agency and responsibility are attributed to *either* the self or to other, bounded selves (1982), i.e., neither to social relations nor spirits.

In cultures where persons are considered as more than mere physical entities, agents are located in one or more of several places *outside* of the physical limits of the person as patient, in family networks or ancestors as in China (Kleinman 1980b) and Japan (Lebra 1976) or in disrupted community relations as among the Ndembu (Turner 1969). All of these examples highlight the conception of the interrelation of self and other, the latter in the form of family and community. The individual, then, is more an *expression* of a larger community than an autonomous "individual".

Primacy of the individual is not to be found in this tradition; the tradition itself, or those aspects of it which are seen as (symbolically) representing it such as marriage, family or life style, are primary. This point lays bare the logic underlying treatment recommendations for the two "problems" mentioned earlier, divorce and homosexuality.

There are other important features to consider as well with regard to the Christian concept of person, most notably, aspects of the personality or dimensions of inner psychological resources such as "strength", "will", "patience", and "endurance". What is important here is that these qualities and resources are seen as the property of an in-dwelling spirit, not as personal qualities of an individual *qua* individual. Success or luck (good or bad) are seen as ultimately stemming from a spiritual source, i.e., outside the domain of personal responsibility. These ideas, these assumptions, may be seen to have some import for clinical praxis among Christian psychiatrists, including diagnosis and therapeutic activities.

CLINICAL PRAXIS

It is of central importance to recognize the hermeneutic, interpretive nature of clinical practice. Just as all illness episodes must be seen as essentially semantic or meaningful episodes (Good 1977), so too much clinical interactions be seen as essentially hermeneutic or interpretive encounters (Good and Good 1981:4). Diagnosis should be seen as an interpretation of symbolic elements, not as a reading of signs of distress which have clinical import *sui generis*. One result of clinical interactions is a definition of the nature of the current situation or condition of the patient, that is, the EM of the physician. The condition which is thought to exist is "clinical reality". It is thought to exist as a feature of the patient, as an individual, at the time of presentation in the clinical context (Kleinman 1980b), and as such manifests a referential view of persons.

If the construction, through interaction in clinical contexts, of clinical reality were a mere decoding of signs and not a semantic, hermeneutic encounter, the bringing to bear of different perspectives on clinical reality, especially non-biomedical perspectives, should not alter that constructed clinical reality. However, research indicates that clinical reality can be changed by the introduction in clinical settings of aspects of anthropological science including knowledge, methodology and theory (Good and Good 1981; Gaines 1982b). New information, or a different perspective, can change the clinical reality because it can alter the *meaning* of the signs of sickness, signs which are actually symbols, things which stand for, but do not resemble their referents.

As Schutz pointed out (1967), people interpret current interactional encounters through a process of negotiation based upon their understandings of the meanings of elements (symbolic) brought to and exchanged in those encounters (words, acts, gestures). Their understandings of these events and that of their coparticipants are based upon their "stock-of-knowledge at hand" which is built up or "precipitated" from previous social experience. Here we raise the issue of the meaning of presenting complaints as symbolic complexes for both patient and healer. Phrased in another way, this is the issue of transference in clinical practice (see Good et al. in this volume). Just as (secular) psychiatrists view their patients, in terms of unconscious assumptions such as the corporeal nature of persons, so too do the Christian psychiatrists. As the psychiatrist seeks to treat a disorder believed to be located within the physical boundary of the person, the Christian psychiatrist sees both a physical and a spiritual being before him or her. Whether the patient him- or herself is aware of one's own spiritual nature is not important; the Christian knows that side or dimension is present, existing as an unrecognized vital aspect of being.

Patients, and people in general, are seen and perceived in meaningful terms according to a remembered past and an assumed conception of self (and, hence, of Other). This may be seen in the examples of divorce and homosexuality. The ideal situation for the Christian is dependency, dependence on Jesus. Autonomy, as in the case of a woman seeking divorce, is thus *not* viewed favorably in this tradition as it would be in the dominant (European Protestant) tradition in American culture and psychiatry. The emphasis on this dependent relationship is reflected in the phrase, "believe *on* God (or Jesus)", rather than "in" God or Jesus. Thus, therapeutic or diagnostic action in the Christian tradition may be based upon a notion of the incompleteness of the person, necessitating action to *maintain* dependence, including leaving a situation as is and simply "enduring" it. The primary emphasis on community (including family) fosters a therapy which maintains rather than splinters those units. In their therapy, Christian psychiatrists believe that God is ever-present and is an active agent in the therapeutic process. His role is seen to vary from that of an assistant to that of the sole, prime mover in the process, depending upon the Christian psychiatrist (Gaines 1982c). Since divinity is part of the therapeutic process (and part of the therapist as well), it should not be surprising that elements of the religious socio-centrism would often prevail over the usual ego-centric approach which posits that improvement depends upon individual action, personal efforts which are an individual's responsibilities (see Townsend 1978; Nunnlly 1961).

Several other diagnostic, therapeutic and management activities are undertaken by Christian psychiatrists which *may* not be seen among "secular" psychiatrists. The first activity I will discuss here concerns an aspect of the diagnostic assessment which some Christian psychiatrists may employ.

Spiritual History

A new development among some Christian psychiatrists is the taking of a "spiritual history". This development is clearly predicated upon the belief that people are spiritual creatures. The spiritual history is distinct from the initial interview (for which see Rittenberg and Simons, this volume), the mental status examination and the usual medical history. The users of the spiritual history feel that it is relevant to an understanding of the resources which individuals may draw upon, or have drawn upon in the past, when confronted with a crisis. The spiritual history includes information on the general background of the individual, especially education, church affiliations and attendance and the like. The history focuses on crisis situations in an effort to explore the family, community and specifically religious sources of support which the patient drew upon in the past. The Christian psychiatrist taking a spiritual history would want to know how particular crises were handled, how they were "endured".

In addition to the general background information, information on crises and sources of support, the spiritual history is intended to point up the value of religion in the patient's life, if the patient has been religious, or to sensitize the patient to this potential in his or her life. In fact, I believe that a major reason or goal of the taking of the spiritual history *is* the sensitization of non- or "under"-religious people and the confirmation of the importance of the dependent relationship with divinity which may be helpful in the patient's current situation.

In a presentation by a Christian psychiatrist to a group of Christian mental health workers, a speaker explained the use of the spiritual history and gave an illuminating example. The speaker, a Christian psychiatrist from California, said that the spiritual history was not only for "the religious", but also for the "atheistic". He said that the spiritual history can point up, for the patient and the healer, a certain lack in the patient's life, the satisfaction of which might be helpful in overcoming the current problem.

As an example, the psychiatrist related an episode from his own clinical experience. The case concerned a friend of the speaker, who, it was pointed out, was an atheist and had experienced a life-threatening illness requiring hospitalization and surgical intervention. The patient evidenced marked depressive affect, the recognition of which led to a psychiatric consultation. The patient's interpretation of his illness, his EM, was that his life, as he had lived it up to that point, was over. His active lifestyle was impossible with his condition; regarding this outcome, the patient's EM coincided with that of his physician.

Prior to surgery, a consultation had been called for and a spiritual history taken. Post-operatively, the consulting Christian psychiatrist continued to work with the patient. The outcome was that the patient survived the ordeal and could look forward to a new, though altered, lifestyle, as a "born again" Christian. In this case, the spiritual history was shown to have converted an atheist in crisis, thus demonstrating the proselytic utility of the spiritual history. Also, however, it demonstrated "empirically", the positive benefits for the patient, i.e., his discovery of new meaning and value in his new, previously devalued, inactive lifestyle. This example points up another therapeutic modality which Christian psychiatrists employ — conversion.

Conversion

The use of conversion is neither universally accepted nor employed by Christian psychiatrists. As mentioned earlier, one practitioner has found conversion quite useful as a therapeutic tool for "curing" homosexuality. The use of conversion as a therapeutic goal, which does indeed alter people's lifestyle as long as they do not "backslide", again points to the conception of the person as spiritual, as potentially a part of an animating divinity.

Prayer With and Prayer For

The use of prayer has been discussed elsewhere (Gaines 1982c) and the distinction drawn between *prayer with* and *prayer for*. The former describes prayer involving patient *and* healer in the clinical context. Such activity dramatically symbolizes the presence and interest of divinity in the healing process, His power to influence that process, and the fact that the healing context is not diadic, but triadic. Both patient and healer submit themselves to the ultimate power, thus effacing the individual basis of the relationship as understood in traditional psychiatry. *Prayer for* a patient is that which is done by the physician in the absence of the patient, usually in non-clinical contexts. Christian psychiatrists will pray for all of their patients, regardless of the faith, or lack of it, of those patients. The patient is usually not made aware of these prayers whereas, in the case of the use of *prayer with* a patient, the patient is aware, and must be a party to, the communication with God, the Holy Spirit or Jesus. However, recent data from my informants indicate a new conceptualization of prayer as a therapeutic tool.

Prayer Observed

A new use of prayer by Christian psychiatrists has its analogue in the early use of hypnosis in psychoanalysis. The patient is asked if he or she feels like praying to God about his or her problems and concerns. Unlike *prayer with* a patient, the psychiatrist in this instance observes the prayer but does not participate. The purpose of the observation is to obtain insight into the genuine, conscious and unconscious concerns of the psychiatrist's patient. The underlying idea was summed up by an informant, whom I shall call Dr. Davis. He explained that having the patient pray about his/her problems and feelings allowed the therapist to get to the heart of the matter much more quickly than would otherwise be the case. As he said, "They may lie to me, but they won't lie to God".

Dr. Davis demonstrates a recognition that his patients, whether Christian or not, may not be candid and honest with him. The observation of patients' thus allows him access to feelings, thoughts and beliefs which might otherwise remain concealed from him for some time. The therapeutic process thus moves more rapidly, he says. With one patient, he and his supervisor (Dr. Davis recently finished his residency) believe that the therapeutic process was completed successfully and at least a year earlier than would have been possible without the use of *prayer observed*.

In considering prayer here, we have raised another issue of importance for the practice of Christian psychiatrists. This issue is the meaning of the religious orientation of the patients of these professional healers. Dr. Davis is an example of a Christian psychiatrist who does not expect his patients, even if "born again", to be truthful with him. How deep does such a feeling run, and how general is it among Christian psychiatrists?

Practice and Cynicism

An outside observer, especially an "atheistic" one, might suggest, as have many "secular" psychiatrist informants, that the religious presentations of the patient may be a mask, resistance to the therapeutic process. Surprisingly, Christian psychiatrists wholeheartedly agree. I posed the question to two of my informants because of its relevance to their clinical practice. Both informants, Dr. Lane from my earlier study (1982c) and Dr. Davis, stated categorically that in fact they *assumed*, until otherwise proven, that *any* patient seeking their aid *because* they were Christian psychiatrists was using his/her religion as a mask for other problems. That is, at least initially, the presentation of the patient as Christian to a Christian therapist was assumed to indicate problems submerged under a religious guise.

My informants went on to say that, contrary to others' ideas about them, they do not expect every problem confronted to be a religious one. Informants stated that when they began their residency, they assumed that "all problems were religious" and that they had to "learn to be cautious about employing prayer with patients" and other things. They said they had a tendency to "jump right in" with their religious orientation. Experience, however, made them wary of the veracity of the religious dimension of the problems with which some of their patients presented.

Moreover, none of my informants has any interest in working in a purely Christian environment and several have turned down very lucrative positions in Christian clinics and universities for less high paying positions at other universities which do not have a Christian orientation. Thus, the practice of psychiatry, including training, makes Christian psychiatrists *less* religious in their orientation to patients rather than the reverse. However, this does not affect their notion of the nature of persons or their relationship with the divine. What is affected are their ideas regarding the general utility of religiously influenced diagnostic, therapeutic and management strategies.

SYMBOLIC GROUPS:
SUMMARY AND CONCLUSIONS

The foregoing account has provided some clues about the nature of psychiatry as a profession, about professions in general and about anthropological theory as it attempts to comprehend such collectivities, in terms of their defining features of belief and action. I have considered psychiatrists and Christian psychiatrists in terms of their defining features of belief and action including their respective conceptions of persons. In looking at the defining characteristics, which would seem to delimit the boundaries of groups, the distinctiveness of the groups begins to blur and the groups seem to lose their individuality.

For example, not all Christians who are psychiatrists are Christian psychiatrists. Not all secular psychiatrists are uninterested in religion in their practice and, as noted above, Christian psychiatrist through experience come to define many, if not most, of their patients' presenting complaints in non-religious terms. There are individuals with religious training, such as bible college, who do not practice a personal version of Christian psychiatry. Many "secular" psychiatrists were shown to be believers (American Psychiatric Association 1975) rather than "atheistic". And we even see reference to the Lord and His power in the core of Biomedicine, internal medicine, by a practitioner who most likely does not regard religion as central or even relevant in his medical work (Hahn, this volume).

The Christian ideology of my informants is held by others both non-professionals and professionals; the latter includes members of such organizations as the Christian lawyers' association or that of Christian realtors. Christian psychiatrists' beliefs do not actually distinguish them from all other psychiatrists or non-psychiatrists; the boundaries of the "group" are thus quite indistinct. A specific religious orientation employed in their practice is likewise without uniqueness, for I am aware of practicing priest psychiatrists and rabbi psychiatrists in the northeastern United States.

In terms of training, there are at least two American psychiatric residency programs which offer, within the context of secular state-supported medical education, Christian psychiatric residency training much as any other subspecialty training would be offered. Residents for these programs are recruited by advertisements placed in Christian journals and magazines, as well as through informal channels. At least one program provides a rotation in a Christian hospital for both Christian and secular residents. The patient population of the hospital is largely Christian (e.g., Evangelical and Fundamentalist Protestant).

In looking at help-seeking, some differences emerge in the ways in which Christian psychiatrists obtain their patients. However, the means by which patients find their way to Christian psychiatrists are not wholly dissimilar to those of other psychiatrists. As I have pointed out, "secular" psychiatrists, and other specialists, do receive and make referrals to Christian psychiatrists inspite of the tendency for intra-faith referrals. In fact, many of the patients received by Christian psychiatrists doubtless come from "secular" sources. Here again we find a lack of distinctive corporateness.

Two forms of sickness in the Christian tradition, divorce and homosexuality, seem at first blush to distinguish this "group" of healers. Divorce, however, *is* considered by secular psychiatry to be a stressful event as it causes major life disruptions, some positive and some negative, as well as engendering very strong emotions such as loss, frustration, guilt, anger, abandonment and the like. While secular psychiatry may locate a disease, e.g., depression, *in* a person which is a *result* of divorce, there is clearly considerable overlap in the secular and Christian viewpoints, especially if one notes feelings of guilt, or failure (of culturally defined roles). For both, there is a close relationship between divorce as illness and disease.

Homosexuality, while considered a sin and as such both an illness and a disease in the Christian tradition, has only recently been perceived very differently by secular psychiatry. DSM III (American Psychiatric Association 1980) makes the new distinction between ego-syntonic and ego-dystonic homosexuality with the latter only being a psychiatric disease; and most lay people still believe either form to indicate serious problems. It is certainly not long ago that homosexuals were handed over to the mental health industry for "cures". So again, the difference between "born agains" and "seculars" turns out to be more apparent than real.

This article has also argued for the centrality of the concept of person for an understanding of EMs of patient and healer and for understanding clinical praxis. But I hasten to point out, as is implied in the foregoing, that while we can contrast the conception of person among Christian psychiatrists with that of secular psychiatrists, neither conception is unique. The Christian view is that of the people of the Mediterranean, or "Book", originally; it is shared with the vast majority of the patients attending Mason Medical Center which is located in the "Bible Belt". Also recall that some 30–40% of Americans say they have experienced something equivalent to being "born again". A key belief in terms of Christian psychiatric clinical practice does not distinguish them from some other professionals and non-professionals in the wider society.

Among those called Christian psychiatrists, then, we find, as we do among secular psychiatrists, a wide range of beliefs and practices. For example the use of conversion as a therapeutic tool is found among Christian psychiatrists, but so far as I am able to determine, its use is quite rare among them. Of my six informants, only one uses conversion as a tool; the other informants all strongly *disavow* its use in their practice. I earlier pointed out the variety of beliefs about the role of divinity in the therapeutic process and the differing views of prayer with and prayer for (Gaines 1982c), as well as the innovation of the observation of patients' prayer.

In the use of conversion and prayer as therapeutic modalities, Christian psychiatrists represent the beliefs and values of their cultural tradition, just as do practitioners of other branches of Western Biomedicine (Gaines and Hahn 1982; and this volume), thus falsifying assertions that "only in tribal societies are values unseparated from medical facts" (Taussig 1980). We also note that psychiatric ideology, whether secular or Christian, is widely shared *vertically* in the social body. Ideas in medicine may be more refined, but they are nonetheless cultural ideas at base which are shared with culture-mates of various social categories.

More importantly, just as some in medicine (and others outside of it) adhere to an "empiricist theory of language" (Good and Good 1981), others seem to adhere to an empiricist theory of medicine (Taussig 1980; Illich 1975) and medical practice. Research presented in this volume and elsewhere in recent years points up the cultural basis of medical practice, medicine as a cultural system, the great heterogeneity of belief and praxis within specialties of medicine, and the overlap in belief and practice with folk and popular sectors of local health care systems (Kleinman 1980; Townsend 1978; Lock, this volume; Gaines 1979, 1982a, b, c).

Diversity of opinion and practice characterizes the ideology and praxis of any medical specialty. The same ideas and practice may be found among other specialties in whole or in part, often in different guises. For example, psychiatrists treat mental sickness, but so do general practitioners, psychologists and the clergy. Psychotropic drugs may be, and presently are, given by other medical specialists and psychotherapy is provided by any number of professional and quasi-professional mental health workers. What are the qualities of a good psychiatrist which distinguish him or her from other medical specialists? Sir Denis Hill (1978), after considering all of the aspects of psychiatric practice, teaching, administration, leadership, treatment, research, etc., could conclude that the qualities of good psychiatrists are "empathy", "responsibility for patients", and "open-mindedness". Such characteristics hardly distinguish psychiatrists, even good ones, from other physicians, not to mention laypersons, concerned with the ill (e.g., folk healers, even family members).

I suggest, then, that the reality, the existence in reality "out there", of Christian psychiatrists or secular psychiatrists or any other such group is a function of empiricist theories of groups as coherent, distinctly labeled social entities which can be contrasted with other such entities, much as the notion of person is conceived in Northern European Protestant tradition. The reality of psychiatry is a matter of abstract conceptualization as are the 'realities' of such entities as human "races" and social classes; these exist in researchers' minds, not "out there". Further, such conceptions are cultural products. We must, therefore, apprehend social and cultural complexity in our research rather than abstracting neat social categories, labeling them, and thereby giving them the cloak of reality such that we can then go about "explaining" them or comparing and contrasting them with other "realities".

I have tried to move back and forth between demonstrating the distinctiveness and, therefore, "groupness" of Christian psychiatry and effacing the view of a group reality so constructed. The complexity of social and cultural realities of Biomedicine suggests that we would do best not to resort to stereotypic, and generally distorted, *macro* critiques of a putatively monolithic and ideologically and behaviorally distinct social group, whether such critiques come from the left (e.g., Taussig 1980; Navarro 1976) or the right (e.g., Illich 1975; Szasz 1961).

A second point I wish to make is more straightforward. The concept of person of professionals and laypersons is of critical importance to an understanding of health-related action, though the conception is neither conscious nor directly germane to sickness episodes. The formulation of the cognitive construct of EMs by Kleinman (1980b) is an important step in understanding lay and professional thinking about sickness (as well as being an important pedagogical device). The model is a clinician's conception of aspects of conscious knowledge which are germane to particular sickness episodes. I would suggest that much thought relevant to clinical contexts or sickness episodes is unconscious and involves understandings, conceptions and assumptions which are not easily articulated as they form the foundation upon which other thoughts, such as the conscious EM, are built. Thus, the interpretation of illness realities for patient and healer occur within broad cultural semantic domains, in what Good has discerned as Semantic Illness Networks (1977). We may say that broad cultural conceptions, such as that of person, *anchor* understandings and knowledge about function and dysfunction, significance and insignificance of specific experiences of symptoms and illness (and define them as such), and also provide nodes of attachment for webs of significance such as Semantic Illness Networks. From these understandings and cultural knowledge are drawn models (EMs) about specific illness episodes.

Sickness befalls persons. But persons are not construed as identical entities cross-culturally. The statement that "a person is sick" is an explanation rather than a description precisely because the meaning and the references of each of the terms vary with the cultural context (Conner 1982; Gaines 1982a; Lee 1959; Shweder and Bourne 1982). What a person is or is not greatly shapes what are thought to be the possibilities of sickness, its cause, outcome and processes. This in turn shapes the conception of sickness, the experience of it and what is deemed appropriate and sufficient therapeutic action in lay, folk and professional circles as individuals manipulate elements of their particular symbolic domains to deal with sickness.

In approaching the meaningful elements of sickness cross-culturally, we need to address the symbolic nature of distress and the symbolic construction of relevant social sectors concerned with the alleviation of it. Without such a perspective, we may miss the meaning of sickness, healing, patients, healers and their symbolic relationship to one another and to the wider domains of human cultural thought and behavior.

ACKNOWLEDGEMENTS

I would like to thank Drs. Robert Hahn and Jan van Breman for their helpful comments on earlier drafts of the present paper.

NOTES

* A version of the present paper was read at the University of Amsterdam Sociology and Anthropology Centrum, May 1983, and that version was published (1983) as 'Person and Practice . . .' Working Paper No. 1, University of Amsterdam Sociology and Anthropology Centrum, Amsterdam, Holland.
1. The existence of a Mediterranean culture area, which includes groups both contiguous and non-contiguous with the Sea, is one of the most significant recent conclusions derived from the anthropology of Europe (see Boissevain 1979; Davis 1975; Gaines 1982a; Gilmore 1982).

REFERENCES

American Psychiatric Association (APA)
  1975 Psychiatrists' Viewpoints on Religion. Washington, D.C.: American Psychiatric Association.
  1980 Diagnostic and Statistical Manual (DSM) III. Washington, D.C.: American Psychiatric Association.
Boissevain, Jeremy
  1979 Toward an Anthropology of the Mediterranean. Current Anthropology 20:81–93.
Conner, Linda
  1982 The Unbounded Self. *In* A. J. Marsella and G. M. White (eds.), Cultural Conceptions of Mental Health and Therapy. Dordrecht, Holland: D. Reidel Publishing Co.
Davis, J.
  1975 People of the Mediterranean. London: Routledge and Kegan Paul.
Devereux, George
  1982 Ethnic Identity. *In* George De Vos and Lola Romanucci-Ross (eds.), Ethnic Identity: Cultural Continuties and Change. Chicago: University of Chicago.
Gaines, Atwood
  1979 Definitions and Diagnoses. Culture, Medicine and Psychiatry 3(4):381–418.
  1982a Cultural Definitions, Behavior and the Person in American Psychiatry. *In* A. J. Marsella and G. M. White (eds.), Cultural Conceptions of Mental Health and Therapy. Dordrecht, Holland: D. Reidel Publishing Co.
  1982b Knowledge and Practice. *In* Noel Chrisman and Thomas Maretzki (eds.), Clinically Applied Anthropology. Dordrecht, Holland: D. Reidel Publishing Co.
  1982c The Twice-Born: 'Christian Psychiatry' and Christian Psychiatrists. Culture, Medicine and Psychiatry 6(3):305–324.
Gaines, Atwood and Robert Hahn (eds.)
  1982 Physicians of Western Medicine: Five Cultural Studies. Special Issue. Culture, Medicine and Psychiatry 6(3).
Geertz, Clifford
  1973 The Interpretation of Cultures. New York: Basic Books.
  1977 On the Nature of Anthropological Understanding. *In* Annual Editions in Anthropology. Guilford, Conn.: Dushkin.
Gilmore, David
  1982 Anthropology of the Mediterranean Area. *In* Annual Reviews in Anthropology. Palo Alto, California: Annual Reviews, Inc.
Good, Byron
  1977 The Heart of What's the Matter. Culture, Medicine and Psychiatry 1(1):25–58.
Good, Byron and Mary-Jo DelVecchio Good
  1981 The Meaning of Symptoms. *In* L. Eisenberg and A. Kleinman (eds.), The Relevance of Social Science for Medicine. Dordrecht, Holland: D. Reidel Publishing Co.
Hahn, Robert
  1982 "Treat the Patient, Not the Lab": Internal Medicine and the Concept of 'Person'. *In* A. Gaines and R. Hahn (eds.), Physicians of Western Medicine: Five Cultural Studies. Special Issue. Culture, Medicine and Psychiatry 6(3):219–236.
Hallowell, A. I.
  1955 The Self and Its Behavioral Environment. *In* Culture and Experience, A. I. Hallowell. Philadelphia: University of Pennsylvania Press.
Hill, Sir Denis
  1978 The Qualities of a Good Psychiatrist. British Journal of Psychiatry 133:97–105.
Illich, Ivan
  1975 Medical Nemesis. New York: Pantheon.

Kleinman, Arthur, Leon Eisenberg and Byron Good
1978 Culture, Illness and Care. Annals of Internal Medicine 88: 251–258.
Kleinman, Arthur
1980a Major Conceptual and Research Issues for Cultural (Anthropological) Psychiatry. Culture, Medicine and Psychiatry 4(3):3–13.
1980b Patients and Healers in the Context of Culture. Berkeley: University of California.
Lebra, Takie
1976 Japanese Patterns of Behavior. Honolulu: University Press of Hawaii.
Lee, Dorothy
1959 Freedom and Culture. Englewood Cliffs, New Jersey: Prentice-Hall.
Light, Donald
1976 Work Styles Among American Psychiatric Residents. In J. Westermeyer (ed.), Anthropology and Mental Health. The Hague: Mouton.
Mechanic, David
1962 Some Factors in Identifying and Defining Mental Illness. Mental Hygiene 46:66–74.
Navarro, Vincente
1976 Medicine Under Capitalism. New York: Prodist.
Nunnlly, J. C.
1961 Popular Conceptions of Mental Health. New York: Holt, Rinehart and Winston.
Schutz, Alfred
1967 Collected Papers I: The Problem of Social Reality. M. Natanson (ed.). The Hague: Martinus Nijhoff.
Shweder, Richard and Edmund Bourne
1982 Does the Concept of Person Vary Cross-Culturally? In A. J. Marsella and G. M. White (eds.), Cultural Conceptions of Mental Health and Therapy. Dordrecht, Holland: D. Reidel Publishing Co.
Szasz, Thomas
1961 The Myth of Mental Illness. New York: Hoeber and Harper.
Taussig, M. T.
1980 Reification and the Consciousness of the Patient. Social Science and Medicine 14B: 3–13.
Townsend, J. M.
1978 Cultural Conceptions and Mental Illness. Chicago: University of Chicago Press.
Turkle, Sherry
1978 Psychoanalytic Politics. New York: Basic Books.
Turner, Victor
1969 The Ritual Process. Chicago: Aldine.
White, Geoffrey and Anthony Marsella
1982 Introduction: Cultural Conceptions in Mental Health Research and Practice. In A. J. Marsella and G. M. White (eds.), Cultural Conceptions of Mental Health and Therapy. Dordrecht, Holland: D. Reidel Publishing Co.

SECTION IV

INTERRELATIONS OF MEDICAL SPECIALTIES

MARY-JO DELVECCHIO GOOD

DISCOURSES ON PHYSICIAN COMPETENCE

INTRODUCTION

Competence in medicine is a salient topic in discourse about and by physicians. Discourses on competence vary with the perspective of the commentator, whether it be from the stance of those within the profession, those who seek its services, or social scientists who study it. The salience of competence talk and the intensity of emotions associated with it by medical professionals and by the lay public suggest the enormity and import of physicians' being and appearing competent. In this paper, three modes of discourse on physician competence will be explored. First, significant work by sociologists who have studied physicians and whose analyses in themselves constitute a sociological discourse on physician competence will be briefly reviewed. Second, "intra-professional discourse" on competence will be analyzed, focusing on physicians in rural medical communities at different stages of structural change. Third, the paper will address the "reflective mode" of competence discourse among individual physicians, who relate the meaning of competence to their own professional and personal lives. Thus the focus of the analysis is on modes of discourse about physician competence rather than on empirical competence *per se*. The social and cultural constructions of these competence discourses will be examined, and the complexity of personal meanings that become infused in competence talk analyzed. The research on which this discussion is based was conducted in rural areas in California.

THE SOCIOLOGICAL DISCOURSE

Competence in the profession of medicine has been addressed by sociologists concerned with the structure and organization of professions, with professional training, regulation of error, and medical uncertainty, and with the source of trust and the fiduciary contract between the profession and the lay public. Parsons (1978) contends that the special fiduciary responsibility of physicians for the health of patients is based on presumptive competence, that is, on the presumption by the lay public that the very status of "physician" implies professional competence. Physician competence for Parsons consists of three components: high intelligence and moral character; technical knowledge and skill, acquired through formal education in the basic sciences and clinical training; and responsibility and willingness to act as genuine trustees of the health interests of patients. Patients, in this model, assume that physicians have these characteristics of professional competence, and they exchange trust for the helping relationship.

Freidson (1970a, 1970b, 1975), over more than a decade of research, has

247

R. A. Hahn and A. D. Gaines (eds.), Physicians of Western Medicine, 247–267.
© 1985 *by D. Reidel Publishing Company.*

argued that the public's trust in physician competence is often unjustified. He holds that presumptive competence has enabled the profession to dominate health services and to monopolize legitimized and licensed medical care without ongoing explicit regulation of the technical competence of practicing physicians. He maintains there is a conspiracy of silence, which emerges from a lack of active and aggressive peer review (also see Paget 1982). The silence of the profession regarding the errors of its members sustains professional dominance. Structural features in the organization of medicine, including the entrepreneurial structure of solo and group practice, the economic dependency of specialists in referral networks, the professional isolation of many practicing physicians, and the limited opportunities for and personal resistance to exchanging information on the incompetence or errors of physician colleagues all contribute to the limits of self-regulation of the profession.

Bosk (1979) delves into the domain of academic medicine where technical and moral competence is taught and rigorously overseen. In his study of surgeons-in-training and their clinical teachers or "attendings", he explores the meanings of the failure to perform competently and argues for distinguishing between technical and moral errors (1979:168). Within the context of a prestigious training hospital, moral errors, which include failure to show proper dedication, interest, thoroughness and responsibility, are far more grievous than errors of medical judgment or technique. Moral errors violate the ethical standards of the discipline and the profession and threaten the very basis of the physician-patient contract; thus they are harshly punished (1979:169—190). Technical errors, given the proper moral stance, are regarded as opportunities to learn, mistakes to be remembered and forgiven (1979:37—45).

The positions taken by Parsons and Freidson on presumptive competence both fail to account for the widespread public questioning of the competence of physicians. Fox (1980:18—19) contends that the very "fundamental and impressive advances in biomedical knowledge" in the last half-century have "uncovered and created uncertainties and risks" previously unknown. Medical uncertainty has thus heightened both professional and public preoccupation with what constitutes physician competence. In the popular domain, doctor shopping, medical gossip, patients' comparisons of their experiences with physicians, the self-care and popular health movements, and malpractice suits create complex conceptions of physician competence among the public. Structural changes in medical disciplines, in medical research and education, and in the power structure and organization of specific health care delivery systems contribute to conflicts within professional medical communities, and, therefore, to informal as well as formal scrutiny of physician performance. Thus, concepts such as "presumptive competence" and "professional dominance" based on the "conspiracy of silence" present incomplete and potentially misleading perspectives on the range of discourse on physician competence.

Bosk's analysis mentioned above, addresses the nuances of the meaning of physician competence within academic medicine and is therefore a corrective to

Freidson's limited perspective, one which purposely neglects the interpretations by the profession. Bosk is thus able to examine the complexities of the limits of professional control of physician performance. The professional solidarity of a working group of physicians-in-training, which may be perceived as contributing to silence on the technical errors of individual residents, is contrasted with the comprehensive responsibility for the group's performance assumed by the "attending" (i.e., supervising) physician. Successful self-regulation of the profession within the training setting, which assures high standards of practice and instills in trainees a high degree of professional self-control (Bosk 1979: 182), is contrasted with the failure of the profession to regulate its practicing members beyond the bounds of academic medicine. Bosk argues that the individualistic orientation in the moral education of physicians provides an inadequate foundation for corporate regulation of the internal affairs of the profession. However, physicians do express concern over the technical and moral performance of colleagues, and these concerns do emerge as salient issues among communities of practicing physicians. Thus, we are led to ask when and why such concern becomes expressed, and what it means for the profession and for individual professionals.

The analysis of physician competence within sociological discourse has followed a clear logic defining a limited set of issues for inquiry. Members of the medical profession, according to this logic, have both real and presumed competencies, special knowledge and skills, and an ethic of conduct that provides the foundation for their organization as a profession. Research within this sociological tradition has focused on uncovering the inherent contradictions and discrepancies from the ideal — on the development of competence through medical mistakes (Bosk 1979; Paget 1982), on the maintenance of the image of competence when it is lacking in reality (Freidson 1970a, 1970b, 1975), and on the discrepancy between presumed competence and growing public uncertainty (Fox 1980). The sociological discourse thus focuses to a large extent on competence as a real attribute of physicians. Yet, while assuming "competence" to be an empirical reality, the sociological tradition also provides the basis for the study of "competence" as a symbolic domain.

It is my intention in this paper to develop an alternative focus by substituting for "physician competence", "the discourse on physician competence" as the object of analysis. This basic shift in the object of inquiry brings into focus new problems for analysis. It is grounded in an alternative to the "positivist-pragmatist" conceptualization of language and discourse (Fabian 1971). In the following analysis, I assume that particular modes of speaking, particular languages (discourses), have not only a "representative" function (they refer to other elements in a situation), nor simply a "pragmatic" function (they affect some aspect of the situation), but that they are "constitutive". Particular human realities are uniquely constituted in discourse and through discursive interactions, even as they articulate with structural features and empirical realities outside of language (White 1976). This understanding of discourse affects the way questions are framed for analysis.

The central question is not "How competent are physicians?" (a representative analysis), nor "How do physicians use competence language to convince the public they are competent even when they are not?" (a pragmatic analysis), but more fundamentally "What is 'competence' as a social and meaningful reality in the world of physicians?"; "How is the experience of practicing physicians articulated through the language of competence?" "How is this discourse invested with the anxiety physicians associate with failures and errors, their need to feel competent in the face of uncertainty, as well as their personal strivings for power and economic gain?" "What role do structural conditions play in producing the discourse on competence, and how do structural developments produce changes in it?" "How and why are structural changes negotiated through the language of competence? How is the competence of physicians, as a social reality, produced, maintained or challenged through lay discourse, and what personal experiences and meanings of patients are articulated through discourse on the competence of their doctors?"

MODES OF DISCOURSE ON PHYSICIAN COMPETENCE

I will discuss two primary forms of discourse on physician competence: the intra-professional discourse and the reflective model of discourse. The intra-professional discourse on the competence of professional colleagues is but partly an articulation of concern about quality of technical skill, medical expertise, moral performance and character, and ethical behavior expected within the profession. Such discourse also provides the vehicle through which cleavages and conflicts within the medical community are articulated and the crises arising out of structural changes of the health care system negotiated. Intra-professional competence discourse appears to be generated by structural changes within medical communities and to be influenced by the production of new medical knowledge and expertise at major medical centers. The structural transformation of medical communities in rural areas, with the influx of recently trained "primary care physicians" and highly trained specialists educated in university residency programs, has frequently jostled professional relationships and introduced new potentials for questioning the performance of physician colleagues. Advances in Biomedicine, which have contributed to the state of flux of the specific content of medical expertise, technical competence and standards of clinical practice, and thus to medical uncertainty, become expressed in intra-professional discourse and conflict. The differential power of specialized expertise and training within the profession and the sheer economic and demographic limitations on the proliferation of medical practices in rural areas contribute to what one physician referred to as "a battle over turf and territory." Interphysician rivalry over "turf and territory" commonly arises between older physicians and newly trained practitioners and between specialists and generalists; it is often voiced and negotiated in competence language.

The reflections of individual physicians on competence suggest why competence talk is such a powerful vehicle for expressing conflicts generated by structural changes and new medical knowledge. Among practicing physicians, this reflective mode of discourse on professional performance articulates intensely experienced personal and professional concerns. It is a mode of discourse through which physicians reflect on their own skills, limitations, and sense of professional and personal worth. This form of competence discourse becomes activated for physicians when they encounter their own professional errors and limits, as well as when they acknowledge their own skills and expertise; when they have to deal with errors and limits of colleagues, when they experience unforeseen medical catastrophes and the limits of medical knowledge, and when they become privy to or involved in colleagial battles which are couched in competence language. It is a mode of discourse that weds personal meanings associated with competence to professional performance, to professional values, and to broader social and cultural interpretations of what constitutes competence.

Other forms of discourse on physician competence, which I will not explore in this paper, are salient in American culture and attest to the American fascination with the medical profession. These include lay talk about physician competence, as well as competence talk among health planners, government regulators of the profession, and health administrators. Popular discourse often takes a critical mode coupled with expressions of high regard for the profession. The ambivalence expressed in this mode of discourse is related in part to the unique role of the medical profession as providers of scientific medical care and as significant actors in patients' experience of illness, birth and dying; ambivalence in part derives from the structure of the professional-lay relationship. Variations on popular discourse are developed by diverse health subcultures in a community, and by health care groups such as the holistic and women's health movements. The social location of speakers, whether lay or professional, may also affect the mode and content of discourses on physician competence, thus infusing each discourse with cultural, social and personal meanings.

SETTING

The data for this paper are drawn from a larger study of health care in rural communities in northern California. A significant differentiating characteristic of rural communities is the extent to which the medical system has been transformed and become more complex by incorporating certain features of urban medicine. Increases in medical specialization, the introduction of new medical technologies, and the sheer rise in the number of physicians available to the patient population occur at different rates throughout these communities. Some formerly isolated communities, which have attracted many new physicians (as well as urban migrants and retirees), have begun to develop fairly complex medical communities, and concomitantly, hospital settings with considerable medical technology.

Other communities, particularly those with low population densities and limited financial resources, remain lightly touched by products of urban medical centers; they retain few physicians in residence and support but limited hospital facilities. However, as in much of the rest of the country, the trend in California is toward growing complexity of rural medicine, as professionals seek alternatives to urban life and as rural populations increase their demand for up-to-date medical services.

Most of the material presented in this paper was collected in two rural regions, one on the North Coast and one in the Central Valley of California. It has been augmented by data from other rural regions in Northern California. Each of the two primary research communities consists of a central market and administrative town, with populations of approximately 6000, plus associated smaller towns. Over half of the population of both regions lives in sparsely populated rural environs — on ranches, small farms, and homesteads.

The economic bases for the coastal region are the seasonal industries of lumber, fishing, and tourism, and a small amount of commercial agriculture. The central valley region is a major center of agribusiness. Both communities constructed hospitals in the early 1970s, each with approximately fifty acute care beds. These hospitals are the sole providers for acute in-patient care in the hospital district or county. Although the coastal community has experienced far more rapid growth of its permanent medical staff, both research sites experienced an influx of physicians and specialists after the construction of the hospitals. The coastal region is considerably more isolated from major metropolitan medical centers, in terms of ease of access and general road conditions, than is the central valley region. However physicians resident in each locale provide the majority of medical care for their respective communities.

Initial contacts with physicians in each of these primary research sites (as well as in other rural communities studied more briefly) indicated that talk about physician competence was rampant in some portion of each medical community. Conflicts between "old docs" and "new docs", between specialists and generalists, were expressed to the researchers in the powerful language of competence talk, often with a good deal of passion. My interest in competence discourse was sparked by these initial remarks, as well as by a concurrent accreditation crisis at the university medical center with which I was associated. Freidson's notion of the medical professional's "conspiracy of silence" clearly had its limitations. Why? What did this talk of physician competence mean? Research on this issue has continued during the past three years. Interviews with physicians, observations of medical politics, and interviews with non-physicians, both in and out of the health professions, constitute the data base for the cases and analysis presented below.

THE INTRA-PROFESSIONAL DISCOURSE ON COMPETENCE

Structural Changes: Old Docs vs. New Docs

Since I came to this town, the new doctors who have recently arrived are all specialists, although the internists and pediatricians call themselves family practitioners. Practicing medicine here used to be really great. Here you are on your own. There is something new all the time. It is more challenging than academia. When I first arrived here, we were all GPs, and two surgeons, and we'd all help each other out. Everyone was helpful and supportive. Now with these new internists, everyone is out for himself. It is not the same. The first internists we had – and I was really instrumental in bringing them here – were fantastic. If you had a problem or thought you were missing something, they'd explain it to you. But these guys! We could learn so much from these guys .... But these guys are trying to drive all the old guys out.

There's real hostility between the old guys and the young guys. I think the old guys are good. Like Dr. *T*, he's a nice guy and very competent. He's up to date. I have my boards in Family Practice and spend more than fifty hours every year in CME (Continuing Medical Education) ... so I don't know why this move to revoke hospital privileges, to proctor us. I don't know what it is, ... why this has happened. We've asked but they won't tell us. I would like to know what it is. – A rural family physician.

Interphysician rivalry and conflict within professional medical communities is amazingly common in rural regions. The past decade has witnessed an influx of physicians into previously underserved rural areas (Williams et al. 1983). This has resulted in structural shifts in the organization of professional communities and in the emergence of cleavages between "old docs", who had been the primary providers of care, and the more recently and highly trained "new docs". The dismay expressed by this rural physician, stated within the context of a discussion of changes in the medical community of one rural region, highlights the relationship between structural changes in the organization of rural medicine, interphysician rivalry, and competence discourse. His comment illustrates the intense personal feelings that are aroused by not only interphysician rivalry, but by the expression of that rivalry through disparaging the competence of "the old guys".

Although interphysician rivalry is not necessarily a new phenomenon in rural medical communities, it has taken on a new form and has been intensified by the influx of board certified specialists and newly-trained, board certified family practitioners. In the communities in our study, this structural change has created boundaries between "old docs" and "new docs" and between specialists and generalists. The coastal community initially experienced this cleavage among physicians ten years ago, and although remnants of the conflict are evident, most serious rivalries along this dimension have been resolved or quieted. The valley community remains in the throes of interphysician rivalry between old and new docs and between specialists and generalists. Common characteristics of these conflicts, including their expression through discourse on physician competence, are well illustrated from the perspective of these two communities. Additional illustrative material from other communities in our study will also be included.

The inherent hierarchy of expertise and knowledge within medicine, manifested in the conflict between specialists and generalists even within major medical teaching centers, becomes expressed in derisive language and terms for the old rural physicians. Physicians with speciality training, especially young graduates, refer to the general practitioners who have served these rural areas for many years as "LMDs", or "Local Medical Docs". LMD is a term of derision; it implies that a physician is of questionable competence, and it distinguishes newly-trained specialists and family practitioners from the "old time" generalists.

General practitioners are aware of the attitude that specialists and new primary care physicians hold towards them. Although many make peace with certain specialists and new physicians, others appear wounded. They counter the questioning of their own competence by specialists with arguments, often conveying anger as well as hurt, that they have a greater breadth of knowledge and technical skills, and, most importantly, that they have had years of experience as opposed to mere training. "Experience" lies at the basis for their claim of competence. In their view, the new specialists lack breadth, are inexperienced, and often fail to provide appropriate consulting services or are generally unavailable as colleagues. One general physican, while reflecting on this challenge remarked:

When I first came to this town, I didn't have people to talk to except other GPs, and I used to do things then that I wouldn't do now what with this malpractice thing. But I never got into any trouble. Everything I did came out all right. If you had trouble, you'd get a consult. I did a fine job on a kid with multiple fractures, fixed him up right . . . . Well, I would never touch that today . . . . These internists present a challenge to my own sense of competence, they are always taking pot shots. But there are a lot of things that they can't do that I can, such as setting small fractures . . . . That's the unpleasant thing. We welcomed those guys in and as far as we knew we were going to be a great working group here.

Another older general practitioner, who had received considerably more training than others of his generation and is regarded as a competent physician and a good colleague of many of the specialists in the county, still expressed bitterness toward many specialists in his community. He commented, "The specialists here set themselves up as God. For them, nobody else knows a damn thing. They stick together, no matter what." His frustration with the division in the medical community was grounded both in his personality and in his view of how members of a community of physicians should relate to one another. Although he had reached professional maturity in a commuhity in which there was endemic interphysician rivalry, because there were two camps of physicians each owning a competing small hospital, he still felt that the new divisiveness between specialists and generalists (expressed in competence talk) was harmful to medicine.

COMMUNITY HOSPITALS: ARENAS FOR COMPETENCE DISCOURSE

New sole-provider community hospitals are frequently the stage on which interphysician rivalry is played out in rural communities. These hospitals become centers where physician competence is reviewed and monitored, and where political conflicts are manifested and expressed in competence discourse. In both communities in our study, hospital privileges and positions of power and authority in staff committees came to be contested and expressed through competence discourse. The actions of specialist staff physicians as well as of hospital administrators set the tone for these conflicts.

North Hospital, a community operated non-profit institution, was built with the intention of attracting newly trained physicians to a remote and isolated region. The region was considered to be medically underserved at the time. The complexion of the medical community had begun to undergo significant changes prior to the opening of the new hospital a decade ago, as older general practitioners who had owned the rural private hospitals retired. A small group of physicians with speciality training, two internists and two surgeons, had recently moved into the area. Four other general practitioners, with a range of years of community service, constituted the remainder of the more permanent medical community. Recruitment of newly trained specialists for the hospital staff was spearheaded by the specialists already in residence, as well as by prominent lay leaders of the community who were anxious to bring medical care in the region up to metropolitan standards.

The Emergency Room Service

The nuances of the growing cleavage between generalists and specialists and between old docs and new docs in this community came to be expressed in the language of physician competence and performance. Both camps used this language in their struggle to control medical staff privileges in the new hospital and to maintain or attain economically viable practices. The old guard generalists made their first stand against the specialists over the issue of emergency room coverage. Prior to the opening of the new hospital and the closure of the out-dated private hospitals, all physicians with staff privileges rotated emergency coverage. Being available for this activity, being on-call to one's patients, and being technically capable to provide basic emergency services were considered standards of performance by this faction of the medical community. After the new hospital opened, emergency coverage was reviewed. The Chief of the Medical Staff, a generalist, argued that all physicians with hospital privileges should participate in emergency coverage. The specialists contended that certain newly arrived physicians, in particular doctors with very narrow sub-speciality training, should be excluded from this requirement. The generalists perceived this as unnecessary special treatment. If a physician's competence was so limited as to exclude the ability to perform in the emergency room should any hospital privileges be granted? For the old guard, breadth of technical skills constituted competence and was an expected part of normal physician performance.

In this particular incident, the generalists lost their battle to the specialists. The Chief of Staff resigned over the disagreement, and the structure of emergency care changed dramatically, with some unexpected consequences. Newly arrived physicians, both generalists with but one year of internship and board certified specialists, began to staff the emergency services as the new medical staff chose to hire out emergency coverage rather than maintain the traditional shared rotation among the staff. Emergency room work provided these new physicians with an economic base in the community and gave them opportunities to build new practices with patients acquired from initial contacts in emergency services. This policy not only opened the area to new physicians by making their move into the area economically feasible, it also further threatened the monopoly on general practice of the old guard doctors. The policy also contributed to the process of redefining quality physician performance. This was among the earliest conflicts that indicated the process of realignment and restructuring of power within the medical community.

The influx of newly-trained, board certified specialists provided the structural basis for new challenges to the dominance and prestige of the old general practitioners. These challenges were voiced principally in competence language, and the arena for these challenges was the new hospital. The challenges threatened the professional and personal sense of worth of the older general practitioners as well as their economic livelihood. The following example of the restructuring of obstetrical and gynecological services illustrates several facets of these complex challenges and the structural changes within the medical community which generated them.

Obstetrics and Gynecology

Before the opening of the new hospital, obstetrical and gynecological services had been provided to the community either by general practitioners resident in the area or by specialists several hours away. Shortly after the new hospital opened, a young, university trained obstetrician-gynecologist was recruited to the area. His reflections on the state of obstetrical practices in the community at the time of his arrival exemplify common themes in the competence discourses of new specialists. In his evaluation of the performances of the old docs, there are judgments on both technical and moral performance, and on the interface between the two domains of competence. He said:

> When I got up here, there definitely was a difference between the general practice community, at that time, and the specialist community . . . . I certainly received no encouragement at all from the general practitioners. I think I was seen as a threat to them. But all three specialists encouraged me to come up. . . . I was the first and only Ob/Gyn to come up, which means in a way that I was the expert and could do what I wanted. I wasn't coming into a situation with established interests, with many docs who did things in a certain way . . . . The reputation of obstetrical care here was not good. The basic medical reputation of the whole region was not good . . . . If you got ill, you left – quickly. And you can see from some of the practitioners of that time and the facilities that it was a well-deserved reputation. And it was probably a reputation of a lot of small rural areas, that had physicians that were trained a good while ago, that were overburdened, overworked, didn't have a chance for continuing education, didn't have facilities, and were seeing many patients a day. They handed out antibiotics right and left, really not taking or not having the time for diagnosis, maybe being a little burned out. For routine things, they could take care of them, or it would take care of itself. But if someone was really ill, they would leave for a larger center. It took a lot of years to turn that reputation around. (The reputation has been dramatically changed during the past eight years.)
>
> You see I practiced a whole different type of medicine. I had been through a fairly good residency with the luxury of being a specialist and having time, putting aside the time, to see patients. I think a lot of general practitioners, especially in small communities, get themselves into real big binds early. They come into a community, there're not a whole lot of docs, there is a need for care, so they develop a very big practice. And all of a sudden, they're seeing forty patients a day. If you see forty patients a day, there is no way you can give them an exam. And beyond that, they get real tired. So it's medicine from the doorway.
>
> Anyway, I became Chief of the Ob-Perinatal Department, such as it was. And I took the opportunity to start a review of the charts . . . just to get some feeling for what was going on. And I was amazed at the things I saw. . . . I found (failures to give appropriate medications to women with RH negative blood type) that; I found a number of cases of just really neglected labors . . . just really poor care under any circumstances. And almost no records.

Two incidents of obstetrical patients neglected in labor occurred following initial chart review. Both cases involved older general practitioners whose competence and charts had been questioned by the young specialist. In each case, the Ob Chief took over management of the deliveries in order to prevent excessively long labors and fetal death. The Ob Chief was incensed not only at poor patient care evidenced by these cases and by chart review, but also by the failure of the old generalists to appropriately consult him in difficult cases. He acted swiftly following these two incidents and suspended the obstetrical privileges of the two general practitioners involved.

Other older general practitioners responded angrily and threatened legal action against this newly arrived specialist — this young physician who, "wore Birkenstocks, had a shaggy beard, and looked like a hippy" — who had the audacity to question the competence of physicians who had long practiced in the community. Some general practitioners viewed the efforts of the new specialist to curtail obstetrical privileges of the general practitioners as motivated by personal interest in economic gain, by an inflated sense of the importance of specialized knowledge, and thus by the specialist's expectation to regulate and control those professional colleagues who practiced within his domain of expertise. It was a conflict focused on "turf and territory".

The Ob service in the hospital was restructured under the direction of the young specialist, who eventually recruited several partners, also Ob-Gyn specialists. A new birthing center was established that was unique in the country. It was a homestyle birthing center that allowed family members and friends to attend births and it later became a model for centers eventually instituted in several metropolitan university hospitals. General practitioners were still allowed privileges for uncomplicated vaginal deliveries; however, the specialists usurped other obstetrical procedures. The older general practitioners either left the area, died, or phased out their obstetrical practices. New generalists (without residency training), many of whom "practiced very good medicine" in the eyes of the Ob Chief and "who consulted appropriately", were allowed to practice without challenge to their competence.

Although the conflict in the medical community was perceived by those on both sides of the dispute as a battle between specialists and generalists, and although the Ob Chief received most of his support from other specialists in his efforts to curtail obstetrical and gynecological hospital privileges of the old general practitioners, the cleavage among the professionals was a good deal more complex. First, age, combined with lack of speciality training, appeared to be important in placing the general practitioners in an embattled position. Not all specialists were newly trained physicians, and the competence of young, newly arrived generalists, without residency training or a board certification in family practice, was rarely aggressively addressed. (This appeared to be the case even when the technical competence of particular new physicians gave other colleagues cause for concern.) Minimum privileges in medicine, surgery, and obstetrics were given to licensed physicians who applied to the hospital's medical staff. The differential treatment of the old generalists and the new generalists appeared to be a response to the willingness of the new generalists to acknowledge the particular expertise and authority of the specialists within the medical community.

Second, the style of practice of the older general practitioners, who relied on experience and failed to consult with local specialists when the specialists deemed it appropriate, led to an intensification of the conflict and to the heightening of competence discourse. Lay midwives, who practiced home deliveries in the more remote areas of the county, were not challenged by the obstetricians who felt that they "consulted early and appropriately". This suggests that the specialists are less likely to question the competence of general practitioners, even those without medical licenses, if the generalists duly recognize the specialists' expertise, special skills, and professional dominance. Clearly, the older general practitioners whose competence was most vocally questioned by the specialists were those who, in the eyes of the specialists, "did not know their limits", and did not acknowledge the hierarchy of medical expertise.

Third, the differences between the old doc generalists and the new specialists were paralleled by contrasts in life style that sharpened and focused the cleavage. During the period of the most radical restructuring of this rural medical community, the area experienced a major influx of young people with alternative life styles. Sometimes referred to as the counter-culture (by long-time residents and by the national press), their dress, back-to-the-land efforts, and political stances contrasted sharply with the more traditionally rural and working class character of the region. Many of the new physicians, specialists and generalists alike, appeared to be members of this counter-culture in their life style, their dress, and their medical politics. (Most refused to join the county medical society.)

These newer physicians also set up practices that were unusual, that contrasted with the large open practices of the older general physicians. They restricted the size of their practices and sought to structure their office schedules to allow time for other than professional activities. Many older general practitioners were initially scornful of what they perceived to be "hippy" doctors, and they questioned their competence and the quality of care they delivered. They wondered at the "morality" of limited availability, and perhaps indirectly, of an alternative life style. Thus, it was particularly difficult for them to cope with the challenges to their own competence by these newcomers and to the withdrawal of their hospital privileges.

The personal meanings of the competence discourse, which was generated by their specialist colleagues and which engulfed the older general physicians as their hospital privileges were first reviewed and then suspended or limited, appeared to be intense and potentially devastating. One physician left the community and joined the Air Force after his competence was questioned. Another moved his practice to a remote rural region across the country. Lay members of the community recalled that one physician had some personal difficulties with alcoholism or drug abuse, although few people considered these doctors as being notoriously incompetent. A third physician, who first had his Ob privileges and then all his hospital privileges suspended, maintained an office-based practice in the community.

However, he continued to come under professional scrutiny and was reported for patient abandonment and for prescribing medications without appropriate examination. While under investigation, this physician committed suicide. It was not known by his colleagues whether his professional difficulties were directly associated with his death. In the case of all three of these physicians, both their technical and moral performance were questioned by the specialists in charge of hospital privileges. To many of their patients and to several older general practitioners, these physicians were considered to be hard working doctors, who were accessible to their patients.

The professional life cycle of physicians is unique among the free professions, in that age and experience are not necessarily associated with increased technical competence. Competence is gained through training, and the more recent one's training and the more specialized one's knowledge, the more likely one is to be perceived as technically competent within the profession. The rapid advances in medical knowledge, the extraordinary changes in standards of practice and care, and the dominance of professionally recognized expertise by major metropolitan medical centers, contribute to the willingness of recently trained specialists to question the competence of older rural physicians. From the perspective of many younger specialists, a good older general practitioner is one who knows his or her limits, who consults appropriately, and who willingly relinquishes areas of practice as board certified specialists in those fields move into the medical community. From the perspective of the older generalists, this attitude of the specialists is often perceived as disconfirming their professional life and the years of experience — and thus knowledge gained through experience — that they have accrued.

Intra-professional discourse on physician competence was clearly generated by structural changes that disrupted relationships of power and expertise among rural physicians. Structural changes in the rural medical communities studied were affected by processes occurring in the profession at large as well as by processes indigenous to the communities themselves. Advances in biomedical knowledge and technique, and therefore in the content of training, have restructured the entire medical profession along the lines of increasing specialization. New knowledge and revised standards of practice, as well as a more sharply defined hierarchy of expertise, have been brought to rural areas through the influx of newly trained physicians during the past decade. The replacement of physician-owned rural hospitals with publicly-owned modern facilities was encouraged by state programs to bring higher quality medical care to rural areas. The new hospitals not only attracted more highly trained medical staff, but also provided arenas in which cleavages between specialists and generalists, between old and new docs, and conflicts over "turf and territory" were played out. The discourse on competence among physicians has thus played a critical role in the ongoing reconstruction of interphysician relationships in rural communities.

THE REFLECTIVE MODE OF COMPETENCE DISCOURSE: PERSONAL
MEANINGS OF COMPETENCE AND PROFESSIONAL SELF-WORTH

Although competence talk among physicians articulates cleavages within medical communities, as noted in the examples discussed above, its power within institutional and professional contexts derives in part from the meaning competence holds for individual physicians. The reflective mode of competence discourse links personal experience to professional values, and private meanings to clinical experience. As discussed in the introduction, when physicians reflect upon competence in relation to their sense of professional self, they often describe emotionally-powerful encounters with the limits of medicine, unforeseen medical catastrophes, their own expertise and errors, and those of their colleagues. The reflective mode of discourse reveals how the meaning of professional competence is invested with personal concerns and experiences.

Most physicians become reflective and quiet when asked about how they deal with error, with questions of their own competence, and with issues involving error or incompetence of colleagues. (See Paget 1983.) Willingness to invest effort in mulling over these issues appears to depend little on how technically skilled a physician actually is and more on personality differences and the personal meanings the individual attaches to issues of competence. When asked about the meaning of competence, physicians often begin by discussing their relationships with other practitioners — their view of the competence of others, challenges to their own competence by their colleagues, and situations in which they must negotiate the responsibility for treating a patient and the appropriate limits of what they or their colleagues are competent to do. This often leads to further reflections on situations that lead them to question their own competence and self-worth.

Consultation settings are extremely sensitive for the negotiation of competence. The consultant often has the power to validate or disconfirm the sense of competence of the practitioner requesting the consultation; at the same time, his or her own competence is on the line. One consulting physician, who recently moved to a rural community, and who was little aware of the depth of the cleavage between generalists and specialists that had characterized the medical community a few years previous to his arrival, commented on physician competence in a magnanimous manner.

Ah, competence. Now that is a very difficult issue and a difficult situation to be in (as a consultant). I have a lot of mixed feelings about it. The model I have for a community of physicians is a monastery model. Your job (as a consultant) is to support your brothers and to help them out. Rather than a competitive model, one in which you are trying to get business. Most people who came up here came for reasons other than to make money, for different reasons. That is the reason that I tend to like this group of doctors better than those in the city. They are nicer people. My approach is as a real consultant. I want to convey to them "you can do this". I want them to feel they can handle it, but also give them the feeling that I'm available. Ninety percent of the problems are resolved through diplomacy. If you get someone who is really bad (a really bad practitioner), then you have a real problem. I'm the new boy on the block now, so people look to me for the latest techniques and information.

Even though certain practices are not quite what they are supposed to be (such as medications prescribed), my method is to allow this knowledge to pass down via percolation and not to rush it.

The discourse on competence for this young specialist raised questions about the appropriate way he should relate to physicians in the community who were less skilled and up-to-date than he. It did not immediately raise issues about his own competence, although he reflected on uncertainty in his own medical practice in other contexts. His self-assuredness in part appears to stem from his recent training in highly prestigious medical centers and the high regard in which he is held by colleagues in the medical community.

Extraordinary clinical events, unforeseen medical catastrophes, the "acts of God" that impress upon physicians the limits of medical knowledge and the innate uncertainty of their art are particularly powerful in activating the reflective mode of competence discourse. Separating out medical errors and mistakes in technique or judgment from events that are beyond the control of standard medical practice of today's physician constitutes a painful component of personal reflection on uncertainty in medicine and on concerns about competence (Fox 1980). Such events may also trigger coping responses from physicians that are geared toward reestablishing their sense of control and mastery, their sense of competence and professional self-worth and esteem (see Bosk 1979).

The following case illustrates modes of coping and reflective responses to un-expected medical catastrophes. A family practice physician, who strove for excellence in her performance and who was deeply concerned with being and appearing to be a competent physician, encountered what she referred to as "the existential issue in medicine" when one of her patients gave birth to a highly distressed infant who died shortly after delivery. The physician was in attendance with two mid-wives with whom she shared her obstetrical practice. In reflecting on the infant's unexpected death, she grappled with uncertainty and was compelled to review her own performance.

It just never occurred to me because it has never happened to me, that if I took super good care of someone and was really there, that things wouldn't go well. I am not saying that I haven't had acts of God before, I certainly have. But none of them have been fatal. In fact, I would say that on the whole, acts of God are a hell of a lot fewer than one would think. A lot of what pass for acts of God are people not paying attention at an energy level – which was certainly not true in this case. You cannot imagine the shock, assuming the baby is fine because the parameters are fine, totally different from knowing that I have a distressed baby and preparing for the worst, which I've done before. Knowing a baby is compromised and getting ready for it – who likes that? But I accept that as part of my work. Thinking that the baby is normal and having it come out almost dead is just not to be believed . . . . I have never seen that happen; I have seen babies with low fetal heart tones come out normal. I have never seen a baby with normal fetal heart tones come out distressed, not even a little.

The physician and her colleagues responded both professionally and emotionally to the infant's death. Their professional reaction was to explain what did happen and to exert greater professional control over future birthing situations. First, obstetrical procedures and practices were reviewed, not just those practiced in this delivery but in all the deliveries in the practice. Decisions were made to increase use of medical technologies and interventions. (In this case, greater use of the fetal heart monitor was adopted instead of a doptone, an external monitoring device.) This was a remarkable decision for the physician, because her philosophy about child-birth, supported by her extensive experience, emphasized the healthiness to mother and infant of limited medical intervention in the birthing process. Patients sought care from this physician *because* of this philosophy.

Second, the physician and midwives turned to professional colleagues, to the pathologist and to the obstetrical specialists to comment on the case. These consultations were at first informal, but were followed by a formal case review, when several similar cases that had been experienced by the obstetricians were reviewed along with this case. The pathologist's report confirmed the women in their competence and judgment and proved to be professionally and emotionally supportive.

The third professional coping response of the physician was less typical and required unusual personal effort. Several months after the infant's death, she arranged to return to a university medical center where she spent several weeks as a participant-observer with Ob-Gyn specialists as they practiced high technology medicine.

These three professional modes of coping were highly instrumental actions, oriented to reestablishing a sense of competence and mastery, of control over medical uncertainties. They were coupled with a good deal of talk, of self-reflection, and eventually of attempts to integrate what had happened into professional as well as personal experience.

The responses of the physician — her choice to return to a medical center for additional training with Ob-Gyn specialists involved in surgery in practicing high technology medicine, and in increasing use of sophisticated interventions and invasive techniques — make sense when the personal meanings she attaches to competence are explored. Six months prior to the infant's death, she talked at length about competence.

Competence is very important to me. I have always half intended to go back and do another residency. What I really wanted to do when I was an intern, the only residency that I looked at and went "oh yum" was a surgery residency. I had two small children . . . . I knew there was just no way, so I did a much shorter residency in Family Practice. About two years ago, and intermittently since then, I have had attacks of doing surgery residencies. I realized from (mulling over) this issue of competence that one of the appeals a surgery residency has for me is that I still have this myth that . . . a good surgeon . . . is the epitome of competence.

I am still being run by, without realizing it, my old myth of what competence is. And it's true that many things I used to be really good at have fallen away because I have chosen to go in other directions. And I feel the loss quite keenly. I used to be really good at operating, and now having done less and less over the years, I've gotten more and more incompetent.

It's just so intimately connected with my strong feelings about competence and my myths about what competence is . . . I realize that I have newer, for me as an individual, newer values for competence. The best thing about a good surgeon is not doing; but the next best thing is doing. I think my old myth around competence was doing. It was . . . something you could see. It was big and dramatic . . . also VERY male. All the things I used to value before . . . that is how I was before. My style was very out there, very concrete, very doing, very dramatic. Not in the sense that I was dramatic, but that the activity I was engaged in was dramatic.

I've been working on bringing out other parts of me for a long time . . . . What I've been engaged in by choice, for very conscious reasons are other things. They are quieter . . . more intuitive . . . not as dramatic . . . much more inward, and I think, female. Much more nurturing.

But now, I am beginning to think, that that real drive, that resurgence, that strong drive, stronger than ever to do a surgery residency, is at least in part (a reaction to) that polarity . . . . It is (in response to) a loss of part of myself. It is a loss of part of myself, my skills, my competence that I value; it is a valuable part in me . . . . It's so interesting to view this desired activity of mine through the peephole of the issue of competence. It was a whole new light . . . (that helped me feel) less grief and more understanding. Less grief at the loss, more wisdom, more understanding . . . more acceptance.

The reflective mode of competence discourse for this physician brought into focus intensely personal as well as professional issues. In part because she is a single parent, she had not pursued a subspecialty; the course of her own professional development had thus deviated from her model of the idealized physician, "the good surgeon". The contrast between what she now valued in herself, professionally and personally, and her previously held "myth" of what epitomizes professional competence for physicians, paralleled major changes in her professional and personal life. Her move from a highly intense and exhausting primary care practice in an urban area to a more low-keyed, somewhat alternative, practice in a rural area, her newer emphasis on acting as a catalyst for patients to bring themselves to wellness, her reluctance to use excessive biotechnology and her caution over aggressive medical interventions in natural processes such as childbirth — all characterized the newer values and directions she had sought to pursue in the past five years. And yet, this physician's "myth" of what epitomizes professional competence, her image of the ideal physician, which may have been acquired through socialization in medical school, continued to be extraordinarily powerful in her assessment of her personal and professional self and in her understanding of her conflicting professional drives. When the newborn's death led her to question her professional performance most seriously, she sought to reassume selected characteristics of her "myth" of what epitomized competence in medicine.

The personal meaning of competence to physicians also articulates with psychological issues that have deep roots in the personal growth and development of individual physicians. The reflective mode of competence discourse often brings forth preprofessional and childhood associations. This same physician, in reflecting on why competence was a "life issue for me", recollected her childhood associations.

Competence was extraordinarily important to my father. He was an engineer, and he was very good at it. My mother was in some respects incompetent. I was always revolted by her incompetence . . . . As long as I can remember, it has been important to me to do things well . . . . It's a real compulsion. I would like to see it become just a part of me and not so compelling. I'm sure competence was one of the big issues in my own family as a child . . . . I think my father, overtly in his words, validated my competence. My mother validated my competence by her incompetence. She probably validated my father's competence by her incompetence. And she left me with a real rage about incompetent women. A disgust that is male, that is absolutely male. Maybe a travesty of the male, but absolutely male.

Gender-related imagery as associated with the reflective mode of the competence discourse, especially for female physicians, characterizes in part their perceptions of themselves and of their own competence *vis-à-vis* other, particularly male, physicians. The personal meanings of professional competence thus become imbued with cultural meanings associated with gender. For this family practice physician, maleness was associated with competence, both in her childhood as well as in her early professional career. And yet her current goals as a family practice physician, with a very large portion of obstetrical patients, are to develop herself into a competent, female physician, with professional qualities that are not only competent but also "female". Clearly, these professional goals entail overcoming her childhood associations of femaleness with incompetence.

The male-female dicotomy in this physician's competence imagery also captured the essence of her early conflicts with the male specialists in the community. She noted how she had begun to change in her relationship to other physicians in the medical community as she came to view her own professional competence in a new light. She recounted:

I think (that) for a long time, I tried to increase my competence, or my vision of myself as competent, or other people's visions of me as competent, at the expense of other physicians' competence. I think that's what a lot of doctors do. It is like there is only so much competence in this world. If I have more, they have less. If they have more, I have less. I think I am just getting to where I don't have to influence people's view of me as competent or my own view of myself as competent, by taking away from somebody else's competence. The mythical part ... has been my tremendous need to be competent. The reality part is that I am more competent ... because I am smarter, I care more, I pay more attention; but I am getting to the point, thank God, finally, where I am willing to be competent and there is no necessary comparison. And I am even beginning to speak ... to someone else's competence .... I've eased up on other men, other professionals. I think I had a need to put all that out there on someone (disagreements over what constituted competent medical practice but generated by personal as well as professional concerns). And what better than on my *male* colleagues who are *specialists*! If I were a specialist too, I am sure I would have less need. But I am beginning to appreciate them much more. I still disagree with them a lot, I think there is stuff they miss, but I am not interested in fighting about it. And they are more accepting ... they are just not as critical of me.

The extraordinarily articulate reflections of this physician illustrate the multiple structuring of the meaning of competence to physicians in private practice. First, there is the cultural construction of the meaning of competence which becomes personalized for the individual physician. Thus, for this physician, both the notion of the surgeon who epitomizes professional competence in medicine and the dichotomized values of competence in gender imagery articulate with the culture of American Biomedicine and with broader cultural images and associations with maleness and femaleness, with active intervention and with intuitive nurturing.

Second, the personal meaning of professional competence is formed by and in turn forms professional relationships within a medical community. Concern over one's own competence, competitive desires to be viewed as competent, and rage or disgust over the incompetence of others within one's professional community, have the potential to generate professional and personal conflicts. Maturity and an assured sense of professional worth and professional competence may otherwise ease colleagial relationships and contribute to a responsible mode of coping with both personal and colleagial errors, mistakes, and with medical uncertainty. The reflective mode of discourse on competence may also come to express structural cleavages within the medical community, as does the more public mode of competence discourse among medical professionals. However, when physicians indulge in this mode of competence talk, they are much more likely to express the nuances of the cleavages and the multiple, at times publicly masked and hidden, reasons that generate conflict.

Third, the personal meaning of professional competence is in part structured by pre-professional experiences, by childhood socialization, by the personality and psychological factors of the individual physician. These psychologically potent meanings are most commonly and sharply revealed in the reflective mode of competence discourse.

CONCLUSION

Analysis of two primary modes of discourse on physician competence, the intra-professional mode and the reflective mode, has focused on "competence" as a symbolic domain. This approach has as its object of inquiry "the talk about", "the language of", "the discourse on" physician competence and professional performance. It is distinguished from the sociological tradition represented by the work of Freidson (1970a, 1970b, 1975) in that it is less concerned with *empirical competence of physicians* and more concerned with the *meaning of competence to physicians*. Although various meanings of competence have been explored in the sociological discourse on physician performance and professional dominance (Bosk 1979; Fox 1980; Freidson 1970a, 1970b, 1975; Paget 1982; Parsons 1978), the primary object of reference has been competence or the components of competence *per se*. Bosk's work (1979) is noteworthy for its attention to the structuring of those components of competence through the training process and for its symbolic perspective on competence talk in the training setting. Fox (1980) has also utilized the symbolic perspective in her fine analysis of "uncertainty" in medicine.

The analysis of the discourse on physician competence has led to questions of not only what, when and why such discourses arise, but also what meanings are associated with competence talk. Clearly, for the communities of physicians in this study, competence talk weds intensely personal meanings to public and professional values. Competence talk is provoked by particular structural situations in the medical community and by personal experiences. Analysis of the discourse on physician competence reveals the complexity of these structural situations and of the cultural and personal systems of meaning in contemporary medicine.

Freidson's analysis, which focuses on how physicians fall into a conspiracy of silence with regard to the competence or incompetence of colleagues in order to maintain professional dominance, is too simple in its handling of the meaning of competence. It is because competence is such a powerful symbol — publicly, professionally, and personally — that such an extraordinary amount of emotional energy is required to challenge a colleague's competence. And yet, there are certain structural situations which are conducive to such challenges. The personal potency of the symbol "competence" also helps to explain why discussions of competence that do arise in disputes over hospital privileges or in consultation settings generate such intensity of emotions. It is ironic that known incompetence among physicians is often left unchallenged, while in the same community conflicts among physicians are voiced in talk of competence as a key and fundamental issue.

The analysis of discourse on physician competence has enabled inquiry into how competence talk articulates structural changes in rural medical communities, professional values and public interpretations, and personal meanings and psychological experiences. The analysis of both professional and popular discourse on competence, the focus on potent terms and discourse within or about the profession of medicine, provides an alternative approach to further explore the symbolic structure of medicine in American society.

ACKNOWLEDGEMENTS

The author would like to thank the physicians who participated in this research and who were so very generous with their time and reflections. The research on which this paper is based was funded by the National Institute of Mental Health, grant number IT24 MH 16463—01, Center for Mental Health Services, Manpower Research and Development. The research was conducted jointly by the author and Byron J. Good. The author wishes to thank him for his critical comments and editorial assistance.

REFERENCES

Bosk, Charles L.
    1979 Forgive and Remember: Managing Medical Failure. Chicago: University of Chicago Press.
Fabian, Johannes
    1971 Language, History and Anthropology. Philosophy of the Social Sciences 1:19—47.
Fox, Renée C.
    1980 The Evolution of Medical Uncertainty. Milbank Quarterly 58:1—49.
Freidson, Eliot
    1970a Professional Dominance: The Social Structure of Medical Care. New York: Atherton Press, Inc.
    1970b Profession of Medicine: A Study of the Sociology of Applied Knowledge. New York: Dodd, Mead, and Co.
    1975 Doctoring Together: A Study of Professional Social Control. Chicago: University of Chicago Press.
Paget, Marianne
    1982 Your Son is Cured Now: You May Take Him Home. In Atwood D. Gaines and

Robert A. Hahn (eds.), Physicians of Western Medicine: Five Cultural Studies, Special Issue. Culture, Medicine and Psychiatry 6(3):237–259.

Parsons, Talcott
  1978 The Sick Role and the Role of the Physician Reconsidered. *In* T. Parsons, Action Theory and the Human Condition. New York: The Free Press.
White, Hayden
  1976 The Fictions of Factual Representation. *In* A. Fletcher (ed.), The Literature of Fact. New York: Columbia University Press.
Williams, A. et al.
  1983 How Many Miles to the Doctor? New England J. Med. 309:958–963.

THOMAS M. JOHNSON

CONSULTATION-LIAISON PSYCHIATRY: MEDICINE AS
PATIENT, MARGINALITY AS PRACTICE

INTRODUCTION

It is difficult to wear simultaneously the hats of clinical anthropologist and theoretical anthropologist, but being the only nonphysician medical anthropologist
reported to be employed directly on a psychiatric consultation-liaison service
(Tilley 1982:267) offers a unique opportunity both to apply anthropology in
clinical medicine and to examine clinical medicine anthropologically. Work in
the clinical setting as an anthropologist presents pressure both to "plunge in"
uncritically and to "stand back" analytically. There are "clinical" obligations to
medicine: teaching medical behavioral science to housestaff and medical students
in the clinical setting (Johnson 1981b), interacting therapeutically with practitioners
and patients throughout the hospital (Rhodes n.d.), and conducting collaborative
research projects and publishing clinically relevant material for health professionals
(Johnson 1981a; Johnson and Murphy 1984; Johnson and Kleinman 1984). On the
other hand, there are "theoretical" obligations to anthropology: acknowledging
the privilege of participation in a complex social system in which activities revolve
around the most intense human life crises and in which professional rituals are
usually hidden from public view; observational data-gathering with an ethnographer's objectivity, and theoretical reformulation to advance anthropological
understandings of medicine as a "cultural system".

The purpose of this chapter is to honor this last obligation to advance anthropological understanding of American medicine. Based on over three years of clinical
work in consultation-liaison psychiatry, it is an attempt to focus on the relationship
between the dominant biomedical and marginal psychosocial "traditions" within
our plural medical "culture". Its principal thesis is that consultation-liaison psychiatry bridges these two traditions, and that a thorough understanding of this
subspecialty of psychiatry, as it confronts the issue of marginality, is crucial to an
understanding of this critical clash of traditions in medicine.

THE NATURE OF CONSULTATION-LIAISON PSYCHIATRY

Consultation-liaison psychiatry is a hospital-based practice in which psychiatrists
(and often other mental health specialists such as psychologists, psychiatric social
workers and nursing specialists), in response to requests from other medical
specialists for assistance in the care of patients, work directly with patients and
physicians on other medical services. A consultation-liaison psychiatrist provides
several kinds of assistance. Although trained to assess traditional psychiatric problems such as psychosis, depression or drug overdose, these psychiatrists are also

269

R. A. Hahn and A. D. Gaines (eds.), Physicians of Western Medicine, 269–292.
© 1985 by D. Reidel Publishing Company.

commonly consulted when patients deviate from expected or normative behavior during illness and recovery, for example, when they experience "too much" (or "too little") pain, express "too much" hostility, or otherwise disrupt hospital routine. Many patient problems which precipitate a "psych consult" are socio-logical, being directly attributable to patients' interactions in the unfamiliar and highly stressful hospital milieu. Such problems include staff-patient relations, family responses to a hospitalized member and adaptation to hospital "rules" and routines. Intrastaff conflicts unrelated to patient problems may also be displaced onto patients, resulting in consultation requests which appear to focus on patient problems, when problems are actually at the staff level. Thus, a consultation-liaison psychiatry team not only deals with patients, but also with their families and the staff which treat them.

It is important to distinguish between the process of consultation, on one hand, and liaison activities on the other. As a consultant, the psychiatrist is like any other specialist in the hospital with a specific area of expertise. Much as an internist requests a consultation from a radiologist when detailed information about a patient's internal anatomy is needed, the consultant psychiatrist is asked to examine patients and offer suggestions for treatment without necessarily provid-ing ongoing care. Thus, consulting activities typically consist of brief interactions with patients and other specialists on a wide variety of clinical services in which psychiatrists evaluate and make recommendations for dealing with specific "patient problems".

In contrast, in liaison activities the psychiatrist participates as an active member of the treatment team on a specific medical or surgical service, engaging in activities such as ward "bedside rounds", inservice training for staff, and collaborative research. Liaison activities also frequently involve coordinating "support groups" or "psychotherapy groups" for staff or for patients' families. Thus, liaison activities are distinguished from consultation by the intensity of involvement with patients and other practitioners, and the increased collegiality between psychiatrists and other specialists which this involvement fosters.

TRADITIONS IN THE CULTURE OF CLINICAL MEDICINE

As anthropologists have begun to study Western medicine, it has become clear that the "culture" of this ethnomedicine must be conceived of not as homogeneous, but as highly pluralistic, with great diversity among its various specialties (Gaines 1979; Gaines and Hahn 1982). With the increased emphasis on technology in medicine over the past 50 years, the dualistic Cartesian perspective of Biomedicine has become the more dominant of two major traditions within the culture of American medicine. Recently, however, renewed interest in primary care specialties has been accompanied by a resurgence of the psychosocial tradition, which empha-sizes social and emotional factors in illness and treatment. Medicine, in general, is taking note of this emphasis; but it is within psychiatry, the medical specialty most maligned by other physicians and mistrusted by the public, that concern with the psychosocial aspects of medicine has been most prominent. There are profound differences between these two traditions within clinical medicine: in diagnostic and therapeutic techniques, in the structure of professional social networks and patient-practitioner relationships, and in underlying value orientations and "Explanatory Models" (Kleinman 1980).

Through systematic examination of consultation-liaison psychiatry, this juxtaposition of traditions within medicine becomes particularly clear, for it is this subspecialty which operates at the interface between psychiatry and medicine. Moreover, it is the consultation-liaison psychiatrist who must grapple with the complexities of biopsychosocial problems in patient care, and simultaneously, with the problems of his or her professional impotence which derive from the marginality of the psychosocial tradition in medicine.

THE HISTORY OF CONSULTATION-LIAISON PSYCHIATRY

The history of consultation-liaison psychiatry is not well documented. One author (Hackett 1978:2) traces the beginnings of consultation-liaison psychiatry to the Massachusetts General Hospital where, in 1873, a young neurologist interested in nervous and muscular disorders was referred all "crocks", patients for whom no physical cause for maladies could be found. In 1920, a psychiatrist was appointed to the Department of Medicine at the Massachusetts General Hospital to study patients who developed mental disorders in conjunction with endocrine disturbances. The 1930s witnessed the immigration of psychiatrists from Europe who had trained in psychosomatics and the mind-body relationship, a tradition much more of European than of American medicine. These refugee leaders of psychosomatic medicine stimulated professional and popular interest in America in psychophysiology and psychiatric medicine. Consultation-liaison psychiatry also has roots in the community mental health movement of the 1960s, but psychiatrists quickly delegated responsibility to other mental health professionals and engaged in private office practice, or worked in psychiatric institutions.

More recently, particularly in academic medical settings, psychiatrists have become interested in the whole range of social and emotional concomitants of illness and treatment in hospitalized patients. Examples of such interests include anxiety and pain in burn wound debridement, depression secondary to myocardial infarction, and family problems associated with terminal diseases. The presence of at least two major journals, *Psychosomatics* and *General Hospital Psychiatry*, is evidence of this resurgence of interest in collaboration between medicine and psychiatry. A 1966 survey of psychiatry residency programs revealed that 75% of 202 programs offered some training in consultation-liaison psychiatry (Mendel 1966). However, a survey of the major psychiatric journals and the programs of the national scientific meetings prior to 1970 reveals little in the way of consultation-liaison topics (Hackett 1978:1). In a 1975 study (Schubert and McKegney 1976), 96% of medical school departments of psychiatry reported teaching programs in the subspecialty.

There are many speculations concerning the causes of the burgeoning interest in consultation-liaison psychiatry, including a growing interest in primary care associated with an increased recognition of the importance of psychosocial factors in clinical practice. Other factors promoting the growth of consultation-liaison psychiatry include grant support for training programs from the National Institutes of Mental Health, an increased emphasis on collaborative research on diseases which involve the interface between psychosocial and biophysiological processes, and the response to an increasing involvement in hospital care by nonphysician mental health practitioners such as psychologists and social workers (Lipowski 1974). In short, many historical forces have shaped the current structure and process of consultation-liaison psychiatry, leading some psychiatrists to disavow traditional careers in private office psychotherapy or in the psychiatric hospital setting, to work more directly with patients and staff in the general hospital.

Historically, there has been a shift in emphasis in consultation psychiatry. Earliest psychiatric consulting activities, dating back to the 1930s, were "patient-oriented" (Henry 1929; Schiff and Pilot 1959). In this traditional model the consultant psychiatrist responds to requests for assistance by focusing on "what is wrong with the patient" through chart review, patient evaluation and formal communication of diagnostic impressions and treatment recommendations in a chart consultation note. Today, some consultation requests are dealt with on this level, and the consultant psychiatrist relies primarily upon expertise in psychiatric diagnosis. Unfortunately, both historically and contemporarily, this approach to consultation has proved to have certain negative features from a psychiatric perspective: consultees are seen as frequently "noncompliant" with consultant recommendations, and also are viewed as inconsistent in requesting consultation.

Problems with the "patient-oriented" approach led many psychiatrists to adopt a "physician-oriented" approach, in which the focus of consultation became the physician-patient dyad. This approach reflects a conviction that a large proportion of consultation requests stem from difficulties in physician-patient relationships, which are revealed in the process of consultation requests (e.g., ambiguous or unclear purpose for requests, or affective statements about the patient by the consultee). Although this approach expands the focus of consultation beyond the patient, it shares with the patient-oriented approach a primary reliance on traditional psychiatric skills.

More recently, the continuing expansion of focus in consultation psychiatry has embraced a "situation-oriented" approach (Schwab 1968), in which the consultant psychiatrist views consultation requests as stemming as much from difficulties in the hospital milieu (with nurses, hospital regulations, etc.) as from the patient's psyche or the interaction between patient and physician. In this approach, the consultant attempts to "diagnose" difficulties in the ward milieu and to "treat" them by working as much with the staff as with the patient (Greenbert 1960; Meyer and Mendelson 1961). This new focus led to a proliferation of liaison activities in which consultant psychiatrists began to interact more intensively with staff and other physician colleagues in attempts to better understand and influence the clinical settings generating consultation requests. Such liaison activities have been the subject of great debate (Strain 1983; Neill 1983; Mohl 1983), both promoted as opportunities to "educate" other physicians about psychosocial issues and condemned as

an overpromise, the promulgation of the 'idealistic biopsychosocial' model. . . . Its zealotry and missionary stance to 'convert the heathens', lack of formal support from the rest of medicine, lack of cost-benefit studies, and general lack of success (Strain 1983:209).

Despite this reticence to engage in liaison activities, which are an almost manda- tory part of the "situation-oriented" approach to consultation, an even more "macro" approach has recently been advocated. "Systemic consultation" (Tarnow and Gutstein 1982) derives from both the biopsychosocial approach in medicine (Engel 1977, 1980) and general systems theory in the behavioral sciences (Buckley 1968). This approach takes an even more "social" view of psychiatric consultation, deriving from a belief that the appropriate role for a consultant psychiatrist is to help create "a psychologically healthy milieu for all individuals (patients, families, staff) who interact in the hospital" (Tarnow and Gutstein 1982:166). It advocates that psychiatrists develop intervention strategies which carry the potential of altering the structure and function of the hospital as a social system.

Regardless of approach, the growing involvement of psychiatrists in consultation and liaison activities has served to increase contact between psychiatry and medi- cine. But the biomedical tradition, as embodied in internal medicine and the surgical specialties, remains the dominant tradition within the culture of medicine. This hierarchy reflects the Cartesian derivation and atomistic character of Bio- medicine, emphasizing quantitative and mechanistic analysis of the workings of the human body. In this view, the body is seen as a collection of interacting organ systems; the soma is a primary focus of interest and the psyche, seen as distinct, is essentially epiphenomenal (Hahn, this volume).

The knowledge and technology peculiar to this biomedical tradition have become the heart of medical practice; the dyadic, contractual character of the structural interrelationships of biomedical practitioners and patients is the archetype; and it is the biomedical belief system which indelibly shapes the *prima materia* that is the student-physician in the process of professional enculturation (but see Townsend 1975a, 1975b; Gaines 1979). An examination of consultation-liaison psychiatry brings into focus the marginality of the psychosocial tradition in all three spheres: technological, structural, and ideological.

TECHNOLOGICAL MARGINALITY

Some of the marginality of psychiatry is rooted in its basic "technology", which is viewed as "unscientific" from the perspectives of Biomedicine. Although its practitioners also use some simple diagnostic and therapeutic techniques, medical practice has become most commonly identified by its enormously complex diagnostic and therapeutic armamentarium such as computerized axial tomography

(CAT scans), microvascular surgery, organ transplantation, and radioimmunoassay. While psychiatrists diagnose and treat conditions such as depression, dementia, anorexia, and suicide, and evaluate treatment technologies and their outcome by patient behavior which is difficult to quantify, other specialists diagnose and treat conditions such as hypertension, emphysema, hepatitis, and anemia, with outcomes validated by laboratory results (blood pressure, pulmonary function, BUN level, hematocrit, serum amylase).

These different outcome measures delimit two classes of data: the qualitative, nominal, "soft", "nonscientific", "untreatable"; and the quantitative, numerical, "hard", "scientific", "treatable". Although medical students and nonpsychiatric residents are admonished to "treat the patient, not the lab" (consider other variables besides single, specific laboratory results) (Hahn 1982; this volume), a common practice in internal medicine is "trolling the patient through the lab to see what bites" (running every test possible in the hope of finding "hard data" upon which to formulate a treatment strategy). In short, medicine tends to eschew "talk" therapies and diagnostic approaches in favor of other techniques, despite the assertion by many biomedical specialists that from 50% to 80% of diagnoses should be derived from the patient's "history" (talking) alone.

In contrast, psychiatrists regard their own diagnostic techniques as extensive and varied: for example, history taking, mental status examination, chart review; procedures such as pentobarbital and dexamethasone suppression tests; such therapeutic techniques as behavior modification, pharmacotherapy, hypnosis, relaxation, individual psychotherapy of various sorts, family therapy, milieu therapy, and community care. With a few exceptions, however, the diagnostic and therapeutic techniques of psychiatry are foreign to the other medical specialties, whose view of psychiatric techniques is severely truncated. When asked to describe what psychiatrists do, other medical specialists usually respond "talk with patients", "give patients drugs", or "shock patients". Thus, although their view is not generally shared by other specialists, psychiatrists view their data gathering strategies as highly differentiated, specialized, and systematic, despite not being immediately convertible to numerical equivalents.

By talking to patients, psychiatrists also regard diagnosis as a part of therapy and therapy as a part of diagnosis, an interdependence usually not explicitly recognized by nonpsychiatric physicians. Within psychiatry, for example, history-taking is equally viewed as "rapport-building", the initial step necessary for successful treatment (Brody 1980). While the mental status assessment of a patient by a nonpsychiatrist usually involves a gross statment about the patient's mental functioning ("He's not very well oriented", "She seems a little paranoid", "This patient is a typical cardiac cripple", "This patient is crazy as hell!"), mental status evaluation by a psychiatrist is usually highly formalized (see Rittenberg and Simons, this volume), and includes an evaluation based on parameters such as appearance, mood, affect, orientation, memory, judgment, etc. Psychiatrists see the reliance on laboratory data by other physician specialists as often unnecessary, dangerous to the patient, costly, and unproductive.

In the diagnostic interview with patients, most psychiatrists explore a variety of social and psychological variables, eliciting detailed information on birth and early childhood development, family interaction and child-rearing practices, adolescent adjustment and sexuality, education and employment, current living situation, personality and kind of present adjustment, social support and life stress, and others. In the tradition of Biomedicine, on the other hand, the social history generally consists only of alcohol and tobacco use, occupation, and marital status. It is perhaps noteworthy that on standard hospital forms used for recording data elicited from the patient during the history and physical examination, the amount of space allocated to "social and family history" is very small, usually no more than three lines on the page. The space allocated for physical examination and laboratory data is much greater.

Thus, although there is some overlap in technique between the traditions of Biomedicine and of psychiatry, the technical modes which are central to medicine are marginal to psychiatry, and conversely, those which are central to psychiatry are marginal to medicine. Psychiatrists tend to gather a large amount of social and psychological information which is of little apparent interest to other physicians, while other physicians put priority on purportedly more "objective" physiological data obtained by laboratory evaluation and physical examination, despite the fact that the interpretation of any laboratory result is anything but straightforward, with sources of error in specimen collection and analysis, as well as problems of test specificity and sensitivity (Gambino and Galen 1975).

The use of drug therapy and a small number of diagnostic procedures are two areas of technical convergence between the traditions of Biomedicine and psychiatry, and their use thus provides a shared medium of exchange for consultant psychiatrists. When considering drug therapy the consultant psychiatrist is put in a double-bind: although a recommendation for drug therapy would more likely be accepted by the consulting physician, there has been both professional and lay criticism of psychotropic overmedication, and such drugs are not free of side effects. Further, fewer than one-half of all consultation requests involve a condition in which drug therapy is indicated (Perez and Silverman 1983). The majority of consultations concern psychosocial concomitants of disease (*illness*) or staff-patient conflict.

Consultant psychiatrists are tempted to recommend drug therapy not only for the manifest function of serving patient needs, but also for the latent and symbolic function of increasing the probability of acceptance of psychiatry by nonpsychiatric physicians, thereby reducing status marginality. Consultant psychiatrists typically say to each other, for example, "let's try the patient on ... (e.g., an antidepressant drug). ... it will probably do no harm, and it will keep the surgeons interested in his depression". In this manner, the psychiatrist's recommendation for drug therapy may be based not only on a patient's condition, but also on the degree to which there is a perceived need to enlist the support of a consulting biomedical specialist and for the psychiatrist to be seen in his or her own right as "legitimate".

Occasionally, consultant psychiatrists perform clinical diagnostic "procedures" such as amytal interviews, pentobarbital tests, or dexamethasone suppression tests (tests in which a drug is injected and the patient's response monitored either behaviorally or physiologically; used as a means to determine the etiology of certain psychiatric conditions such as catatonia, drug abuse, and depression). For example, when asked to see a patient and to render an opinion as to the cause of a catatonic state (organic vs. functional), consultant psychiatrists may conduct an amytal interview to assist in the differential diagnosis. The procedure involves the use of injections, intravenous equipment, "crash carts" (resuscitation equipment), and other paraphernalia which are part of the *materia medica* of Biomedicine.

Consultant psychiatrists enjoy such opportunities because a "procedure" will attract the attention of other physicians, who otherwise ignore or devalue psychiatric "talking" activities. When such procedures actually provide solutions to diagnostic dilemmas, they are viewed by psychiatrists as enhancing the status of psychiatry within medicine. Following such procedures, psychiatrists have been noted to say, "This amytal interview ought to raise our stock at least twenty points with the medical folks!" and, "That impressed the medical people more than anything we've done all year!"

Thus, although the traditional techniques of psychiatry and Biomedicine are divergent, consultation-liaison psychiatrists confront the problem of marginality by simultaneously asserting the importance of their approach and, whenever appropriate, utilizing procedures which most closely conform to those of the biomedical tradition; appropriateness is judged both by the condition of the patient and by the "secondary gain" of interspecialty influence. There is a perceived benefit derived from mimicking the biomedical approach, if not for patients, at least for psychiatry and the psychosocial tradition in its relationship to medicine.

Technology has important symbolic, as well as purely instrumental, functions in medicine. The manipulation of symbols in consultation-liaison psychiatry reveals much about the marginality of psychiatry and the psychosocial tradition. The white coat, for example, has a long-recognized symbolic significance in medicine: its color as a representation of purity of purpose; its various lengths as markers of relative status within the academic medicine status hierarchy; its use as a clear discriminant of professional and patient status.

Although it is standard practice for biomedical specialists to wear the white coat in the hospital (indeed, almost all hospital personal including nurses, dietary staff, laboratory technicians, and even anthropologists are now mimicking this practice by wearing some variant of a white coat), many psychiatrists have interesting ambivalence about its use. Some refuse to do so, particularly those psychiatrists in private practice from the community with only marginal ties to academic medicine, who express disdain for the "insecure psychiatrists who feel the need to assert their professional status" (by wearing a white coat). Actually, inpatient psychiatry units in the hospital are noted for their lack of "uniforms", perhaps a vestige of the emphasis on "deinstitutionalization" within mental health during the past decades. Psychiatrists who train in such psychiatry units have been socialized to reduce the use of overt symbols of the distinction between patients and staff, and the coat becomes a source of conflict as a symbol of the distinction between the psychosocial and biomedical traditions in medicine.

In academic teaching hospital settings, white coats are typically embroidered with a name, degree, and department. Some consultation-liaison psychiatrists request that "Psychiatry" not be put on their coats because it "invites people not to pay attention to you", while others assert that it should be included on the coat so that the "importance of psychiatry in medicine can be asserted".

The stethoscope and otoscope-ophthalmoscope are also central symbols of bio-medicine. Indeed, careful observation leads to the conclusion that the prominence with which the stethoscope is displayed when not in use, is directly related to the need to appear "medical". (Thus, medical students early in clinical work typically carry their stethoscopes prominently draped over the neck and shoulders, while older "attendings" keep theirs tucked away in a coat pocket.) Although most psychiatrists do not carry such equipment, because they are rarely actually needed, some do wear safety pins in their coat lapels (a clear symbol of neurology, a field in which pins are used to test sensation). There are rare occasions when it might be appropriate for a consultant psychiatrist to examine a patient, and "attendings" on the consulting service do admonish residents to "go listen to a chest" or "check the eyes" as part of more general assertion of the importance of understanding the biophysiological in addition to the psychosocial ("We actually need to know *more* than the medical people.").

In short, although instrumental technology in psychiatry is marginal to that of Biomedicine, and *vice versa*, it is interesting to note how consultation-liaison psychiatrists manipulate some of the technology of Biomedicine for the symbolic effect of reducing status marginality.

STRUCTURAL MARGINALITY

In addition to technological marginality, consultation-liaison psychiatrists must fight structural marginality. One element of that marginality derives from the hospital geography. Patients seen by psychiatric consultants are scattered on dif-ferent wards throughout the hospital, each with a specialized nursing and medical staff, with whom psychiatrists generally have less frequent interaction than the medical specialists whose patients are concentrated in one or two wards. Psychiatry residents training in consultation-liaison work are frequently told to "spend as much time as possible out in the hospital" because it will "increase visibility". Becoming accustomed to such "foreign territory" is a difficult process, and the inclination of consultation-liaison residents is to spend more time in the familiar surroundings of psychiatry offices. In fact, a major locus of interaction between consultation-liaison psychiatrists and other medical specialists is the cafeteria, "neutral territory", in which discussion about consultation issues frequently occurs.

More important than spatial considerations, consultant psychiatrists are marginal to the structural core of medical practice, the physician-patient dyad. In this relational *sine qua non* of medicine, physicians speak of "having" a patient and patients similarly speak of "having" a physician, a metaphor which reflects a complex, nonreciprocal relationship of possession with moral, legal, emotional, and therapeutic facets (Hahn 1982). Consultant psychiatrists do not "have" patients in the same way as do their counterparts in Biomedicine or their psychiatric colleagues in private practice. In consultation work the normal physician-patient dyad is opened to include the patient's physician and other caretakers as well. A common goal of consultation-liaison psychiatrist is the mediation of misunderstandings between patients and practitioners, so that the "object" of their care may be a network of people.

Typically, when conversing about patients, consultation-liaison psychiatrists refer to "Dr. Jones' patient" or "the burn unit patient" rather than "my patient". In this way, the consultant psychiatrist expresses his or her marginality to the core structure of medical care, even if very much involved in a particular patient's care. Although this structural arrangement is common in many consultant relationships, such as that between a referring internist and a radiologist, when the two physicians involved are both potential "possessors" of a patient the norms of professional practice dictate that great care be taken not to be seen as being "in competition" for a patient. Consultant psychiatrists are particularly vulnerable to this charge, given the aforementioned fact that many consultations are a direct result of a poor relationship between patients and their physicians.

It is only after working with another physician and patient for a long time, or after a consulting physician has formally transferred responsibility for a patient to psychiatry (a rare event which only occurs by mutual agreement of physicians, and sometimes with the agreement of the patient), that the psychiatrist begins to talk about "my patient". A formal transfer to responsibility to psychiatry usually occurs only after all "medical" options have been exhausted. The transfer may be termed a "dump" or "turf", revealing much about the structural position of psychiatry. Significantly, the special structural relationship of consultation-liaison psychiatrists to patients and their physicians is a departure from that usually taught and learned about in medical school; comfort with consultant status by psychiatrists emerges slowly in the course of professional maturation.

Consultation Approaches

As mentioned earlier, psychiatrists display varied approaches to consultation: *patient-oriented* (what is wrong with the patient?); *physician oriented* (what is causing the physician difficulty?); or *system oriented* (what is going on in the situation which leads to the consultation?). Although these are not logically exclusive, they may be separately practiced. Consultation approaches in psychiatry have been in flux for the past several years, moving from an emphasis on dyads (Weisman and Hackett 1960; Bibring 1956) to emphasis on general systems within the hospital (Miller 1973; Tarnow and Gutstein 1982). Unlike nonpsychiatric consultants, who are typically "patient-problem oriented", hospital milieu or social system variables, including the orientation of the consulting physician, are usually of equal importance in understanding patient problems for consultant psychiatrists.

Inexperienced or insecure consultation-liaison psychiatrists tend to be more patient-oriented in their approach, betraying the biomedical bias of their medical school training and their prior cultural experience. More experienced psychiatrists tend to approach consultation requests form a general systems perspective, "diagnosing" problems in the relations of their biomedical colleagues and in the hospital environment. Although formal medical training provides no precedent for this consultation approach, such as organizational development and systems theory, or for employing "marketing strategies" for increasing perceived benefits of psychiatric intervention in the hospital setting (Guggenheim 1978), experience in consultation-liaison work leads some to recognition of the effectiveness of such an approach.

The Consultation Process

While seldom perfectly executed in reality, the ideal consultation process is a highly ritualized set of activities. The process may be described as follows. After receiving a consultation request, the consultation-liaison psychiatrist attempts to contact the referring physician in person. In talking with the physician, the psychiatrist collects psychosocial information that the physician may know about the patient. Information is also collected on the physician-patient relationship (length and duration of the relationship and the physician's feelings about the patient), and the patient's physical condition. The consultation also clarifies the expectations of the consulting physician, which are often only implicitly stated in a written consultation request.

Although overtly gathering information about the patient, the consulting psychiatrist simultaneously "diagnoses" problems in the physician-patient relationship (such as negative feelings on the part of the physician toward the patient). At this time also, the psychiatrist establishes whether or not the patient has been told that his or her physician has requested a psychiatric consultation. This helps to further assess the physician-patient relationship, and also avoids the awkward situation of attempting to interview a patient who may be unaware of the request for psychiatry and disinclined to talk to a psychiatrist.

Following discussion with the consulting physician, the consultant psychiatrist contacts staff in the patient's ward to elicit a description of patient problems. The initial source of the consultation request is also ascertained. In many cases, nursing staff will ask a physician to "request a psych consult" because of patient behaviors which are disrupting or disturbing to nurses, but about which the physician may have no personal knowledge.

Preliminary interaction between consultant psychiatrists and others in the system (nurses, physicians, family, etc.) not only serves the patient care functions of problem definition and data gathering, but also the "promotion" or "marketing" of psychiatry and the psychosocial tradition. The psychiatrist who is interpersonally skilled and enthusiastic, and who communicates competence without arrogance, will not only gather more and better information in such an interaction, but will also increase demand for future services.

After discussions with ward staff, the patient's chart is reviewed for additional data. The patient is then interviewed and specific data are elicited regarding the immediate circumstances of the hospitalization, past social and medical history, and mental status. The psychiatrist also elicits the patient's perspectives an why the attending physician requested a psychiatric consultation, as well as the patient's "Explanatory Model" of his illness. Following the patient interview, family members may also be contacted for information. The psychiatrist then constructs a "consultation formulation" which summarizes the situation, writes a formal consultation note on the patient's chart, and communicates findings verbally to the attending physician. Again, the style with which impressions are reported to consultees is a critical consideration. Residents are taught to "package" their reports to maximize attractiveness to consultees: such techniques include avoidance of psychiatric jargon, concentration on problems which are most immediately resolvable (even if they are not the patient's most critical problems from a psychiatric perspective), and "openness" to the use of drug therapy.

If consultation-liaison psychiatrists can provide explanations and treatment recommendations which are intelligible, concrete, and likely to succeed, they are much more likely to be accepted by biomedical specialists, who will more likely request further consultations. Diplomacy in consulting is also critical. It is not uncommon for a consultant psychiatrist to uncover a clear biophysiologic problem overlooked by a physician consultee, or to recognize errors in judgment which contribute to the patient's problem; these situations must be dealt with diplomatically because, as one resident noted, "there's nothing the medicine people hate more than psychiatrists telling them now to practice medicine".

Thus, unlike the orientation of the traditional physician-patient dyad, the primary orientation of the consultant psychiatrist is toward the referring physician rather than the patient. At times this is difficult, as psychiatrists have been heard to comment, "I may know perfectly well what to do for the patient, but the biggest problem will be to convince his physician!" Additional evidence of the basic physician-to-physician orientation of the consultation process is the practice that both a written and verbal report be given to the physician requesting a consult. This is, "because there are some things that can be said to another physician that should never be written on a patient's chart". An example of such "unwritten" data is an assessment by the consultant psychiatrist that another physician "has lost interest in a patient because the patient's problems are no longer a challenge" or "has difficulty dealing with an assertive patient who appears to question physician authority". Such assessments may be broached orally with the referring physician, but never included as part of the written record. Such a "public" discussion of physician disagreement about patient care, or negative feelings toward patients, would be a serious breach of professional ethics. Thus, much of the focus of consultation-liaison work never appears on the chart in a direct fashion.

In short, the consultation process can be viewed as an exchange in which the manifest function is patient care but in which the latent, and perhaps equally important function, is the establishment and maintenance of professional social organization and the proselytizing of the psychosocial tradition within medicine. The process, with formal emphasis on patient problem-solving but with informal yet acutely deliberate emphasis on interaction between consultation-liaison psychiatrists and other health professionals, serves to cement the interprofessional relationships which comprise the social structure of the health care professions. It should also be noted that consultation psychiatrists serve a "therapeutic" function at the institutional level, mediating in disputes between various elements in the hospital bureaucracy such as nursing, medical staff, and administration.

IDEOLOGICAL MARGINALITY

The consultation process, in which the traditions of Biomedicine and psychiatry come into contact, provides insight into the plural beliefs, value orientations, and other aspects of ideology in the "culture(s)" of medicine (Hahn and Kleinman 1984). For example, in the ideology of the consultation-liaison psychiatrist, there are several criteria for a desirable consultation. "Good" consultations are those in which "you can really understand what the referring physician wants", there is enough information provided by the physician, the physician has no apparent covert intentions for the consultation (such as "dumping" or "turfing" a patient), and diagnostic or therapeutic success is possible or likely. Good consultations are also those in which the problem is not exclusively either "medical" or "psychiatric". Consultation-liaison psychiatrists value working on patient problems which overlap the traditional boundaries between psychiatry and medicine, and which offer opportunities for investigation of complex interrelated factors from the microbiological to the social level. Other good consultations are those which are requested early in a patient's treatment (avoiding the appearance that psychiatry is an "afterthought" or a "last resort"), in which the psychiatrist can contribute to the overall treatment plan, and in which continued involvement or a clear-cut opinion or service is requested. Finally, the opportunity to "teach" other physicians and medical personnel about psychosocial factors is another criterion of a good consultation.

"Bad" consultations are those in which "you end up doing the work the other physician should be doing". Typically, this involves talking with family members of patients and providing them with information or listening to their concerns about the patient's illness. From the psychiatric point of view, biomedical physicians typically spend far less time in these activities than they should; consultation-liaison psychiatrists negatively value consultations in which they see their primary role as patching up poor physician-patient relationships, particularly if this is perceived as brought about by negligence on the part of another physician. Another type of consultation which is devalued is that which precludes collaboration, particularly those in which the patient is viewed as being "dumped" on psychiatry.

In the biomedical tradition, "crocks" (patients with suspected "functional" problems because no organic basis for complaints can be found) are clearly devalued,
especially when compared to "fascinomas" (patients with complex problems
which still offer a diagnostic challenge). Psychiatrists dislike consultation requests
for "crocks" in part because of the implications of a "dump", but also because
of a general feeling that biomedical physicians are all too quick to assume non-
organic causes for problems and that functional problems are as much "medical" as
organic.

Consultation requests for patient problems which by tradition are made to
psychiatry (evaluation following drug overdose, chronic pain, etc.) are less negatively valued by consultation-liaison psychiatrists; they are viewed as a part of
medical practice which "belongs" to them, and as "just part of a normal day's
work".

In responding to consultation requests, professional "posturing" may come
into play. For example, in response to offhand remarks from surgeons that they
"have a patient who could really use psychiatry" or that they "have a case psychiatry would really be interested in", psychiatrists say to each other, "If they
want us to be involved, they will have to write it as a formal request". Although
this is explained as a medical-legal imperative, there are other times when psychiatrists say, "A verbal request for a consultation is the same as a written one!"
The formal approach is reserved for those surgeons who are perceived to be least
interested in psychiatry or the psychosocial tradition; in such cases, the act of
writing a consultation request symbolizes an acknowledgement of the marginal
tradition. Similarly, in reporting findings from a consultation to a consultee, the
insistence on verbal contact by the psychiatrist is seen as a way to have greater
impact on physicians viewed as intransigent and overly invested in the biomedical
tradition.

In short, in categorizing the variety of consultations which are made to psychiatry, "good" or "bad" consults appear to have as much to do with the implications
of the consulting activity for the relationship between the consulting physican
and the psychiatrist as with the patient. Consultation requests are "good" if the
process defines the relationship of the psychiatrist to other physicians and nurses
as an ongoing and interactive process, and which are interpreted by psychiatrists
as indicative of a high level of mutual professional respect.

Despite the fact that the positive or negative value of a consultation request is
in large part determined by the implications for the relationships between psychiatrists and referring physicians, even when that relationship is good, consultation-
liaison psychiatrists are troubled if they perceive overt neglect of patient problems.
When talking about physicians on another service with whom they have poor
relationships, psychiatrists will say, "Whose problem are they asking us to treat?
We should make sure that we're being asked to treat the patient's problem, not
the staff's!" For example, requests for psychiatric consultation to prescribe anti-
anxiety or sedative-hypnotic medication for sleep may be perceived by psychiatrists
as attempts to keep patients from disturbing the normal routine of the ward; such

disruption may only mildly inconvenience the staff, for example, when a patient remains awake after the nursing shift change at 11:00 pm. Such situations illustrate the inherent ambiguity about 'the subject of the consultant psychiatrist's work — patient, staff, or the medicine itself.

Just as consulting activities and attitudes toward this process reveal much about the interaction of psychiatry and medicine, liaison activities provide further evidence that the latent function of patient care activities is the cementing of professional relations between psychiatrists and other physicians. As noted earlier, consultation almost always involves identified patients with specific problems, but the focus of liaison activities is primarily interspecialty, with patient care a common but not a necessary catalyzing element. In liaison activities, psychiatrists participate in the ritual activities of other specialties such as early morning "work rounds", in-service training for staff, support groups for staff, and collaborative research. By participating in such ritual activities psychiatrists essentially penetrate the "subcultures" of the other specialties, understanding their language, activities, and rhythms. This "fieldwork" also serves to increase the visibility of psychiatry to other medical disciplines. Thus, through liaison activities there is less likelihood of misunderstanding or stereotyping because there is more shared discourse.

For consultation-liaison psychiatrists involved in the liaison process, the same issue of written (formal) or verbal (informal) consultation requests arises. Psychiatrists prefer the formal process and encourage it. Informal consults may be regarded as "afterthoughts" which are "not even important enough to be included in the patient's record". Biomedical physicians often request informal consultations by psychiatrists because they suspect their patients will "reject psychiatric care"; psychiatrists interpret this as further denial of the importance of psychosocial issues, and an abrogation of responsibility on the part of Biomedicine to "convince" patients that "emotional" problems are as legitimately "medical" as are "physical" ones. In this interspecialty posturing, the patient's perspective may or may not be solicited.

In order to maintain active liaison relationships, however, psychiatrists accept informal consultations. Informal consults are viewed as an inevitable consequence of the liaison process; they are accepted as part of an exchange in which "dropping by to see a patient" will either increase the likelihood of getting more formal consultations in the future, or decrease the number of "bad" consultations. The psychiatrist involved in liaison activities, then, is caught in a double-bind in which informal consultations are necessary to validate relationships with other physicians, but in which formal consultation requests are seen to reaffirm the relevance of psychiatry for medicine. A confounding variable is the fact that informal consultations preclude the possibility of financial reimbursement. In the strongest liaison relationships, psychiatrists may have *carte blanche* (term for "standing orders for consultation on all patients") to work with patients on another service.

In general, liaison activities are viewed positively by psychiatrists because in the liaison process they can introduce psychological or social topics and demonstrate their validity on another specialist's "turf". Liaison activities allow the psychiatrist to assume a proselytic posture in an effort to get the psychosocial issues they believe to be an important part of medicine attached to, if not incorporated into, the biomedical conceptualizations of other specialists.

A significant feature of consultation-liaison work is the fact that psychiatrists view the other specialists as "patients" as they attempt to introduce psychological and social issues in the diagnostic and therapeutic process of medical practice. The same communicative dynamics which occur between psychiatrists and their patients occur between liaison psychiatrists and other specialists, including overt and purposeful communication of caring and empathy. For example, in an attempt to encourage another physician to consider family dynamics in the etiology of a particular problem, a psychiatrist may approach the physician by saying, "I know this is a very difficult patient to work with, but . . ." or "You seem to be having some trouble with this patient; is there something going on that I could help you with?" In this way the psychiatrist assumes a "therapist" role for another physician, who is thereby placed in a "patient" role. In talking with each other, psychiatrists refer to a surgeon's insensitivity to psychosocial issues in terms which reveal an assumption that most biomedical physicians are unwitting "victims" of the current medical education system and should not be "blamed" for the biases with which they are "afflicted"; with proper "care" or "treatment" they might "get well". This assumption of a "therapeutic relationship" with colleagues serves to enhance the status of psychiatrists, at least in their own eyes.

Once a liaison relationship has been established, psychiatrists may actually request that physicians in other specialties ask for consultations on specific patients. Psychiatrists will initiate consultation requests to themselves when there is a patient problem of particular personal interest or when there is a perceived opportunity to teach residents about psychosocial issues. Such requests are also made as a test of the strength of the liaison relationship. Again, patients do not necessarily participate in the decision to involve psychiatry in their care.

In short, liaison activities differ from other consultation activities in that they tend to reduce the social distance between psychiatry and nonpsychiatric specialties by encouraging an elaboration of interactional modes: in addition to meeting about a particular patient's problem, there will be participation in rounds and research together, as well as informal socializing in the cafeteria. These encounters offer opportunities for refining status/role arrangements (at least as perceived by the participants themselves). Liaison activities are also valuable to the committed psychiatrist because of the opportunities presented for educating other health professionals about the psychosocial tradition and because they provide a way of including psychosocial variables in basic biomedical research and practice.

It should also be noted that there is real benefit derived from the therapeutic posture which consultation-liaison psychiatrists adopt toward other physicians. Many of the stresses of medical practice result in repressed or displaced frustration and hostility; these may be given vent through these informal arrangements, in which needed mental health care is provided to a group of professionals who traditionally both seek and receive very little. Most significantly from an anthropological perspective, liaison activities increase psychiatric participation in the ritual activities of other medical specialties; they can be viewed as rites of intensification which reaffirm the basic kinship of psychiatrists and other physicians.

SOCIALIZATION AND MARGINALITY

Traditionally, anthropologists have learned a great deal about the belief system of a culture by looking at its socialization process, and the same is true for the "culture" of medicine. The differences between the psychosocial and biomedical traditions, and the marginality of the former *vis-à-vis* the latter are apparent when one looks at medical education (Coombs 1978) and residency training (Light 1980). In general, studies show that the negative evaluation of psychiatry increases as students proceed through their formal education (Sharaf et al. 1968). While more than 50% of students in their first year of medical school indicate a strong interest in psychiatry, and 20% list psychiatry as a possible specialty choice, fewer than 10% of medical students actually specialize in psychiatry for their residency. In their training, students see psychiatry as poorly taught, lacking discernible purpose, poorly organized, and lacking coordination with clinical exposure (Castelnuovo-Tedesco 1967). When students talk about faculty influence on career decisions, professors of internal medicine are six times as likely to be recalled as influential and nine times as likely to have shaped students' views of medicine. Psychiatrists are seen by medical students as more likeable but less competent than surgeons and internists (Coker et al. 1960).

Residents on medicine and obstetric services are of the general opinion that psychiatry residents have very little to offer. They may say, "Psychiatry residents are so strange!", referring either to the belief that many psychiatry residents are foreign medical graduates who, regardless of specialty, have low status within the culture of medicine; or referring to the demeaning but widely shared belief that psychiatrists "must be a little crazy themselves" to be interested in psychiatry. Residents from nonpsychiatric services may also say, "They (psychiatry residents) don't really do anything for the patient!", betraying the biomedical bias that getting patients to "feel better" is not essential to "curing" them. In addition, psychiatry residents are denigrated by residents of biomedical specialties as not "having to make the tough decisions" or "having to put in the long hours on call" that other residents do — potent "rites of passage" into physician status. One gets the impression not only that there is a type of professional envy or jealousy of psychiatry residents, but that there is also contempt, anger, and hostility.

Such negative bias, reflecting general physician attitudes toward psychiatry, is much stronger among residents. As neophyte converts to their respective fields, residents have even stronger needs to defend themselves than their more secure elders. Because nonpsychiatric residents tend to be less comfortable with psychosocial aspects of patient care, psychiatry residents serve as constant reminders of their area of professional "inadequacy" or "incompetence" at a time when the need to escape the liminality of student status and assert professional competence is most strong.

Psychiatry residents typically have some difficulty in the initial stages of their consultation-liaison rotation, in part because psychiatry residents view this service somewhat negatively. Like residents in other specialties, psychiatry residents also need to feel competent and "professional" (they are usually senior residents about to complete their training), but in consultation-liaison activities they feel very much in "foreign territory" and threatened with "rejection" by the rest of medicine. The normal physician defense of self-assured arrogance is singularly counterproductive on a consultation service, leaving psychiatry residents in an uncomfortable position.

In addition, participating in the ritual activities of another specialty (such as 7:00 am rounds on the surgery service), crucial for liaison work, is seen as both medically unnecessary ("It's absolutely unnecessary for surgeons to make such early rounds, and definitely not in the patients' best interests!") and personally unrewarding ("It's hard for me to justify getting to the hospital so early to watch those other residents waking patients up and mistreating them!"). Psychiatry residents are also angry at subjecting patients to lengthy psychiatric interviews at the request of another service, only to have resultant recommendations "ignored". Therefore, for a number of reasons, psychiatry residents on consultation-liaison service are initially reluctant to interact with residents on other specialties (and *vice versa*); much of this initial interaction involves symbolic or ritualistic assertions of personal competence (see Delvecchio Good, this volume) and of the professional appropriateness of psychiatry in medicine.

The comments of residents to students are both a powerful socializing force and revealing of the marginal status of psychiatry. Residents on other services subtly but clearly convey to medical students their belief that psychiatry has little to offer or is not really a part of medicine. Comments to students such as, "We've done all we can. . . . let's ship the patient up to the fourth floor (psychiatry ward)!" or "Let's call the shrinks. . . . at least it can't do any harm!" are illustrative of this attitude and its inculcation in the process of professional socialization. On the other hand, a more experienced Ob-Gyn resident, from a team with a liaison psychiatrist, was heard to admonish a medical student by saying, "The reason you think that patients on the internal medicine service don't have psychosocial problems is because the docs up there don't bother to look for them". This defense of psychiatry (or at least the psychosocial tradition in medicine) is evidence of the ultimate impact of psychiatry and the acceptance of the psychosocial tradition which may result from strong liaison activities.

Family medicine residents are generally more accepting of psychiatry and the psychosocial tradition, but even in a family medicine setting the style of the consultation-liaison psychiatrist is as important as the substance of psychiatric intervention in influencing perceptions of psychiatry. Family medicine residents value a psychiatrist who "knows exactly when to get involved and when to stay out . . ."; they prefer a psychiatrist who allows them to try to solve problems on their own, but "is always ready to back us up when we really need help", and whose style of teaching about psychosocial issues is very low key. Also valued is a consultant psychiatrist who is "good with patients" and "willing to see patients whenever requested". But even family practice residents reflect the pervasive view of the dichotomy between psychosocial and biomedical traditions when they note that there are "some good psychiatrists who really know medicine, as well".

In short, there are some clear structural constraints which inhibit collaboration between psychiatrists and other medical specialists at the residency level. These constraints tend to reinforce some of the stereotypes that psychiatrists and other physicians have incorporated into their belief systems. Under the worst of circumstances, psychiatry residents are contemptuous of residents in other specialties for their constricted view of medicine, and psychiatrists are denigrated by other residents for their inability to "do anything" for patients. Because the use of drugs is so significant, both actually and symbolically, in medicine the psychiatrist is viewed most positively as a psychopharmacologist, and less positively as a psychotherapist.

In working together, psychiatric and nonpsychiatric residents may come to at least mutual toleration; there are settings in which the consultation-liaison psychiatry residents become valued members of other specialty teams. Psychiatry residents, despite some frustrations, find several things about the consultation-liaison service appealing. Not only does it give them the opportunity to make use of their biomedical training, which they would "otherwise forget", but it also allows them to maintain greater contact with the other specialties of medicine and to apply their special expertise in the psychosocial realm within those contexts.

The professional socialization of the consultation-liaison psychiatrist involves not only internalization of values, maturation of self-image, and construction of clinical reality, but also the elaboration of "survival strategies" for interaction in nonpsychiatric medical subcultures. Residents on consultation-liaison service are taught, for example, that the psyche, soma, and society significantly interact when the patient is sick, and that intervention efforts must be directed at all three spheres no matter what the disease. Biomedical physicians, on the other hand, see disease as primarily either "in the mind" or "in the body", though they agree that serious physical problems can lead patients to be depressed. While other physicians feel that social and psychological factors are important, they do not construe them as part of the core clinical reality or as one of the many variables which are amenable to medical treatment. While other specialists see patients as either "medical patients" or "psych patients", psychiatry residents are taught that this dichotomization should be resisted. For example, psychiatry residents are taught to react negatively to the common statement that a depressed cardiology patient is "medically clear". From the psychiatric perspective, as long as a patient has emotional problems, these are still "medical" problems which should be defined as a part of medicine and medical treatment.

Psychiatry residents on consultation-liaison rotation are also taught the importance of maintaining identity as psychiatrists, while simultaneously making efforts to collaborate with other specialists. If other physicians are "difficult" and disregard the psychiatrist's advice ("noncompliance") or fail to consult the psychiatry service at all ("denial" or "resistance"), the psychiatry residents are taught that other physicians know that the position of psychiatry is correct but "are threatened by it because of their own obvious lack of training or ability" to work in the psychosocial realm. They are taught that such difficulties are "symptomatic of what is wrong in medicine" or that the other physicians are innocent "victims" who have not yet "see the light" which would expand their reductionist view of patients.

Most importantly, consultation-liaison residents are taught that it is their role to teach other physicians about psychosocial factors in clinical settings. In terms of self-image, this is a powerful message indeed: being a teacher of another physician is a status-enhancing posture analogous to the high-status role of "physician's physician". In this way, the self-image of the consultation-liaison psychiatrist emerges as a physician who is at the forefront of modern medicine, combining the best of biomedical technology with social and psychological expertise, with a mission of expanding the conceptions of clinical reality held by other medical specialists to include issues central to the psychosocial tradition in medicine.

THE FUTURE OF A MARGINAL TRADITION

Conflicting constructions of clinical reality underlie and influence the activities of the consultation-liaison psychiatrist in interaction with other specialists; these differences in clinical reality are reflected in differences in lexicon, ritual activity, and symbolic representations in the clinical milieu. In each of these, psychiatry is distinctive from the dominant tradition of Biomedicine, representing a marginal tradition and attempting, through consultation and liaison activities, to change the practice of clinical medicine.

And yet, although presented as such here, the psychiatric subculture itself should not be viewed as homogeneous. Despite a general commitment to the psychosocial tradition, there is a theoretical and practical pluralism within psychiatry in which practitioners may subscribe to any one of several philosophical emphases including biological, psychodynamic, behavioral, family, and community perspectives (Lazare 1973; Gaines 1979). There are also profound differences among psychiatrists with respect to involvement with other specialties. There are psychiatrists who so abhor the biomedical tradition and the practice of clinical medicine, and who feel so uncomfortable in the hospital setting, that they only practice psychotherapy with patients who, they believe, have to "physical" disease. At another extreme are those who feel that there is no such thing as "mental illness" (Szasz 1960). There are also psychiatrists who risk the charge of reductionism from within their own ranks by asserting that most psychiatric problems result from biochemical disturbances. This latter group is currently in great favor within medicine, one might conclude, not only because of empirical data from clinical practice and research, but also because their perspectives parallel so perfectly those of the biomedical tradition which dominates American medicine. Indeed, it is interesting that many such psychiatrists are abandoning the social science perspectives which formerly were the hallmark of the discipline just as the other medical specialties are "rediscovering" social and cultural factors in sickness.

Many consultation-liaison psychiatrists truly want to change American medicine. In the minority, even within psychiatry, and marginal to medicine in so many ways, it is a lonely quest. It demands an exhausting eclecticism to move back and forth between individual and social system foci, particularly with an ambiguous status which can be highly distressing. One psychiatrist quit consultation-liaison work because he "found consultation-liaison activities very lonely . . . cut off from traditional psychiatry in situations where other physicians do not speak the same language". Such activity has also been described as "overwhelming", "hopeless", "demoralizing" (Auerbach 1975), and "devalued by medical colleagues" (Mendelson and Meyer 1961). Even if such feelings can be tolerated, unless supported by an academic department in a medical school it is difficult to make a living as a consultant only, and there is no revenue-generating analog to liaison work in private practice (Fenton and Guggenheim 1981). There is also a growing sense of the futility of trying to influence Biomedicine. A prominent consultation-liaison psychiatrist has recently expressed the opinion that, despite the missionary zeal of some, psychiatrists have had so little success at influencing the perspectives of the biomedical tradition through liaison activities that the effort should be abandoned (Hackett 1982). Consultation-liaison psychiatrists must also deal with the recognition that many problems they are asked to resolve are outside the practical purview of any health professional, and that the solutions to such problems are political rather than medical. As one psychiatrist colleague put it, "The health care system is sicker than our patients!"

Nonetheless, there is a general resurgence of psychosocial interests among primary care general internists and family practice physicians, and there has been an expansion of research on stress, compliance, psychosomatics, and psychopharmacology which promotes interaction and diffusion of ideas between the biomedical and psychosocial traditions. One aspect of consultation-liaison psychiatry work which calls for further exploration is its relationship with natural "allies" such as hospital social work, clinical psychology, psychiatric nursing, and perhaps even medical anthropology, in promoting the perspectives of the psychosocial tradition. While there is a history of some competition among these fields, collaboration might be mutually beneficial.

Finally, it is important that the role of patients in this clash of traditions in medicine be more fully appreciated. Although there is little question that competent, professional care is rendered to patients by both psychiatrists and other physicians in clinical practice, it is also clear that the clinical milieu is a social setting in which the interaction between psychiatrists and other physicians may become as much a battle for professional status and ideological supremacy as for the health of patients. Physicians must be sensitive to the possible unintended consequences for patient care of such internecine struggles.

REFERENCES

Auerbach, O.
  1975 Liaison Psychiatry and the Education of the Psychiatric Resident. I. R. Pasnow (ed.),
        Consultation Liaison Psychiatry. New York: Grune and Stratton.
Bibring, G.
  1956 Psychiatry and Medical Practice in a General Hospital. New England Journal of
        Medicine 254:366–372.
Brody, H.
  1980 Diagnosis is Treatment. Journal of Family Practice 10:445–449.
Buckley, W.
  1968 Modern Systems Research for the Behavioral Scientist. Chicago: Aldine.
Castelnuovo-Tedesco, P.
  1967 How Much Psychiatry are Medical Students Really Learning? Archives of General
        Psychiatry 16:668–675.
Coker, R. et al.
  1960 Patterns of Influence: Medical School Faculty Members and the Values and Specialty
        Interests of Medical Students. Journal of Medical Education 35:518–527.
Coombs, R.
  1978 Mastering Medicine: Professional Socialization in Medical School. New York: The
        Free Press.
Engel, G.
  1977 The Need for a New Medical Model: A Challenge to Biomedicine. Science 196:129.
  1980 The Clinical Application of the Biopsychosocial Model. American Journal of Psy-
        chiatry 137:535.
Gaines, A.
  1979 Definitions and Diagnoses. Culture, Medicine, and Psychiatry 3(4):381–418.
Gaines, A. and R. Hahn (eds.)
  1982 Physicians of Western Medicine: Five Cultural Studies. Special Issue. Culture, Medi-
        cine and Psychiatry 6(3).
Greenbert, I.
  1960 Approaches to Psychiatric Consultation in a Research Setting. Archives of General
        Psychiatry 3:691–697.
Gambino, A. and R. Galen
  1975 Why Are Clinical Laboratory Tests Performed? When Are They Valid? Journal of
        the American Medical Association 233:76.
Fenton, B. and F. Guggenheim
  1981 Consultation-Liaison Psychiatry and Funding: Why Can't Alice Find Wonderland?
        General Hospital Psychiatry 3:255–260.
Guggenheim, F.
  1978 A Marketplace Model of Consultation Psychiatry in the General Hospital. American
        Journal of Psychiatry 135:1380–1385.
Hackett, T.
  1982 Consultation Psychiatry Held Valid, Liaison Held Invalid. Clinical Psychiatric News,
        January, p. 36.
  1978 Beginnings: Liaison Psychiatry in the General Hospital. I. T. Hackett and N. Cassem
        (eds.), Massachusetts General Hospital Handbook of General Hospital Psychiatry.
        St. Louis: The C. V. Mosby Company.
Hackett, T. and N. Cassem (eds.)
  1978 Massachusetts General Hospital Handbook of General Hospital Psychiatry. St. Louis:
        The C. V. Mosby Company.
Hahn R.
  1982 "Treat the Patient, Not the Lab": Internal Medicine and the Concept of 'Person'.
        Culture, Medicine, and Psychiatry 6(3):219–236.

Hahn, R. and A. Kleinman
1984 Biomedicine as a Cultural System. *In* M. Piatelli-Palmarini (ed.), The Encyclopedia of the Social History of the Biomedical Sciences. Milan: Franco Maria Ricci Publ. Co. (In press.)
Henry, G.
1929 Some Modern Aspects of Psychiatry in General Hospital Practice. American Journal of Psychiatry 86:481–499.
Johnson, T.
1981a Interpersonal Skill in Physical Diagnosis. *In* J. Burnside (ed.), Physical Diagnosis: An Introduction to Clinical Medicine. Baltimore: Williams and Wilkins.
1981b The Anthropologist as a Role Model for Medical Students. Practicing Anthropology 4:8–10.
Johnson, T. and J. Murphy
1984 Psychosocial Adaptations in High Risk Pregnancy. Chapter *In* R. Knupple and J. Drukker (eds.), Care of the High Risk Pregnant Patient. New York: W. B. Saunders.
Johnson, T. and A. Kleinman
1984 Cultural Concerns in Consultation Psychiatry. *In* M. Weiner and F. Guggenheim (eds.), Handbook of Consultation and Emergency Room Psychiatry. New York: Jason Aronson.
Kleinman, A.
1980 Patients and Healers in the Context of Culture. Berkeley: University of California Press.
Lazare, A.
1973 Hidden Conceptual Models in Clinical Psychiatry. New England Journal of Medicine 288:345–351.
Light, D.
1980 Becoming Psychiatrists: The Professional Transformation of Self. New York: Norton.
Lipowski, Z.
1974 Consultation-Liaison Psychiatry: An Overview. American Journal of Psychiatry 131:623–630.
Mendel. W.
1966 Psychiatric Consultation Education. American Journal of Psychiatry 123:150–155.
Meyer, E. and M. Mendelson
1961 Psychiatric Consultations with Patients on Medical and Surgical Wards: Patterns and Processes. Psychiatry 24:197–220.
Miller, W.
1973 Psychiatric Consultation: I. A General Systems Approach. Psychiatr. Med. 4:135–146.
Mohl, P.
1983 What Model of Liaison Psychiatry Meets Whose Needs? General Hospital Psychiatry 5:213–215.
Neill, J.
1983 Once More Into the Breach: Doubts About Liaison Psychiatry. General Hospital Psychiatry 5:205–208.
Perez, E. and M. Silverman
1983 Utilization Pattern of a Canadian Psychiatric Consultation Service. General Hospital Psychiatry 5:185–190.
Rhodes, L. A.
n.d. Reflections on the Anthropologist as Institutional Analyst. Paper presented at the Annual Meeting of the American Anthropological Association Meeting, Chicago, 1983.
Schiff, K. and M. Pilot
1959 An Approach to Psychiatric Consultations in a General Hospital. Archives of General Psychiatry 1:349.

Schubert, D. and F. McKegney
    1976 Psychiatric Consultation Education – 1976. Archives of General Psychiatry 33:
        1271–1273.
Schwab, J.
    1968 Handbook of Psychiatric Consultation. New York: Appleton-Century-Crofts.
Sharaf, M. et al.
    1968 Psychiatric Interest and Its Correlates Among Medical Students. Psychiatry 21:
        150–160.
Strain, J.
    1983 Liaison Psychiatry and Its Dilemmas. General Hospital Psychiatry 5:209–212.
Szasz, T.
    1960 The Myth of Mental Illness. American Psychologist 15:113–118.
Tarnow, J. and S. Gutstein
    1982 Systemic Consultation in a General Hospital. International Journal of Psychiatry
        in Medicine 12:161–185.
Tilley, D.
    1982 A Survey of Consultation-Liaison Psychiatry Program Characteristics and Functions.
        General Hospital Psychiatry 4:265–270.
Townsend, J. M.
    1975a Cultural Conceptions and Mental Illness: A Controlled Comparison of Germany and
        America. Journal of Nervous and Mental Diseases 160:409–421.
    1975b Cultural Conceptions, Mental Disorder, and Social Roles: A Comparison of Germany
        and America. American Sociological Review 40:739–752.
Weisman, A. and T. Hackett
    1960 Organization and Function of a Psychiatric Consultation Service. Int. Rec. Med.
        173:306–311.

CECIL G. HELMAN

DISEASE AND PSEUDO-DISEASE:
A CASE HISTORY OF PSEUDO-ANGINA

INTRODUCTION

One of the most useful contributions of medical anthropology to the study of health and ill-health in different cultures, has been the analytical distinction between "disease" and "illness", between the perspectives of the Western-trained clinician and that of the patient. Various writers on this theme, such as Cassell (1976), Eisenberg (1977), Fábrega (1973, 1975), Lewis (1975), and Kleinman (1978, 1980) have all pointed out the differences and the complex interrelationship between these two perspectives. In their view, "disease" refers to "objective" abnormalities of the structure and function of body organs and systems, which can be grouped into named pathological entities such as diabetes and tuberculosis. By contrast, "illness" refers to the subjective response of the patient to being unwell; how he, and those around him, perceive the origin and significance of this event; how this event effects his relationships with others; and the steps he, and they, take to remedy the situation. Unlike disease, illness has psychological, moral, and social dimensions, and is part of the wider spectrum of misfortune in general. In the view of Engel (1980) and Cassell (1976), these wider dimensions of misfortune cannot be dealt with within the biomedical model of disease, which they see as characterised by mind-body dualism, and a view of the complexity of ill-health merely "reduced to physico-chemical terms" (Engel 1980: 536).

One problem with this disease/illness dichotomy is that the biomedical model, that is, the medical perspective on ill-health, is often assumed to be a homogeneous, internally consistent, and rationally scientific body of knowledge. It is also assumed that the diseases which comprise this model are consistent, scientifically defined entities that are unchanged in whatever context they appear. This view of the unitary, universal, and scientific nature of Biomedicine is held by most clinicians, and appears to be shared by some anthropologists (e.g., Press, 1978:71–72). Fábrega (1973:218–219) notes that in Biomedicine, disease is seen as "an abstract entity with specific properties and a recurring identity"; it is "universal in form, progress, and content; and it can in fact be logically divided into stages, each with a beginning and an end point". To Kleinman (1980:77), too, "disease commonly has a typical course and characteristic features that are independent of setting. Illness is always more or less unique". In comparing medical and lay 'Explanatory Models' – that is, "the notions about an episode of sickness and its treatment that are employed by all those engaged in the clinical process" (1980:105), Kleinman contrasts medical Explanatory Models based on "single causal trains of scientific logic" with lay models characterised by "vagueness, multiplicity of meanings, frequent changes, and lack of sharp boundaries between ideas and experience" (1980:107).[1]

293

R. A. Hahn and A. D. Gaines (eds.), Physicians of Western Medicine, 293–331.
© 1985 by D. Reidel Publishing Company.

Studies of pluralistic health care systems in Third World countries — where Western biomedicine is just one of the therapeutic options available to ill people — also give the impression of the consistent, homogeneous, and scientific nature of Biomedicine (e.g., Kimani 1981; Sussman 1981).

However, a closer examination of the biomedical model — its theory and its practice — suggests that far from being homogeneous, it is rather a cluster of Explanatory Models which vary greatly according to speciality, context, audience, and type of condition, as well as the personal characteristics of the physician, and his or her position in a professional hierarchy. The Goods (1981:177) have pointed out that any physician or medical discipline has a repertoire of interpretative models — biochemical, immunological, viral, genetic, environmental, psychodynamic, family interactionist, and so on, each with its own "structure of relevance". Eisenberg (1977) has noted that in psychiatry the perspective on psychoses includes "multiple and manifestly contradictory models", such as behavioral, psychodynamic, and social models; in practice, physicians employ both 'tacit' models based on personal and everyday knowledge, *and* explicit, more scientific Explanatory Models. To some extent, both context and audience (whether medical colleagues or a lay audience) determine which model is used. In a previous study (Helman 1978) I suggested that general practitioners often use a lay or folk idiom of diagnosis or treatment which "makes sense" to their patients, rather than the "official" scientific models employed more commonly in hospital medicine. One can differentiate therefore, not only between different *theoretical* models used by physicians, but also — as Kleinman (1980:110) has pointed out — between these more "scientific" models and the observable *clinical* ones that they actually employ in their day-to-day practice. This in turn has its effect on the Explanatory Models used by patients, and there is often — over time — a complex interrelationship between these two sets of models, each of which has a varying amount of influence over the other as diagnosis and treatment take their course.

To illustrate the relationships between lay and medical models, I describe here the case of Mr. Harry White,[2] a patient in a family practice in a southern suburb of London. While Mr. White's experiences are not necessarily typical of those of the majority of British patients, an account of them does, I think, illustrate a number of themes: (1) the plurality of medical models employed by physicians, and especially the differences between models used by hospital doctors, private specialists, and general practitioners; (2) the complex nature of "disease" in the biomedical perspective; (3) the problems of "illness without identifiable disease", and the "mimicry" of disease by illness; (4) the interrelationship between lay and medical models of ill-health; and (5) the problem of iatrogenic, or doctor-induced, ill-health.

CASE HISTORY: MR HARRY WHITE

Harry White is a 46-year old advertising executive. He is married and has two children aged four and one year old from this — his second — marriage. He consulted his National Health Service (NHS) general practitioner (GP) during a busy evening clinic for two episodes of pain on the left side of his chest, each lasting about five minutes. He was worried that the pains "have something to do with my heart". He admitted to the GP that he had been "under a lot of stress recently", from problems at his business, various financial difficulties, the illness of his elderly father, the long drive to work every morning, and the lack of sleep caused by the crying of his younger child during the night. He was briefly examined by the GP who found no physical abnormality, but sent him up to the Casualty Department (emergency room) of the local General Hospital for further tests. He was told by the GP "I'm sure there's nothing seriously wrong, and it's just due to strain, but we'd better be sure and have a few tests". At the hospital, Mr. White saw a Registrar (resident) who did an electrocardiograph and took blood tests. A half-hour later, to his alarm, Mr. White was admitted to the Coronary Care Unit; this admission was, he said later, a "traumatic shock". For three days he was kept in bed, and forbidden to undertake any activity. He was constantly examined by doctors and nurses; his temperature and blood pressure were monitored every two hours; and he had daily electrocardiographs and blood tests. He was told by several of the junior doctors that he had had "a slight heart attack". He was then transferred to another ward where everyone else was "a heart case" — usually those who had had a myocardial infarction; he was here for ten days. For the first three days in this ward, he was forbidden to walk, and could only go to the toilet in a wheel-chair assisted by a nurse; he was then allowed to slowly resume walking and other activities. During this period he was told by the Senior Registrar that all the tests taken were normal, that he had *not* in fact had a "heart attack", but that "you probably have angina". He was prescribed Nifedipine (Adalat), a drug commonly used for angina, and discharged from hospital, having been told not to work for six weeks. During his hospital stay and thereafter, his wife became increasingly anxious about his health and prognosis, and about her ability to cope with the two young children in the future. After his discharge, Mr. White "felt physically shattered" and extremely anxious as well; he also continued to have left-sided chest pain which increased in severity, and sometimes lasted up to eight hours. He was afraid to exert any effort, and was easily tired and worried about the "pressure" in his chest; he was "nervous about doing things" — especially as the hospital had given him no advice on how much he could do. He became more and more apathetic, and repeatedly questioned his own capability to lead a normal life in the future.

The general practitioner was informed by letter from the House Officer (intern) in charge of Mr. White's hospital treatment that he had had a "myocardial infarc-tion"; later a second letter arrived from the Senior Registrar saying that Mr. White had had "chest pain . . . thought to be anginal in origin", but that *all* tests done in the hospital were "negative". To clear up this apparent discrepancy, Mr. White was referred two weeks after his discharge from hospital to an eminent cardiologist, whom he saw privately (i.e., outside the NHS, and therefore paid for directly). The cardiologist examined him thoroughly, did various tests including several electrocardiographs, and found no abnormalities whatsoever. He also elicited the facts about the sources of "tension" in his daily life, and said that this was responsible for his "hyperventilation", i.e., rapid over-breathing — something he had never noticed as a problem before — and that this caused his symptoms and could easily be treated by breathing into a brown paper bag. He prescribed no medication, and strongly reassured the patient that "there is no evidence of ischemic heart disease"; he did not suggest further blood tests because, as he wrote to the GP, "I thought it much more important for him to leave here without any reservations remaining to be settled". On hearing of the new diagnosis, Mr. White's wife reported that her husband "looked 20 years younger". Mr. White described the cardiologist as having "put my mind at rest".

He consulted his GP again a few days later, saying that he now had "hyperventilation" and "would like to have it treated"; he wanted "treatment for breathing". He was still having occasional left-sided chest pains, but less severe; which the GP now referred to as "muscular aches". He prescribed diazepam ('Valium'), and suggested to Mr. White that he relax more and reduce his sources of "stress". At the insistence of Mr. White, though, the GP referred him to another private specialist, a Chest Physician with an interest in "hyperventilation" and other "psychosomatic" disorders. He was told by this physician that he had "a classical case of hyperventilation" and not of heart disease, and that he would require "breathing re-training to eliminate faulty habits" (of breathing). Mr. White's version of this diagnosis, told to the GP, was that "I have been breathing incorrectly for as long as I've been able to breathe", that "tension makes it worse", and that "a person who breathes OK gets out of tension easier". He was taught the "proper way" to breathe, using his diaphragm. However, after the consultation, he still felt unwell, still had chest pain, and was increasingly tense about "not doing enough" of his proper breathing exercises.

Two months after he first developed the chest pain, Mr. White was assessed at the hospital Out-Patient Department by an intern for a check-up arranged at the time of his discharge. The intern, who had never seen him before but had access to his hospital records, told him that he definitely had "angina", and that he needed an urgent electrocardiograph (which turned out to be normal, as was his physical examination). For his chest pain he was nevertheless prescribed glyceryl trinitrate (nitroglycerine) tablets — a drug commonly used for angina, and widely known to the public. He found that these tablets burnt his tongue, did not relieve the pain; and, on the advice of his GP, he cancelled all further appointments at that hospital.

A month later he again consulted the GP. He was still attempting to do the "breathing exercises", and occasionally taking the diazepam. He said he was still "under stress", particularly "aggravation with my previous wife", and he now felt that all his recent chest troubles had been because he'd been "all pent up — I've never let off steam — I'm not that type of person". He still feels that "something is radically wrong", that the specialists had still "not done the full job — only helped 70%". According to his wife he is still not well; he "acts like 56, not 46".

He is often pale, has occasional chest pain, is easily tired and fatigued, still tense about "not breathing properly", and has a growing fear of sexual inadequacy. Hr is also nervous about travelling long distances. To his wife he is "a changed person − not himself". The GP has suggested that they consult a psychotherapist for further help, but they are reluctant to take this course of action.

THE BRITISH HEALTH CARE SYSTEM

To put the case-history of Harry White in context, it is necessary to give a brief overview of the British health care system.[3] Since its inception in 1948, the British National Health Service (NHS) has provided free and unrestricted health care to the entire population, at both general practice and hospital levels. Each person belongs to the "list" of a GP in his or her area. If they are dissatisfied, or move to another area, then they can change GPs. Consultations between patients and their GPs are free of charge, and take place at specified times at the clinic or surgery, or by house-call for emergencies at other times. Levitt (1976) has estimated that there are about 26 000 GPs in Britain, each with an average 'list' population of 2347 patients. Levitt estimates that while about 75% of symptoms are treated by patients themselves, the NHS GP is the first point of contact for 90% of those who *do* seek professional medical care. About one-third of a GP's patients will receive some form of hospital treatment per year. GPs can refer their patients to NHS hospitals for a specialist opinion on the case, or for diagnostic laboratory or X-ray investigations. If requested by the patient, they can also refer him or her to a private specialist, outside the NHS.

There is a clear division in Britain between hospital and general practice medicine: they have different historical roots[4] and orientations, and hospital medicine still has a higher professional status and greater NHS expenditure,[5] though this is gradually changing. General practice is essentially home- and community-based in Britain; as Hunt (1964:162) has expressed it, modern general practice "to do its greatest good, must reach patients promptly in and near their homes". The modern NHS GP is part of a "primary care team", which includes district nurses, health visitors, social workers, medical receptionists, and local health clinics. In only a minority of cases are hospitalized patients cared for wholly or partly by their own GP. Out of the 482 782 hospital beds allocated in England, Scotland and Wales in 1976, only 13 665 (2.8%) were "general practitioner beds", of which 5406 (1.1%) were maternity (obstetric) beds (Chaplin 1976:374−377). In 1978, in England and Wales, there were only 350 "cottage hospitals" − i.e., hospitals run entirely by GPs − with an average of 20−40 beds each (White 1978). In British hospitals, although GPs can visit the wards and discuss the management of their patients with hospital specialists, most of the responsibility for the patient's care is taken by these specialists and their junior medical colleagues.

As in other modern industrial societies, British hospitals are divided into specialty departments, though some hospitals specialize in only one condition, organ, or part of the body, such as Heart, Eye or Skin hospitals. In 1974 there were 42 recognized clinical specialities within the NHS hospital framework (Levitt 1976: 99). Because the NHS has so wide a patient constituency, doctor-patient consultations are often more rushed than in private medicine. The average consultation time for NHS GPs is 5–6 minutes (Morrell 1971:454), and there are often long waiting lists for non-urgent operations or out-patient appointments.

Parallel to, though interrelated with the NHS, is the *private* sector of health care, which resembles the American system in many ways. Most hospital consultants (specialists) have private patients – as do many GPs – in addition to their NHS patients. There are private laboratories, clinics, and a few private hospitals. There are two large private health insurance schemes (British United Provident Association, and Private Patients' Plan), and several smaller ones. Most patients who utilize private medicine in Britain are also registered with a local NHS GP, and people move freely between the two systems. What money buys in the private sector is *time, choice*, and *control*: i.e., a longer consultation time with a GP or specialist (with more time for explanations of the patient's condition by the doctor), and shorter waiting time for operations; choice of consultant or hospital; and the feeling (or illusion) of control over the treatment given – if one specialist's treatment is unsatisfactory, then one can always go to another.

These differences – between general practice and hospital medicine, and between the public and private sectors – help explain some of the variation in Explanatory Models discernible in different parts of the health care system.

THE DISTRIBUTION OF MEDICAL KNOWLEDGE WITHIN THE NHS

The types of clinical information about a particular patient or illness episode actually made *available* to clinicians caring for that patient within the NHS vary greatly in both quality and quantity. To some extent this depends on the structural position and context that the clinician occupies within the NHS. This is discussed in more detail below, and is shown schematically in Table I.

A general practitioner, for example, knows a great deal about the social and familial background of a patient on his list; he may have dealt with that patient since childhood, and probably cares for several members of the family at the same time. Unlike the United States, British general practice is more home- and community-based, and visits to an ill patient's home are quite common. As Harris, (1980:27) remarks: "In general practice it is easy to appreciate how a patient's illness and social circumstances are related, because the social circumstances are visible." Such social and familial information, though, is *not* available (at least not in any depth or detail) to hospital doctors dealing with a patient – especially in an emergency situation.

Conversely, NHS GPs can only order certain "minor" tests – both laboratory and radiological tests – from their local NHS hospital. These tests include: hematological (blood counts, hematocrits, etc.), biochemical (serum electrolytes, etc.), virological (e.g., certain antibody titers), and bacteriological tests (such as cultures of blood, sputum, urine, stools, etc.). Certain X-rays can also be ordered, especially

TABLE I

Types of information available to different NHS clinicians faced with a particular episode of ill-health

	General practitioners	Junior hospital doctors	Senior hospital specialists
Social & familial information	▨		
History (reported symptoms)	▨	▨	▨
Examination (physical signs)	▨	▨	▨
Minor tests	▨	▨	▨
Major tests		▨	▨
Specialised experience of certain conditions			▨

▨ = Information available.

of the chest, skull, abdomen, and skeletal system. While some GPs do electrocardio-graphs in their offices, others prefer these to be done in the Casualty Department and interpreted by a cardiologist on the spot. Other, more "major" investigations can only be carried out in hospital, at the request of a hospital specialist; these include certain X-rays such as Barium enemas and arteriograms, certain biopsies, gastroscopy and sigmoidoscopy investigations, and ultra-sound and CT scans. While the information from these "major" tests will eventually reach the GPs – sometimes after a delay of several weeks – they are meant more for the immediate interpretation and use of *hospital* specialists. Both hospital doctors and GPs, though, collect the same clinical information in the consultation – i.e., symptoms elicited by questioning, and physical signs elicited by examination.

A further dimension of the information available to different clinicians is that of *experience* in the interpretation of certain information by a physician, e.g., one specialising in cardiology. This experience is of three types: (1) the physician's own experience gathered during his or her years in a particular speciality; (2) personally transmitted information from his medical colleagues; and (3) the experience of other physicians in the same speciality, as described in the more complex medical textbooks and speciality journals and conferences. This "second-hand" knowledge is of particular importance in modern industrialized society with the "explosion" of scientific knowledge expressed in books, journals, etc. (Toffler 1970:144–149). This explosion limits certain information to specialists in a particular field, and such information is largely inaccessible to busy GPs, and is only beginning to be accessible to junior hospital doctors entering a particular speciality. Also, as Kleinman (1982) has pointed out, professional specialization can influence what information is actually "observed"; a specialist with a particular orientation – who is looking for a particular cluster of symptoms and signs – "sees" the disorder differently from a specialist with another orientation. Thus specialization affects both the availability of clinical information, and the interpretation of that information.

Not all the information available about a patient may be used, though, in determining diagnosis and treatment; this is illustrated later in the case of Mr. White's "pseudo-angina". Even in the presence of "hard" information, such as X-rays, diagnosis and treatment are subject to a continuing process of "negotiation" between lay and medical models, in reaching an agreement as to further courses of action (see Stimson and Webb 1975:972).

In the case-history of Mr. White, the two private specialists consulted have the same information base as the senior hospital specialist, i.e., the Senior Registrar. They have access to the results of both major and minor tests done in the hospital, but also have more time to elicit more social and behavioral information and background. The *time* factor is also important in the distribution of medical knowledge within the NHS. Social and familial information is usually gathered by GPs over several years; symptoms and signs of ill-health are gathered in a much shorter time (in many GP consultations, as noted earlier, in 5–6 minutes); changes in these symptoms and signs are more closely observable on a daily basis in a hospital ward setting than in general practice; and the results of both minor and major tests are available almost immediately for hospital doctors to interpret and act upon, but only reach GPs after a variable period of time, often subject to postal and other delays.

THE RANGE OF BIOMEDICAL MODELS

Mr. White's case-history illustrates some of the different biomedical explanations for ill-health encountered by a single patient in a three-month period. During this time, five different explanations for his condition were given by the different clinicians involved in his treatment. In addition to the GP's own explanation ("muscular aches from stress"), the four specialists each gave a different explanation to the GP for Mr. White's condition. While all five of these sets of explanations were couched in biomedical concepts and language, they differed substantially from one another – consituting a range of different Explanatory Models.

Biomedicine – the Western practitioner's perspective on ill-health – comprises a cluster of Explanatory Models. Following Kleinman's formulation (1978), each Explanatory Model provides explanations for some or all of five aspects of ill-health: etiology, the onset of symptoms, the pathophysiological processes involved, the course or natural history of the illness, and the appropriate treatment to be given. Within Biomedicine, practitioner models vary greatly, and the clinical decision-making process is subject to a variety of influences, as illustrated in Table II.

TABLE II
Influences on the clinical decision-making process

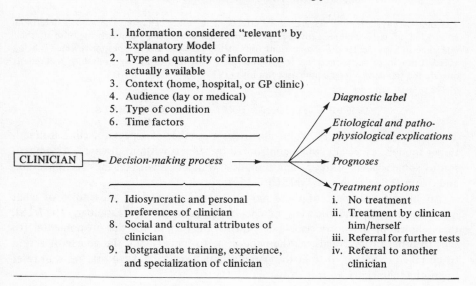

1. Information considered "relevant" by
   Explanatory Model
2. Type and quantity of information
   actually available
3. Context (home, hospital, or GP clinic)
4. Audience (lay or medical)   *Diagnostic label*
5. Type of condition
6. Time factors   *Etiological and patho-*
                                           physiological explications

CLINICIAN ───► *Decision-making process* ───────► *Prognoses*

                                           Treatment options
7. Idiosyncratic and personal   i.   No treatment
   preferences of clinician   ii. Treatment by clinican
8. Social and cultural attributes of   him/herself
   clinician   iii. Referral for further tests
9. Postgraduate training, experience,   iv. Referral to another
   and specialization of clinician   clinician

In any particular episode of ill-health, these influences will include: (1) the clinical information regarded as relevant "data" by an Explanatory Model (see Eisenberg 1977:18); (2) the type and quantity of clinical information actually available to the physician (see Table I); (3) the context of diagnosis and treatment (whether in general practice or hospital, private or public sector medicine); (4) the audience (whether patients or other clinicians, and therefore whether couched in the folk idiom or in biomedical concepts); (5) the type of condition (whether a straightforward condition such as a bone fracture, which is easily understood by patients, or a more complex psychiatric condition requiring a similarly complex Explanatory Model); (6) time factors, as mentioned above; (7) the personal preferences and idiosyncrasies of the clinician — including "pet" or favourite theories or conditions; (8) the social and cultural attributes of the clinician, which may affect his or her interpretation of a clinical situation; and (9) the nature and extent of post-graduate medical or other education, e.g., a residency in surgery or one in psychiatry, and the clinical speciality of the clinician — the models used by psychiatrists are different from, say, those of gastroenterologists, though they sometimes overlap. Post-graduate medical education includes the nature and extent of the clinician's *experience* of similar conditions in his own practice, or in the practices of others, for example, as published in the medical literature.

The context of diagnosis and treatment includes the position that the clinician occupies in the professional hierarchy; for example, the tightly monitored and controlled role of the junior doctor in a hospital.

Whatever Explanatory Models are employed, each one — as Eisenberg (1977) has noted — is a way of constructing reality, of imposing meaning on the chaos of the phenomenological world. He notes:

The models physicians use have decisive effects on medical behavior. The models determine what kind of data will be gathered; phenomena become "data" precisely because of their relevance to a particular set of questions (out of the possible sets of questions) which is being asked. Once in place, models act to generate their own verification by excluding phenomena outside the frame of reference the user employs (1977:18).

FIVE PRACTITIONER EXPLANATORY MODELS

The case-history of Harry White illustrates a number of aspects of clinical practitioner models, especially when confronted by "illness without disease". A comparison of some aspects of these clinical models, which deal with diagnosis, explication, and treatment, is shown in Table III.

An important aspect of these models is *choice*: initially, the choice of what questions to ask, and the type of data to be gathered (see Eisenberg 1977:18); then choice of diagnostic label, of explanation to give for the phenomenon (to self, to other professionals, to the patient, or to family), and the course of action to be taken (whether to treat the patient oneself, call for diagnostic tests, or refer to another clinician).

1. *The General Practitioner Model*

To a large extent, general practice in Britain is as much directed towards the treatment of illness", as towards that of "disease".[6] The minor, self-limiting nature of many conditions seen in general practice, the short consultation times, the access to only a limited range of diagnostic tests, all lead to an emphasis on symptomatic treatment — rather than a more "scientific" and precise diagnosis and treatment (see Helman 1978). In addition, the long-term familiarity of a GP with a patient and his family — in both sickness and health — all lead to an emphasis on the personal, social, and familial aspects of ill-health.[7] In Hunt's view (1964:165), the GP should "put care of the patient's mind before that of his body", and, "the family doctor's awareness of what patients think and feel is vitally important for the whole of his or her work". In general practice, as Harris (1980:27) puts it: "*No* illness can be understood or managed without reference to the unique circumstances of the patient who suffers it", and "all diagnoses have a social component, whether or not there are social problems".

In this setting, the GP is a form of fictive relative, privy to much information about the family dynamics; unlike hospital medicine, the patient — or unit of treatment — is the *family*, not the individual. The physical signs of the patient are only one component of a much wider picture. Unlike hospital doctors, who wear white coats, British GPs usually wear civilian clothes, usually live in the community in which they practice, and often phrase diagnoses and sometimes treatment more in the folk idiom than in "scientific" terms (Helman 1978). Most

TABLE III

Comparison of practitioner explanatory models

	General Practitioner	House Officer (Intern)	Senior Registrar (Resident)	Cardiologist	Chest Physician
Diagnostic label	Muscular aches	Myocardial infarction	Angina pectoris	Pseudo-angina	Pseudo-angina
Etiology	External stressors	Coronary artery thrombosis	Narrowing of coronary arteries	Hyperventilation	Hyperventilation
Predisposing causes	Introverted hypochondriacal personality	Coronary heart disease	Coronary heart disease	Tension	Perfectionist personality, bad breathing habits, tension
Site of physiological malfunction	Musculo-skeletal system	Cardiovascular system	Cardiovascular system	Respiratory system	Respiratory system
Treatment	Reassurance, psychotherapy, tranquillizers	Hospital admission, medication, observation	Hospital admission, medication, observation, follow-up	Reassurance, rebreathing in paper bag	Breathing, re-training and overcoming faulty habits
Focus of treatment	Patient and family unit	Patient	Patient	Patient	Patient

of the conditions seen by GPs are, as mentioned, minor and self-limiting. Levitt (1976:95) quotes a study of the morbidity of 2500 patients in a NHS family practice in one year — 1365 of these had "minor illnesses", 288 "major illnesses", and 588 "chronic illness". Most major diseases are dealt with wholly or partly by the local hospital specialists to whom the patient is referred. Experienced GPs work on the basis of the aphorism "Common things occur commonly", and less common, major diseases are usually referred in a short while to specialists. GPs act as a "screening mechanism", to differentiate illness, which they treat, from major disease — which will be partly cared for by the hospital. Younger GPs, who are nearer to the official hospital "textbook picture of disease", are more oriented towards the use of hospital tests. Levitt (1976:97) estimated that 25% of all GPs — mostly the younger, more recently qualified ones — account for 75% of all requests to hospitals for these tests.

In the case of Harry White, the GP had access to information about his family background which was inaccessible to hospital doctors; e.g., he had known, for several years, that Mr. White was an introspective, introverted individual, with a long history of psychological symptoms such as anxiety, depression, insomnia or loss of libido, as well as "psychosomatic" symptoms such as migraine and tension headaches. His mother had died slowly of Coronary Heart Disease, and he had asked for check-ups of his blood pressure on several occasions (it was always normal). He was under stress from a number of sources: the illness of his elderly father, lack of sleep from the crying of his baby, staff problems at work, business worries, the long drive to work in the mornings, alimony problems with his former wife, and the over-anxiety of his present wife. According to the GP's records, the present Mrs. White had consulted him *12* times in the previous six months complaining of pains on the left side of her chest, and her left breast. On all these occasions no evidence of physical disease was found, either by the GP or by two specialists to whom she was referred. At the time she denied any domestic or other stress.

The GP model, unlike hospital models, included much information of a social or psychological kind, and focussed more on illness than on disease (which could only be conclusively excluded by a specialist). The tensions within the family unit, the hypochondriasis and over-anxiety of both parties, and the frequent resort to somatization were considered the most important phenomena in the Explanatory Model. Like the patient's model, it altered over time as new information was received from the various specialists consulted. The basic GP model of this case is shown in Table IV.

2. *The Junior Hospital Doctor's Model*

The medical staff in British NHS hospitals are organized, in each speciality, into hierarchies known as "firms". Each "firm" usually consists of a Consultant (senior specialist) and under him tiers of junior doctors supervised by him. After graduation, a young doctor becomes a House Officer or Intern (for one year), then Senior

TABLE IV
The general practitioner model

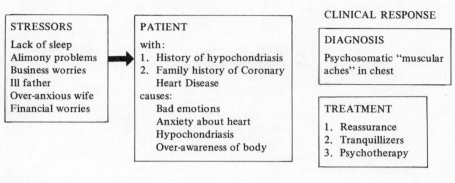

CLINICAL RESPONSE

STRESSORS	PATIENT
Lack of sleep	with:
Alimony problems	1. History of hypochondriasis
Business worries	2. Family history of Coronary
Ill father	Heart Disease
Over-anxious wife	causes:
Financial worries	Bad emotions
	Anxiety about heart
	Hypochondriasis
	Over-awareness of body

DIAGNOSIS

Psychosomatic "muscular aches" in chest

TREATMENT

1. Reassurance
2. Tranquillizers
3. Psychotherapy

➡ = Effecting, or acting upon.

House Officer (for one year), Registrar (one to three years), then Senior Registrar (three to five years), and then eventually a Consultant (Levitt 1976:98).

The hospital is, in effect, a miniature city (Helman 1980), with its own self-contained world and implicit and explicit rules of behavior. In the ward, the patient's behavior is tightly controlled by rigid schedules, fixed meal-times, and treatment schedules, all based on ostensible "scientific" premises. Mr. White's experience in the Coronary Care Unit is an example of this organization. Both nurses and junior doctors (House Officers and Senior House Officers) – i.e., those medical staff most intimately in contact with the patient – can also only act in a circumscribed way, tightly controlled and supervised by their medical superiors (Titmuss 1964:278).

The junior hospital doctor's model of ill-health, based on limited information and experience (see Table I), is closest to the "textbook picture of disease" and his or her constant fear is one of mis-diagnosis – to be led astray by the "clinical minicry" to be described later.[8] In one study, too, quoted by Waxler (1981:294–295), a hospital resident on night duty tended to hospitalize patients to be safe – "because he is unsure of his evaluation and is far less resourceful in planning and implementing an alternative to hospitalization". In that sense, the junior doctor's own anxiety is being treated, as well as the illness/disease of the patient. Mr. White was admitted to the hospital and the Coronary Care Unit "to be safe"; even in the absence of experience and the results of tests, the textbook picture of disease assumes an underlying "somatic referent" until proved otherwise (see Day and Sowton 1976:337). As Short puts it (1981:310), in discussing chest pain from Coronary Heart Disease, "a complete absence of abnormal physical signs by no means excludes the diagnosis" – and this knowledge is bound to reinforce the junior doctor's anxiety about missing an important diagnosis.

The initial hospital letter, written by the House Officer to the GP, shortly after Mr. White's hospitalization, gave the diagnosis as "myocardial infarction", and stated:

TABLE V
The Junior Hospital Doctor's Model

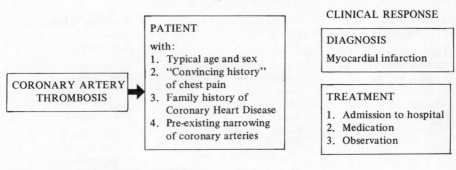

CLINICAL RESPONSE

CORONARY ARTERY THROMBOSIS ➡

PATIENT
with:
1. Typical age and sex
2. "Convincing history" of chest pain
3. Family history of Coronary Heart Disease
4. Pre-existing narrowing of coronary arteries

DIAGNOSIS
Myocardial infarction

TREATMENT
1. Admission to hospital
2. Medication
3. Observation

➡ = Effecting, or acting upon.

Course and Management: No marked enzyme or ECG changes, but in view of his age and convincing history he was treated as an infarct. No complications.

The junior hospital doctor's model is shown in Table V.

3. *The Senior Hospital Doctor's Model*

Senior Registrars are given considerable autonomy in making diagnoses and pre-scribing treatment, though this varies from "firm" to "firm". In the management of Mr. White, the Consultant played little or no part, and final responsibility seems to have been that of the Senior Registrar. Over a ten-day period he had access to a wider range of clinical information (see Table I), than the House Officer who dealt with him on admission, including Mr. White's behavior over time in the ward. As a Senior Registrar specializing in Internal Medicine, his experience of such cases was fairly wide — though probably not as wide as an older cardiologist, who would usually be more familiar with all the possible presentations of Coronary Heart Disease. To the Senior Registrar, there is still the fear of "silent" — i.e., asymptomatic and unidentifiable — Coronary Heart Disease, which is known to occur (see Julian 1977:18). Angina pectoris, as a biomedical conceptual category, is associated with a cluster of dangers — especially in younger men — in the view of a clinician. In this case, despite the absence of "hard" evidence of a myocardial infarction or of Coronary Heart Disease, but faced with the symptoms and be-havioral changes mimicking angina pectoris, the Registrar concluded:

Because of this man's age and the character of his pain, we felt it wisest to exclude M.I. (myocardial infarction) and he was admitted for investigation. Subsequently, serial ECG's remained normal and cardiac enzymes were not elevated. He made an uneventful recovery and was discharged home to convalescence. Our feeling is that if this man did indeed sustain a myocardial infarction it was of a very minor extent. He was discharged home on Adalat 10 mg t.d.s. because he had minor episodes of chest pain during admission which were thought to be anginal in origin.

This explanatory model illustrates some of the "non-scientific" elements of practitioner clinical models. The "if" and "thought to be", in the absence of "hard" data of a physical abnormality, indicate the *subjective* element in clinical diagnosis and treatment, and in that sense their resemblance to lay models of ill-health. Despite the growth of modern diagnostic technology, what Feinstein (1975) sees as the "art" of medicine (i.e., treatment and prognosis) still persists, and even diagnosis is under the influence of subjective and contextual variations (see Stimson and Webb 1975:37).

Unlike the GP model, the models of both junior and senior hospital doctors focused on the patient, rather than his family. The Senior Registrar's model is shown in Table VI.

TABLE VI
The senior hospital doctor's model

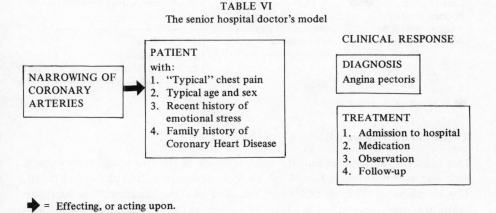

= Effecting, or acting upon.

4. *The Cardiologist's Model*

The cardiologist's model, based on a wider range of clinical information and experience, and not influenced by a position in a hospital hierarchy, offered an explanation for Mr. White's "illness without disease" — the so-called "hyperventilation" syndrome. Since consultation with a specialist in the private sector increases the consultation time, the amount of clinical information available for making diagnoses also increases, and there is also more time for explanations to the patient. The cardiologist elicited some of the "tension" factors in Mr. White's life (though fewer than those known to his GP), which "caused" his hyperventilation, and thus the "pseudo-angina". His tests first excluded any physical abnormality (though an arteriogram was not performed) — the main aim of the consultation — and he was confident enough to rule it out unconditionally. The eventual diagnosis given was based on a loose cluster of symptoms, signs, and behavioral changes, for example:

I had little doubt clinically that he was describing the hyperventilation syndrome to me, and noted that he did tend to sigh deeply, albeit unaware of this, during the consultation.

Unlike the two hospital models, this includes psychological and behavioral information, as well as the absence of any physical abnormality, in reaching the diagnosis of "hyperventilation". The resemblance of "pseudo-angina" to "real" angina was unmasked, and an alternative physical diagnosis was given, with a simple physical self-treatment ("re-breathing into a brown paper bag"). This model can be expressed as is shown in Table VII.

TABLE VII
The cardiologist's model

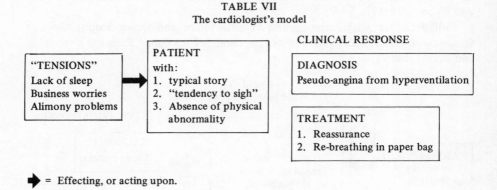

= Effecting, or acting upon.

5. *The Chest Physician's Model*

This model is, to some extent, the most complex of the five practitioner models, including as it does moral, behavioral, social, environmental, and physical elements. The diagnosis of "hyperventilation" resulting in "pseudo-angina" is based on subjective interpretations of a cluster of symptoms, signs, and behavioral changes — in the absence of any clear pathognomonic evidence of a physical disease process (see Lum 1981; Evans and Lum 1977). As Eisenberg has noted (1977:18), models determine the types of clinical information that will be gathered, and will be considered relevant "data". I have suggested that this choice of the information to be gathered is partly determined by idiosyncratic or personal preferences of the physician. These preferences — for a particular diagnosis, disease, or set of symptoms and signs — especially in the absence of "hard" physical data — are one aspect of the physician's clinical construction of reality, embodying also some of his own moral or social viewpoints, rather than testable scientific hypotheses. Like folk Explanatory Models, or those of diviners in non-industrialised societies, this type of approach involves searching for a single unifying principle or identity from the apparent chaos of symptoms and signs that make up the clinical picture. In this case, the unifying principle is that of a *pseudo-disease* (which is described in more detail below); the signs and symptoms are gathered together under a single diagnostic lable such as "hyperventilation" — and given a "typical" or "classic" clinical personality (even though, as Lum [1981:1] notes, this is impossible in hyperventilation which mimics so wide a range of disorders). To the chest physician in this case:

Mr. White presented a classical picture of hyperventilation . . . . The history was typical . . . .
Close enquiry, however, reveals many features typical of hyperventilation, and not of heart
disease . . . . Examination revealed no physical abnormality of heart or lungs but the breathing
was quite typical of hyperventilation.[9]

This model also embodies a theory of personality types; Mr. White "has the typical
perfectionist personality", with "faulty habits" (of breathing). With these "faulty
habits" he is particularly vulnerable to outside "tension". The onus of treatment,
as with the cardiologist, is placed on the patient, who will require "breathing
retraining" to eliminate these bad habits. Some relaxation exercises and auto-
hypnosis were also suggested for his "general tension". Defining the patient by
personality-type also helps shift the responsibility for therapeutic failure to the
patient himself, in a form of "victim blaming". There is a paradox, though, between
this view of "faulty habits" and the "perfectionist" personality of the victim;
while he strives for perfection in his daily life, he has not yet perfected even his
own breathing. Here, the treatment recommended is "hard work" towards recovery
– a work ethic philosophy with strong moral disapproval of "bad habits" and lack
of work; for example (from a letter to the GP after the second consultation with
the chest physician):

He confesses that he is not practicing his breathing exercises as assiduously as he should because
in recent weeks he has been too busy. I managed to get him breathing tolerably well again,
but he will need to put in a lot of work to conquer his bad breathing habits. However he does
realize this, and I extracted a promise that he would work harder at it.

This model implies a view of normative behavior, not only in a social sense, but
including the control of bodily functions such as breathing. It does also include a
cluster of vague symptoms and signs which allegedly reappear when the patient
is made to hyperventilate during the consultation ("Voluntary overbreathing
reproduced a typical bracket[10] of symptoms with which he was quite familiar."),
and in this way an otherwise tenuous diagnosis is "proved" in the eyes of the
clinician, and those of the patient. A summary of the chest physician's model is
shown in Table VIII.

THE PATIENT'S EXPLANATORY MODELS

The five clinical practitioner models mentioned above differ in a number of ways
(see Table III). These include: the diagnostic label, etiology, predisposing factors,
the definition of the patient (the individual, or the family), the locus of responsibility for the illness – and for its treatment, the origin of the symptoms, and so on.
In the three-month period described in Mr. White's case-history, he made contact
with all five of these practitioner models. During this time, his perspective on his
own illness underwent a continuing process of re-definition and re-labelling (see
Amarasingham 1980). Each clinical model he encountered had its effect on his
own definition of the problem, its possible significance, treatment, and prognosis,

TABLE VIII
The chest physician's model

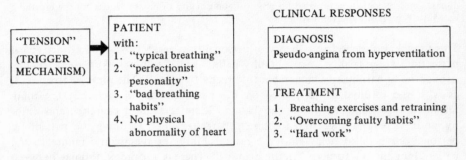

= Effecting, or acting upon.

as well as the behavior appropriate for each diagnosis. In this way, clinical explanatory models may come to create the behaviors they seek to explain.

Each interaction between physician and patient represents a transaction between two Explanatory Models (Kleinman 1980:111), usually through the process of "negotiation" (see Stimson and Webb 1975:48, 119), in which both parties attempt to attain a consensus about the appropriate diagnosis, and the best treatment to be given. The ongoing effect of these negotiations on Mr. White's definition of his illness are shown in Table IX.

The lay models employed in this case represent, therefore, the *interplay* between the five clinical models and Mr. White's beliefs about illness in general, and his own illness in particular; that is, between medical views of "cardiac disease", and lay views of "heart problems". As Kleinman (1980:109) has noted, lay explanatory models can undergo changes fairly often, due to the "diffused" nature of popular medical knowledge, and this is illustrated in this case-history.

It should be noted, though, that lay Explanatory Models do not necessarily include comprehensive theories about the structure and functions of the human body, and the pathophysiological processes involved in ill-health, as implied in some medical anthropological writings. Much of the model is unconscious (see Kleinman 1980:109) and, as I have mentioned elsewhere (Helman 1981:416–417), the patient is *not* an endless theorizer with conceptual models to fully explain every illness event.

Although, in this case, Mr. White's *behavior* changed, becoming more typically "angina-like" after his experiences in the Coronary Care Unit, several interviews with him during this period did not reveal more detailed Explanatory Models than are mentioned in the case-history. He was unable to articulate how the heart functioned, and how it mis-functioned. Mr. White's final Explanatory Model has a more hydraulic, mechanistic imagery: he ascribes all his recent chest problems to having previously been "all pent up. I've never let off steam. I'm not that type of person". He still feels that "something is radically wrong", and that the various

TABLE IX

Negotiations between patient's and clinicians' diagnostic models

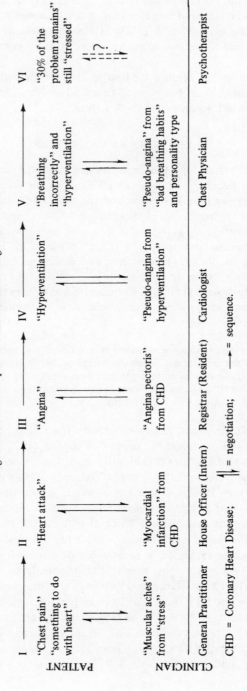

	I	II	III	IV	V	VI
PATIENT	"Chest pain" "something to do with heart"	"Heart attack"	"Angina"	"Hyperventilation"	"Breathing incorrectly" and "hyperventilation"	"30% of the problem remains" still "stressed"
CLINICIAN	"Muscular aches" from "stress"	"Myocardial infarction" from CHD	"Angina pectoris" from CHD	"Pseudo-angina from hyperventilation"	"Pseudo-angina" from "bad breathing habits" and personality type	
	General Practitioner	House Officer (Intern)	Registrar (Resident)	Cardiologist	Chest Physician	Psychotherapist

CHD = Coronary Heart Disease;   ⇌ = negotiation;   ⟶ = sequence.

specialists had still "not done the full job — only helped 70%" (of the problem). While the GP was prepared to refer him to a psychotherapist, it is possible that this remaining illness (the "30%"), is situational in origin, at least from Mr. White's point of view, and therefore unlikely to profit from contact with yet another clinical model.

At each stage in Mr. White's medical treatment, his own model represented a mixture of elements, from both lay and medical sources, and this will be described more fully below in the context of "folk angina".

THE NATURE OF "DISEASE"

In discussing the range of physicians' models, and the distribution of medical knowledge, it is necessary to look more closely at the biomedical perspective on "disease". Several authors have criticized the mind-body dualism of Biomedicine, its reduction of ill-health to physicochemical terms, and its over-emphasis on biological information — as opposed to social or behavioral information — in deciding on diagnosis and treatment (e.g., Cassell 1976; Eisenberg 1977; Engel 1980; Kleinman et al. 1978). Kleinman and colleagues (1978) for example, see biologic concerns as being more basic, "real", and clinically significant to clinicians than social or psychological factors. Good and Good (1981) also note Biomedicine's emphasis on symptoms as being mainly reflections or manifestations of disordered somatic processes:

Symptoms achieve their *meaning* in relationship to physiological states, which are interpreted as the referents of the symptoms . . . Somatic lesions or dysfunctions produce discomfort and behavioral changes, communicated in a patient's complaints. The critical clinical task of the physician is to "decode" a patient's discourse by relating symptoms to their biological referents in order to diagnose a disease entity (1981:170).

Western Biomedicine tends to over-emphasize the role of biological information in the diagnosis and treatment of "disease". Feinstein (1973:212) also sees diseases as "conceptual medical entities that identify or explain abnormalities in the observed evidence". These "abnormalities" imply concepts of "normality" built into the various Explanatory Models. There are, however, several tiers of "normality" and "abnormality" — not all of them based on biological criteria — in the models used by clinicians in this case-history. While the "official" Biomedicine of medical schools and textbooks does adhere more closely to numerical definitions of physical abnormality (e.g., as expressed in measurable deviations from a defined range of "normal values" such as height, weight, hemoglobin level, white cell count, and serum electrolyte levels [Helman 1981:548]), other, *non*-physical definitions of normality are used by most clinicians as part of their (clinical) Explanatory Models. The concepts of "stress" (the GP), "tension" (the cardiologist), and "bad breathing habits" (the chest physician), all imply wider social, psychological or moral (and behavioral) definitions of normality which are not dissimilar to those employed in lay models of ill-health. The "tacit", everyday models — particularly of GPs – based on "commonsense" and their own inherited folk knowledge, all help widen definitions of normality or abnormality beyond the purely biological (see Helman 1978).

Biomedical diagnosis is based on three types of clinical information: (see Table I): the history (the patient's reported symptoms, as well as social and familial information reported by the patient or their family); the examination (the physical signs of disease, as elicited by the clinician in his examination, often with use of special instruments such as a stethoscope or otoscope); and hospital investigations (which in the context of the British NHS include both minor and major tests). There is, of course, an overlap between these three types of clinical evidence. All three, for example, require the subjective *interpretation* of the results by the clinician, as mentioned earlier. In addition, many of the hospital tests can be seen as extensions of the traditional methods of examination: touching, feeling, looking, listening, and smelling, (see Helman 1978:126). X-rays, sigmoidoscopy, endoscopy are all ways of "seeing", echocardiographs a way of "hearing", and so on. Nevertheless, there *has* been a shift in the relative importance of the three types of clinical information.

This shift is from history/examination towards hospital investigation, from "subjective" evidence to supposedly "objective" evidence, the latter usually couched in numerical, easily quantifiable terms. Historically, it seems as though the center of gravity of the Western medical world has moved from community-based general practice towards the hospitals (especially the teaching hospitals) – a process that has been underway in Britain since the 18th-century (see Levitt 1976:88). Parallel with this process, has been the more recent growth in diagnostic technology which can now identify abnormalities of bodily structure or function at the cellular, biochemical, or molecular level. There has therefore been a considerable shift in the types of clinical information available and considered relevant to medical explanatory models, provided that the results of these complex investigations are available to clinicians.

In Feinstein's view (1975), the growth of modern diagnostic technology (particularly in a hospital setting), has had the result that:

With increasing frequency in modern medicine, diseases are diagnostically identified as abnormalities not in a patient's clinical state (such as fever, jaundice, or chest pain) but in a paraclinical entity. The paraclinical abnormalities of disease can be diagnostically cited in such terms as morphologic structure (*coronary heart disease, carcinoma*), biochemical function (*diabetes mellitus, hyperthyroidism*), physiologic function (*atrial fibrillation, malabsorption*) or microbial invasion (*viral infection, meningococcemia*).[11] Although the aid of modern diagnostic technology allows these paraclinical abnormalities to be diagnosed with unprecedented specifity and consistency, the principal "lesion" of each such paraclinical disease has an associated spectrum of diverse clinical manifestations that may not always occur specifically or consistently (Feinstein 1975:4).

The diagnosis of these "paraclinical" entities is a feature of high-technology hospital-based medicine, which has access to the major Tests noted in Table I, in addition to other clinical information. As mentioned above, this represents a shift towards the putatively "objective" and "scientific" types of information, towards "hard" rather than "soft" information. In the days before advanced technological diagnoses were developed (and to some extent in general practice still), diseases were diagnosed by the interpretation of reported symptoms and observable physical signs. The shift towards "paraclinical" disease entities has changed that — at least in hospital medicine — and has led to a new classificatory system of disease, whose units are now *paraclinical disease entities*. This new classificatory system — available to all clinicians now who have access to diagnostic technology — has raised a new series of problems for clinicians.

As Feinstein (1975) points out, while the diagnosis of paraclinical disease entities can now be accurately carried out with the aid of technology, the *clinical manifestations* of such an entity are now increasingly complex and difficult to interpret. Some of these manifestations represent the "primary effects" of the disease's principal abnormality (e.g., angina pectoris is a primary effect of Coronary Heart Disease), while others are "secondary effects or complications" (e.g., congestive heart failure). These primary and secondary effects can appear alone, or in various overlapping combinations, so that, "the disease in a particular patient may occur with some, all, or none of the possible clinical manifestations" (Feinstein 1975:4).

This results in various "subsets" of patients with the *same* (paraclinical) diagnosis, but *different* clinical manifestations (or no clinical manifestations whatsoever — the case of "disease but no illness"), which may result in different treatments and different prognoses. Conversely, patients with identical *clinical* manifestations may have different *paraclinical* diagnoses as revealed by diagnostic tests. This latter case results in the situation I have termed *clinical mimicry*, to be discussed below in the context of Mr. White's "pseudo-angina". To some extent this case represents the widening gap between illness and disease (especially paraclinical disease) in the modern industrialized world.

Since *all* the possible clinical manifestations of a disease cannot be described, what Feinstein (1975) calls the classic "textbook picture of disease", (what I would prefer to call the "official", or standard version of the disease), is usually based on the most common or pathognomonic manifestations of the paraclinical disease. However, there are in effect two tiers of medical textbooks, and of medical descriptions of a particular disease: (1) the "textbook picture" mentioned by Feinstein, which is directed to medical students, or newly-qualified doctors; and (2) the specialist textbooks on a particular disorder, or range of disorders, which list *all* (or at at least most) of the known, possible clinical manifestations of a certain paraclinical disease. Familiarity with this latter kind of textbook is part of the specialized *experience* (see Table I) of senior hospital doctors. It enables them to move beyond the "textbook picture" of a disease and identify all of its possible variants, or to eliminate the other conditions that may exactly mimic its clinical manifestations.

THE MIMICRY OF DISEASE

Specialist textbooks, in particular, usually list a wide range of differential diagnoses — including other conditions that closely resemble or mimic it clinically — for a particular pathological condition. This mimicry can affect both symptoms (e.g., angina pectoris), and signs (e.g., tachycardia), and even the results of both "major" and "minor" investigations. An abnormality in an X-ray or blood test can have several different explanations, for example, and can indicate several different disease processes. The Explanatory Model of the experienced hospital specialist involves fitting together all the information available on a particular illness episode — symptoms, signs, and the results of certain tests (which identify the paraclinical disease process) — to make a definite diagnosis, initiate treatment, and assess prognosis. The assessment of treatment and prognosis, based mainly on clinical criteria, Feinstein (1975:6) sees as the "art" of medicine — unsupported by the more "scientific" information which is used to diagnose the paraclinical disease process.

Most medical textbooks, especially specialist textbooks, warn of the danger of *mis*-diagnosis — of mistaking one disease or symptom for another. This *clinical mimicry* of one condition by another, poses a major problem to the inexperienced diagnostician, or the physician who does not have access to various hospital tests (e.g., the GP in this case). This clinical mimicry can be of two types: (1) the clinical manifestations (or results of tests) of one paraclinical disease may mimic those of another (e.g., pseudo-gout), or (2) the clinical manifestations may classified as "disease" by the biomedical model, though *no* evidence of any organic paraclinical disease is found with diagnostic technology; despite this, the "disease" label persists. This latter group represents the "illness without identifiable somatic disease" group, and includes the psychosomatic disorders, hysteria, certain types of hypochondriasis, and certain folk illnesses which closely resemble known diseases. They are often termed "functional" as opposed to "organic" disorders.

The conditions in group (2) can be of two, overlapping types: (a) symptoms and/or signs that closely mimic a known disease or symptom (e.g., "pseudo-angina"), or (b) more diffuse "diseases" (e.g., hyperventilation, Da Costa's Syndrome) which do not closely resemble a paraclinical disease (though some of its component signs or symptoms may), but whose diffuse clinical manifestations are given a disease "personality" by grouping them under a single diagnostic label. All of these conditions, where there is a discrepancy between the *clinical* presentation (i.e., symptoms and signs) of a disease entity, and the underlying *paraclinical* condition (as revealed by diagnostic technology), I have termed *pseudo-diseases*. In pseudo-diseases, the diagnosis of the disease entity — based on its apparent clinical "personality" — is *not* supported by any "*hard*" evidence (e.g., certain X-rays of laboratory tests) of the appropriate underlying physical or organic abnormality — or indeed of any physical abnormality whatsoever. These conditions illustrate the tenuous connection between models of clinical and paraclinical diseases (see Feinstein 1975:4). The range of conditions covered by the biomedical definition of "disease" is illustrated in Table X.

TABLE X
The range of biomedical "disease"

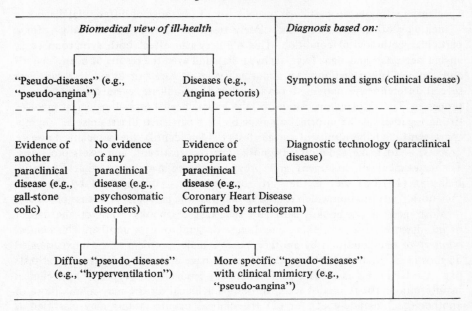

Examples of pseudo-diseases where the clinical picture of one paraclinical disease is mimicked by that of another paraclinical disease are: pseudo-gout (which mimics real gout clinically, but has a different cause), pseudo-fractures (which resemble real fractures on X-ray, but are due to certain changes in the bone itself), pseudo-precocious puberty (not "real" precocious puberty, but due rather to a secretory abnormality of the gonads), intestinal pseudo-obstruction ("a clinical and radiologic picture of acute or chronic intestinal obstruction for which no mechanical cause can be demonstrated"), pseudo-hyponatremia, male pseudo-hermaphroditism, pseudo-hypoparathyroidism, some forms of pseudo-angina, and many others (see Beeson et al. 1975). There is also pseudocyesis or "pseudo-pregnancy", where:

a woman imagines that she is pregnant and accordingly suppresses her menstrual function and develops other symptoms and signs of pregnancy such as nausea and vomiting, breast changes, increases in weight, and swelling of the abdomen. She may even allege that she can feel fetal movements and, ultimately, that she is in labor (Jeffcoate 1975:499).

In the past, when they were more common, both tuberculosis and syphilis were considered great mimics of many other diseases with both being known as the "great imitators" (Brainerd et al. 1969:149, 812).

Faced with the possibility of clinical mimicry, there is an ever-present fear in the clinician's mind (particularly junior, less experienced clinicians) of missed or mis-diagnosis, which can sometimes have fatal consequences.[12] This results in a reluctance to diagnose conditions as "non-organic", "functional" or "psychogenic" unless exhaustive tests have ruled out a physical cause — the "somatic referents" mentioned by Good and Good (1981:170). A common mimic of "real" organic disease, for example, is *hysteria* (see Eisenberg 1977:11–12), whose clinical manifestations can resemble a wide range of diseases including epilepsy or paralysis which can only be ruled out by diagnostic tests. Conversely, McHugh (1979:678–680) warns that some physical conditions such as multiple sclerosis, early acute idiopathic polyneuritis, bulbar myaesthenia gravis, postencephalitic Parkinsonism, and periodic paralysis may all mimic hysteria — particularly as they are characterized by a vague, changing clinical pattern. One example of the biomedical reluctance to diagnose hysteria was the outbreak of abdominal pain in an English village in 1972 which involved 130 children (Smith and Eastham 1973); the children were rushed to hospital and subjected to numerous tests, all of which were normal. Local food was tested, and the environmental searched for weedkiller sprays, gas leaks, unusual temperature changes, viruses, etc., but nothing abnormal was found. The authors concluded:

A diagnosis of hysteria is strengthened if all other factors are examined and possible physical causes eliminated: we believe that hysteria played the main part in the spread of this outbreak (Smith and Eastham 1973:958).

Medical textbooks also warn of the patient who, for psychological reasons,[13] has learnt to duplicate the "personality" of symptoms and signs of certain diseases, and travels from hospital to hospital having repeated tests and even operations; known as the "Münchausen Syndrome", patients with this condition "imitate illnesses so skillfully that extensive investigations and even surgery are undertaken before the diagnosis is suspected" (Hawkins 1975:326).

In addition, patients exposed for prolonged periods to clinical models may "learn" the behavior and symptomatology appropriate to their diagnosis, as in the case of Harry White. This will be discussed later in the context of the social labeling perspective on ill-health.

PSYCHOSOMATIC "DISEASES"

As Eisenberg (1977:13) has pointed out, not all the named "diseases" in the contemporary biomedical model can be identified as organic pathology (he quotes the example of hysteria) — despite the shift towards the identification of underlying physical abnormalities, or paraclinical diseases, mentioned by Feinstein (1975: 4). Given this undoubted shift, how does Biomedicine deal with episodes of "illness without disease" where *no* physical abnormality can be identified by the clinician, despite the use of modern diagnostic technology? One way is to group the collection of symptoms, signs, or behavioral changes associated with the unwell patient — which are often remarkably diverse and variable — into the conceptual entity I have termed a *pseudo-disease*: i.e., to label these clinical manifestations of illness as "disease", despite the lack of "hard" evidence of organic pathology. An example of this form of "medicalization"[14] are the diffuse conceptual entities known as *psychosomatic diseases*. These "diseases" usually derive their disease "personality" from the organ or system where the symptoms predominate. They often closely resemble, and overlap with, both folk illnesses and other biomedical diseases. Examples of these psychosomatic diseases are: "non-organic pelvic pain" (Henker 1979), the "irritable bowel syndrome" (Waller and Misiewicz 1969), "spasmodic torticollis" (Matthews et al. 1978), "pseudo-angina" (Evans and Lum 1977), "Da Costa's Syndrome" (Hurst et al. 1974), and "hyperventilation" (Waites 1978).

Biomedical explanatory models deal with the *etiologies* of these cases of "illness without disease" in a number of ways: (1) by postulating some underlying, but as yet undiscovered, physical cause — often called the "idiopathic" group (e.g., the "irritable bowel syndrome" — "the diagnosis is difficult because, as yet, no organic lesion has been demonstrated" and because "it may mimic other gastro-intestinal diseases" [Waller and Misiewicz 1969:753, 755]); (2) by seeing the condition as "psychogenic", "neurogenic" or "psychosomatic" — i.e., originating in, and caused by, "the mind" or "brain" — such as "neurocirculatory asthenia", "an ill-defined syndrome of psychogenic or neurogenic origin, often mistaken for organic heart disease" (Friedberg 1969:1721); or (3) by multi-causal explanations, such as Lum's (1981:3) explanation of "hyperventilation" as being due to "habitually unstable breathing" in a "perfectionist or mildly obsessional personality", which in turn causes somatic symptoms, which then causes anxiety, more somatic symptoms, and so on. In this view, the focus is on the somatic or biochemical changes which — in the presence of "unstable breathing", a certain type of personality, and an external stressor or "trigger" — cause emotional symptoms such as anxiety.

An example of a diffuse illness entity grouped under a single "disease" label is the *Da Costa's Syndrome* — defined as a "psychogenic" or "functional" disorder. It is a vague cluster of symptoms — several of which "mimic" organic heart disease, such as chest pain, palpitations, or shortness of breath — and which can have a multitude of clinical manifestations. As Friedberg (1969) points out:

Despite the distinctive titles given to this syndrome it is not a nosologic entity. It is nothing more than a moiety of the more general picture of psychoneurosis, which, in the cases under discussion, chances to assume entirely or predominatly the garb of cardiac or circulatory symptoms (1969:1721).

Its multiplicity of presentations is matched by a multiplicity of names, each of which embodies a different perspective and focal symptoms (Eisenberg 1977: 12) — "neurocirculatory asthenia", "irritable heart", "soldier's heart", "effort syndrome", "anxiety neurosis", "cardiac neurosis", "vasoregulatory asthenia", and "hyperdynamic β-adrenergic circulatory state" (see Hurst et al. 1974).

Faced with a particular illness episode characterised by some of the symptoms noted above, the vagueness of the "disease" category is likely — in my opinion — to make clinical explanatory models express more of the "vagueness, multiplicity of meanings, frequent changes, and lack of sharp boundaries between ideas and experience" that Kleinman (1980:107) sees as typical of lay Explanatory Models. Like those lay models, the history of Da Costa's Syndrome shows both cultural patterning and changes over time (Eisenberg 1977:12). And as with other psychosomatic conditions, there are few objective physical signs on examination, and tests such as electrocardiography are all normal; it is a case of "illness without disease".

Good (1977:39), in discussing "heart distress" in Iran, has pointed out that folk illness categories can be understood as "images which condense fields of experience, particularly of stressful experience", and also as "the core symbols in a semantic network, a network of words, situations, symptoms and feelings which are associated with an illness and give it meaning for the sufferer". In a similar way, grouping a series of vague symptoms under a single diagnostic label, can be seen as giving *meaning* to these symptoms in the eyes of the diagnostician — even in the absence of "hard" data of a paraclinical disease entity. Medical models, like lay models, organize clinical chaos into diagnostic order; in instances — like the Da Costa's Syndrome — where a paraclinical disease cannot be demonstrated, and where there are multiple clinical manifestations, the diagnostic category often has social, moral, and psychological elements more often associated with folk illness categories, especially with regard to etiology. For example, sufferers from Da Costa's Syndrome are said to have "a fundamental ego insecurity", with "maternal or familial overprotection" in childhood, often with a history of "serious maladjustments", "nervous breakdowns", or "long absences from school or work", (Friedberg 1969:1721). Situations that precede or cause the symptoms include "emotion-provoking situations, illness, hard physical work, pregnancy, and military service" (Hurst et al. 1974:1553).

Eisenberg (1977) has noted that the same constellation of symptoms and signs can be ascribed to medical causes (as in Da Costa's Syndrome, or "soldier's heart") *or* given a moral quality (e.g., cowardice) if they appear in, say, a battlefield situation. Medical models of psychosomatic "diseases" — because they include social, familial, behavioral, and personality information, as well as biological information (or often, the absence of it) — seem more likely to be *time-* and *context-specific* than models of other diseases. They explain why those symptoms happened to that particular individual, at that particular time. In that sense, they bear a much closer resemblance to the sort of folk illnesses described by Fábrega (1973:218) which are also characterized by the interrelationship of personality, social, familial, and moral factors, and where each illness event, to a significant extent, is unique and "idiosyncratic in form, progress and content". El-Islam (1975), for example, describes such a folk illness, with symptoms very similar to the Da Costa's and "hyperventilation" syndromes, which effects women of Qatar, and which is also imbedded in a matrix of sociocultural factors.

Like Da Costa's Syndrome, *hyperventilation* is a loose and changeable diagnostic category — a "pseudo-disease", or cluster of pseudo-diseases. As Lum (1981:1) has written: "Hyperventilation can fairly claim to have replaced syphilis as the great mimic". It "can manifest itself by bizarre and often apparently unrelated symptoms

that may affect any part of the body and any organ system" (Waites 1978:1700).
Like Da Costa's Syndrome, there are few clinical signs, and tests reveal *no* underlying
paraclinical disease. As a disease category, it does not provide the basis for the
"single causal trains of scientific logic" which Kleinman (1980:107) sees as typical
of medical Explanatory Models when faced with a particular episode of ill-health.
No clear causal or predictive link can be made between the supposed pathophysiological processes involved, "hypocapnia" and "respiratory alkalosis", and the
vast range of its possible clinical manifestations. It has none of the "recurring
identity" associated — at least in the "textbook picture of disease" — with other
diseases, but rather a fluid and unpredictable identity. It is supposed, though,
to be very common, and to account for 6–10% of all referrals to specialist clinics
(Lum 1981:1). Like other psychosomatic disorders, the diagnosis is based on
three factors: (1) the patient's behavioral changes, and reports of subjective symptoms (which are often organised into folk illness entities), (2) the absence of a
clearly demonstrable paraclinical disease after extensive investigation,[15] and (3)
the grouping of the symptoms and behavioral changes under a single diagnostic
label, into a pseudo-disease, which often includes a wide and changeable range
of phenomena. The case-history of Harry White illustrates one such pseudo-disease
— *pseudo-angina* — one of the many manifestations of the "hyperventilation"
syndrome (Evans and Lum 1977).

"REAL" ANGINA, "PSEUDO-ANGINA", AND "FOLK ANGINA"

In the biomedical perpective on ill-health (see Table X), it can be seen that there
are two categories of "angina", "real" and "pseudo". The textbook picture or
personality of the former, *angina pectoris,*[16] first described by Heberden in 1768,
is "a clinical syndrome caused by inadequate oxygenation of the heart, characteristically precipitated by exertion, and relieved by rest or sublingual nitroglycerin"
(Beeson et al. 1975: 994). A key component of this syndrome of "real" angina,
is the patient's subjective experience of a certain type of crushing chest *pain* on
exertion. Fábrega and Tyma (1976) have pointed out the subjective quality in pain:
pain itself cannot be directly observed, but only persons expressing pain and/or
behaving as though they are in pain. The chest pain of "pseudo" angina closely
mimics that of "real" angina, and the range of behavioral changes may be identical.

As a diagnostic category, "real" angina pectoris does not fully cover or predict
all the phenomena within it; rather it is "a variable and impermanent symptom
complex which is subjective in personal interpretation" (Julian 1977:26). As
such, presentation and interpretation are subject to a degree of cultural patterning
— even in the presence of "hard" evidence from diagnostic technology (e.g., electrocardiography or arteriography) of Coronary Heart Disease. In the biomedical
model, anginal pain is "real" in the presence of such evidence of paraclinical disease,
but "pseudo" in its absence. Even with such hard evidence, the link between
paraclinical and clinical elements is tenuous, unpredictable, and often confusing.
Only 80% of "real" angina cases, for example, have the "classic" or textbook form

of chest pain; the rest are "atypical". Similarly, Coronary Heart Disease — and even myocardial infarctions — can occur *without* anginal pain (Oram 1971:441); as Julian (1977:18) notes: "coronary arterial disease can remain silent for many years and indeed forever in the majority of individuals".

The syndrome of "real" angina pectoris can be mimicked clinically by a number of conditions, including gastric or duodenal ulcers, esophageal spasm, reflux esophagitis, gallstone colic, and "hyperventilation" (Julian 1977:61–64) — all of which cause *"pseudo angina"*.[17] In 40% of these "pseudo" causes, its clinical personality is *identical* to Heberden's classic description of ischemic angina (Herman et al. 1973). Nevertheless, even in the absence of "hard" evidence for (paraclinical) Coronary Heart Disease, the diagnostic personality of "angina pectoris" remains as a pseudo-disease: "the syndrome of angina pectoris without identifiable heart or coronary disease is now a well-recognized clinical entity" (Herman et al. 1973: 446). To the biomedical model, searching for somatic referents, there remains "the enigma of patients with angina and angiographically normal coronary arteries" (Day and Sowton 1976:334); these authors are still searching for an organic cause. In some cases of "pseudo" angina, the cause will be found to be other paraclinical diseases (e.g., gall-stone colic), but in others, for example, in the case of Harry White, no organic cause is found (see Table X). In both cases, though, anginal-type pain is viewed as a disease, until proved otherwise.

In addition to biomedical views of "heart disease" in general, and angina pectoris in particular, there is a large body of lay beliefs in Britain about the heart and its various states of health and illness. Like "heart distress" in Iran, which links together a whole field of physical and emotional experiences and "a complex of symbols, feelings, and stresses" into a single potent image (Good 1977:48), the wide range of "heart problems" from the Western lay perspective is also imbued with emotional and social meanings, and with lay notions of causality and treatment. But like "heart distress" in Iran, "heart problems" are not a neatly bounded folk category, but can refer to the illness, to an individual symptom (e.g., chest pain), or to the cause of other types of illness (see Good 1977:47).

Lay beliefs about the heart have deep historical roots; the heart is the traditional focus of emotional expression, and there is a rich folklore of the heart in Britain, as in other societies (see Boyadjian 1980). This inherited folklore is an important component of lay models relating to symptoms believed to be caused by "heart problems". Like heart distress", the range of "heart problems" links together both emotional and physical elements — a linkage which is reflected in language (e.g., "heartsick", "heartsore", "heartful", "heartless", "heartbroken", "hearty", or "he died of a broken heart"). This linkage is also reflected in literature, from the Bible to Shakespeare.[18] Lay beliefs about the etiology of "heart problems" include notions of interpersonal effect ("he broke her heart", "her daughter caused her so much trouble she gave her a heart attack"), and the effect of the environment ("stress gives people heart attacks", "crowded places give me palpitations"). The "building blocks" that help constitute folk illnesses associated with the heart are, as with other folk illnesses (see Helman 1978), based on subjectively experienced symptoms and signs, such as: chest pain, shortness of breath, palpitations, a rapid heart beat, or a flushed face (said to be a sign of "blood pressure"). The interpretation of these signs and symptoms is based on lay theories of how the circulatory system works, and where the heart and major blood vessels are anatomically located.

In Boyle's study (1970:288), a sample of British patients interviewed placed the position of the heart at various points across the chest; 14.9% perceived it as occupying most of the chest volume. These beliefs about the location of the heart obviously affect the interpretation of symptoms arising from the chest. In Harry White's case, his interpretation of his vague left chest pain was as "something to do with my heart". Both his own beliefs, and the experience of his mother who has suffered from Coronary Heart Disease, contributed towards this anatomical assessment.

Lay models dealing with ill-health related to the heart (and on which virtually no ethnographic research has been carried out in modern Britain) have been heavily influenced by the biomedical model, as shown in the case of Harry White. But lay beliefs about such modern biomedical "disease" categories affecting the heart as "angina pectoris", "coronary thrombosis" and "hypertension", though they employ medical labels and terminology, often differ greatly from the biomedical model of these conditions (see Blumhagen 1980, on "Hyper-Tension"), and include moral, psychological, and social elements. Symptoms and signs believed to originate in the heart are sometimes classified under a single label, borrowed from biomedicine, and overlapping with its model to a lesser or greater extent (see Blumhagen 1980:200).

An example of this labeling process is what I have termed "*folk angina*". This is a folk illness category characterized by: certain signs and symptoms (especially pain "over the heart"); a set of beliefs about their origin, significance, and meaning; the sorts of treatment that are believed to be helpful; the probable prognosis; and the types of behavior that are appropriate for a sufferer with this condition. All of these are gathered under the label "angina", often applied for the first time after contact with a clinical model. Like other lay Explanatory Models, "folk angina" is highly idiosyncratic; however, the continuing diffusion of biomedical models into the patient population may make this illness entity more standardized in the future. This is illustrated here; Mr. White's experiences of the Coronary Care Unit, and various clinical models, shape his symptoms and behavior into a pattern closely resembling "real" angina, with chest pain on effort, easy fatiguability, pallor, and gradual limitation of his daily activities.

The clinical "personality" of "folk angina", i.e., the symptoms, signs, and behavioral changes believed to characterize a case of "angina", is derived from a number of sources, including radio and TV programs, "home-doctor" books, novels and films, medical advice columns in newspapers and magazines, and health education propaganda (which describes the characteristics of those most "at risk", as well as the clinical presentation of some conditions, their dangers, and the appropriate behavior of those who suffer from them). A patient advice leaflet on Angina,[19] for example, suggests the limitation of lifestyle in those with this condition, "It is important to lead as normal a life as possible within the limits set by the angina"; "At all times be sensible – do not go beyond the pain barrier". This information is blended with inherited folklore about "heart problems" and their remedies (see Chamberlain 1981:214–215, 223, who says, "Avoid steps and stairs as much as possible"), with subjectively perceived symptoms and physical changes, with the experiences of others with a similar condition (see Chrisman 1977:370), and with ideas derived from contact with the medical model. Several of these processes are illustrated in the case-history of Harry White.

The complex illness entity that results from this blending process can be termed "folk angina" if it is *labeled* "angina" by the patient, or by those around him. "Folk angina" may or may not co-exist with "real angina" and Coronary Heart Disease, or with "pseudo angina" (as in Mr. White's case). But if the two labels *do* co-exist, that is, if the folk label of "angina" is confirmed by a clinician, or originates in a clinical model, and there is *agreement* about the meaning and implications of this diagnostic model between the two parties, then this overlap between the two systems may produce the "cultural healing" described by Kleinman (1980:36). This shared cognitive system between patient and healer, if it exists, is characteristic of the "placebo" effect (Adler and Hammett 1973), and also of its opposite, the "nocebo" (or in this case, iatrogenic) effect (see Hahn and Kleinman 1981; Lévi-Strauss 1967:162; Lex 1977). The negative effects on a patient's health and behavior of a medical diagnosis are illustrated in this case-history. Other research on this topic is discussed below.

IATROGENIC ILL-HEALTH: THE IMPORTANCE OF DIAGNOSTIC LABELS

The case-history of Mr. White, as well as illustrating the plurality of biomedical Explanatory Models, also indicates the importance of diagnostic *labels*, whether these originate in lay or medical models. The case illustrates the interrelationship, and overlap, between these two sources of diagnostic labels (see Table IX), and the iatrogenic (or doctor-induced) effect of medical labels on Mr. White's behavior and self-perception. The iatrogenic effect also results from the patient's experiences of hospitalization (e.g., the Coronary Care Unit), and of the hospital's diagnostic technology.

Contact with clinical models of diagnosis and treatment has an educational aspect; the patient *learns* about his or her "disease", what information to give at each consultation, which information is most significant ("Have you had any of that tightness across your chest again?"), what information is considered relevant by the clinician, and what is not. Clinical consultations and diagnoses help define, condense, and translate the chaos of symptoms and signs into a recognizable biomedical entity; from the patient's point of view, these consultations are also part of the ongoing redefinition of his condition into a biomedical conceptual "shape" (see Table IX), and can have important effects on his life and behavior. This is illustrated by Mr. White, whose behavior and symptoms became more classically "angina-like" after prolonged contact with clinical models.

The impact of diagnostic labels on the individual's life, has been described by Waxler (1981). In her view, medical labels can affect a patient's symptoms, behavior, social relationships, prognosis, self-perception, and the expectations of others. This effect can occur even in the absence of "hard" evidence for a paraclinical disease, either in a case of "illness without disease" (as in the case of Mr. White), or when the label is mistakenly applied to a patient who was previously well. In one study (Waxler 1981:297), a group of farmers who presented no biomedical evidence of heart disease, but who had labeled themselves as having "heart disease" when misunderstanding their doctor's diagnosis, radically changed their life-style — taking more "heart-related precautions" such as frequent naps, stopping smoking, and fitting sun-shades onto their tractors. As Waxler notes:

The label itself — what the farmer or his family *believes* to be the case — has an important effect upon his behavior, even when he has no symptoms and no heart disease (1981:297).

In another study, by Haynes and colleagues (1978), workers in a large industry were screened for hypertension. In those (asymptomatic) patients who were told they had "hypertension", absenteeism from work rose by 80%, greatly exceeding the 9% rise in absenteeism in the employee population during the same period. The context in which medical consultation and labeling occur can have physiological, as well as behavioral effects; in one study, blood pressure readings on a group of apparently healthy men were found to be higher when recorded at a clinic than when recorded later in their own homes (Beckman et al. 1981). The pathogenic effect of belief and labeling, the "nocebo" effect, has been amply described in the anthropological literature (e.g., Lévi-Strauss 1967:161–162), usually in the context of "magical death" or "voodoo" death; an hypothesis on the neuro-physiological etiology of this phenomenon is described by Lex (1977:327–331). The two sides of the placebo/nocebo phenomenon have also been reviewed by Hahn and Kleinman (1981), who point out that "belief kills; belief heals".

If diagnostic labels can have powerful effects on both behavior and health — as suggested in both the biomedical and anthropological literature — then why do these labels tend to "stick" (see Waxler 1981:296), even in the absence of biomedical "disease"? Waxler suggests that the individual may become enmeshed within certain institutions that sustain the label rather than encouraging its rejection. Harry White's experiences in the Coronary Care Unit, the convalescent ward filled with "heart cases", and the outpatient consultation with the intern are all examples of this process. As Waxler points out (1981:297), "Once an individual is labeled as "ill" he is likely to be labeled again". The fear of clinical mimicry, or "silent" Coronary Heart Disease on the part of clinicians, also contributes towards this continued labeling.

From the patient's perspective, "de-labeling" by the physician ("There's nothing wrong with your heart. You don't have angina") may be unsuccessful in convincing the patient that he does not have "heart problems". This may be the result of a number of factors: the persistence of the "illness", that is, of symptoms still in the region "over the heart", as well as the emotional and behavioral changes associated with "folk angina"; the secondary gain from the sick role for the patient; the widely known fact that medical science is still advancing, and what cannot be diagnosed today might be diagnosed tomorrow with better technology; and reinforcement from medical models. Reinforcement may come not only from diagnostic labels ("You probably have angina"), but from experiences of hospitalization (e.g., Mr. White in the Coronary Care Unit). In addition, complex diagnostic *tests* also reinforce the patient's notion that "there is something wrong, somewhere".

These factors may explain why in Ockene and colleagues' (1980) follow-up study of cases of pseudo-angina up to two years *after* they had had normal arteriograms, 44% still believed they had "heart disease", 70% still had chest pain, 63% were still unable to work because of the pain, and 51% still considered themselves disabled. In all cases they had been told, at the time of their arteriograms, that there was no evidence of any underlying physical "disease". Similarly, the factors noted above, as well as the iatrogenic effect of diagnostic labeling, may explain the apparently poor prognosis of a number of other psychosomatic disorders such as "non-organic pelvic pain" (Henker 1979:1132), "spasmodic torticollis" (Matthews et al. 1978:491), "the irritable-bowel syndrome" (Waller and Misiewicz 1969:755), and the Da Costa's Syndrome (Friedberg 1969:1724).

The folk illnesses overlapping with these "disease" categories may survive attempted medical "de-labeling", because they are rooted in a different model, based on a different system of "proof" (mainly the persistence of symptoms and behavioral changes). This folk perspective is, in turn, derived partly from more traditional models of the origin and management of misfortune in general; as such it has powerful social, symbolic, and psychological elements (see Good 1977).

Such folk illnesses may also persist as reactions to continuing stress; in the case-history of Mr. White, a number of stressful factors in his daily life are likely to persist, including his business worries, anxious wife, crying baby, long drive to work, ill father, and the conflicting interpretations of his condition by different clinicians. In addition, there is the residual stress of his hospitalization, especially in the Coronary Care Unit (see Cay et al. 1972). Given a stressful situation, as well as a tendency towards *somatization*[20] due to personal and/or cultural factors, what factors influence the *localization* of diffuse symptoms to a certain part of the body, and its shaping into a recognizable "disease" or "pseudo-disease" entity? Mechanic (1972) has described this situation in the case of "medical students' disease"; here there is a two-stage process, involving the students' emotional reaction to stress (from examinations, anxieties in dealing with new clinical experiences, etc.), coupled with their exposure to specific knowledge about disease, and this provides the students with "a new framework for identifying and giving meaning to previously neglected bodily feelings" (1972:1133). That is:

Diffuse and ambiguous symptoms regarded as normal in the past may be reconceptualized within the context of newly acquired knowledge of disease.

This process of turning "illness" into recognizable "disease" (or in this case pseudo-disease), is illustrated in the case-history. Much of Mr. White's knowledge of "heart disease" was acquired by contact with clinicians, nurses, and other patients in the Coronary Care Unit (see Cowie 1976), so that by the time of his discharge from the hospital his "folk angina" more closely resembled the clinical picture of "real" angina. Further factors in his localization of symptoms were the long-term experiences of his mother who had "real" angina (i.e., Coronary Heart Disease), and possibly the emphasis on the left side of the chest expressed by his wife over several months. Friedberg (1969:1721) has also noted that localization may result from the "inadvertent remark of a physician", or the rejection of an application for life insurance, with the person defined as being "at risk" of a particular condition. Also, certain culturally defined disorders which locate the origin of diffuse symptoms in a particular organ — such as "heart distress" in Iran (Good 1977), or the *Crise de foie* in France — may all influence this localization. The effects of health education propaganda and the increasing numbers of health screening campaigns (see Haynes et al. 1978), need to be assessed in the future; in particular, their possible iatrogenic effects on health, and the spread of folk illnesses which closely resemble medical diseases from this diffusion of medical knowledge into the community.

A final factor in the labeling of vague somatic symptoms as "disease" — even in the absence of evidence for a paraclinical disease process — is what might be termed "the clinician's illness". This is a complex of subjective feelings such as doubt, anxiety, fear or confusion, that may exist, particularly in younger, less experienced clinicians, when faced with a puzzling case of clinical mimicry and "illness without identifiable disease". Faced with this situation, and the strong bias towards locating a "somatic referent",[21] the younger doctor may choose a "disease" label to give the symptoms and signs a biomedical identity (as a "pseudo-disease") and thereby "play it safe" and reduce his or her anxiety.

The case-history of Mr. White illustrates the iatrogenic effect of the plurality of clinical models that he encountered in a three-month period. It also illustrates the dynamic interrelationship of lay and medical models, and the differences between theoretical, "scientific" medical models and the clinical models used by practitioners on an everyday basis.

ACKNOWLEDGEMENTS

I wish to gratefully acknowledge the useful comments of Robert Hahn, Arthur Kleinman, Murray Last, and Tina Posner on a first draft of this paper.

NOTES

1. Kleinman (1982) in a personal communication, has pointed out that while "disease" in medical theory "has a typical course and characteristic features that are independent of setting", in actual practice clinical models are a mixture of popular and textbook models. In that sense "disease" too is a sociocultural construction.
2. Not his real name.

3. For more detail see Levitt (1976) or Stacey (1976).
4. See Levitt (1976:88–94). The precursors of GPs were specialized tradesmen known as Apothecaries. From 1617 they were licenced only to sell drugs prescribed by physicians. By 1703 there were entitled to see patients and prescribe for them. They became the GPs of the poor and middle classes, with no access to hospitals. Physicians had a higher status than surgeons or apothecaries, and for centuries were the only "real" doctors. From 1700–1830 there was the rise of the "great voluntary hospitals", in which both surgeons and physicians practised.
5. See Levitt (1976:179). In England and Wales in 1972, more than half the NHS budget was spent on the hospital sector, even though only 2.3% of patients are cared for annually as hospital inpatients.
6. Especially the treatment of symptoms, rather than causes (e.g., a virus). See Helman (1978).
7. That is, GPs have a longitudinal perspective on illness events, rather than a cross-sectional one.
8. While this paper was being written, a 44-year-old man in the same practice diagnosed by a cardiologist as having only "pseudo-angina" died suddenly of a heart attack a week after this diagnosis was given.
9. See Waites (1978:1701): "Dyspnea is a common presentation, and sensation of inadequate depth of respiration ... . Occasionally, the patient will notice excessive yawning or frequent sighing respirations." Also Lum (1981:2): "Rapid, irregular, sighing respirations ... extravagantly erratic breathing pattern."
10. That is, cluster.
11. Note the similarity to Chrisman's typology of folk etiologies of ill-health (1977:362): mechanical, balance, degeneration, and invasion etiologies.
12. See Note 8 above.
13. Hawkins (1975:326) describes this patient as "a psychopath".
14. Kleinman (personal communication, 1982) has suggested the term "diseasization" for this type of "medicalization", which I find an apt label.
15. Attempts have been undertaken to make the diagnosis of this condition more "scientific"; see Evans and Lum (1977:156): "Laboratory diagnosis was based on a typical spirometric pattern ... low or normal resting $PaCO_2$ ... and, in 50% of patients, reproduction of chest pain by 2–3 min. voluntary hyperventilation".
16. "Angina" from the Greek "anchein", "to choke" (Julian 1977:1–3).
17. "Pseudo-angina" was first described by Sir William Osler in 1892 (Ockene et al. 1980: 1249).
18. E.g., King Lear (Act 5, Scene 3):

> But his flaw'd heart –
> Alack, too weak the conflict to support! –
> 'Twixt two extremes of passion, joy and grief,
> burst smilingly.

19. 'Take Heart: A Booklet for Angina Patients', Stuart Pharmaceuticals, Ltd., Cheadle, England, 1979.
20. See Kleinman (1980:149–158) on somatization.
21. In that sense, doctors too are somatizers. Much of Biomedicine is based on the search for these "somatic referents", as noted earlier.

REFERENCES

Adler, H. M. and V. B. O. Hammett
    1973 The Doctor-Patient Relationship Revisited: An Analysis of the Placebo Effect. Ann. Int. Med. 78:595–598.

Amarasingham, L. R.
    1980 Movement Among Healers in Sri Lanka: A Case Study of a Sinhalese Patient. Culture,
          Medicine and Psychiatry 4:71–92.
Beckman, M. et al.
    1981 Blood Pressure and Heart Rate Recordings at Home and at the Clinic. Acta Med.
          Scand. 210:97–102.
Beeson, P. B., and W. McDermott (eds.)
    1975 Textbook of Medicine. Philadelphia: W. B. Saunders Company.
Blumhagen, D.
    1980 Hyper-Tension: A Folk Illness with a Medical Name. Culture, Medicine and Psy-
          chiatry 4:197–227.
Boyadjian, N.
    1980 The Heart: Its History, Its Symbolism, Its Iconography, and Its Diseases. Antwerp:
          Esco Books.
Boyle, C. M.
    1970 Difference Between Patients' and Doctors' Interpretation of Some Common Medical
          Terms. Brit. Med. J. 2:286–289.
Brainerd, H., S. Margen, and M. Chatton
    1969 Current Diagnosis and Treatment. Los Altos: Lange Medical Publications.
Cassell, E. J.
    1976 The Healer's Art: A New Approach to the Doctor-Patient Relationship. New York:
          Lippincott.
Cay, E. L. et al.
    1972 Psychological Reactions to a Coronary Care Unit. J. Psychosom. Res. 16:437–447.
Chamberlain, M.
    1981 Old Wives' Tales: Their History, Remedies and Spells. London: Virago Press.
Chaplin, N. W. (ed.)
    1976 The Hospital and Health Services Year Book. London: The Institute of Health
          Service Administrators.
Chrisman, N. J.
    1977 The Health Seeking Process: An Approach to the Natural History of Illness. Culture,
          Medicine and Psychiatry 1: 351–377.
Coulter, D. F. and D. J. Llewellyn (eds.)
    1971 The Practice of Family Medicine. London: E. and S. Livingstone.
Cowie, B.
    1976 The Cardiac Patient's Perception of His Heart Attack. Social Science and Medicine
          10:87–96.
Day, L. J. and E. Sowton
    1976 Clinical Features and Follow-Up of Patients with Angina and Normal Coronary
          Arteries. Lancet 2:334–337.
Eisenberg, L.
    1977 Disease and Illness: Distinctions Between Professional and Popular Ideas of Sickness.
          Culture, Medicine and Psychiatry 1:9–23.
El-Islam, M. F.
    1975 Culture Bound Neurosis in Qatari Women. Soc. Psychiat. 10:25–29.
Engel, G. L.
    1980 The Clinical Applications of the Biopsychosocial Model. Am. J. Psychiatry 137:
          535–544.
Evans, D. W. and L. C. Lum
    1977 Hyperventilation: An Important Cause of Pseudoangina. Lancet 2:155–157.
Fábrega, H. and D. B. Silver
    1973 Illness and Shamanistic Curing in Zinancantan: An Ethnomedical Analysis. Stanford:
          Stanford University Press.

Fábrega, H.
1975 The Need for an Ethnomedical Science. Science 189:969–975.
Fábrega, H. and S. Tyma
1976 Language and Cultural Influences in the Description of Pain. Br. J. Psychol. 49: 349–371.
Feinstein, A. R.
1973 An Analysis of Diagnostic Reasoning; Part I and II. Yale J. of Biology and Medicine 15:583–616.
1975 Science, Clinical Medicine, and the Spectrum of Disease. In Beeson P. B. and W. McDermott (eds.), Textbook of Medicine. Philadelphia: W. B. Saunders and Co.
Friedberg, C. K.
1969 Diseases of the Heart. 3rd Edition. Pp. 1721–1727. London: W. B. Saunders Company.
Good, B. J.
1977 The Heart of What's the Matter: The Semantics of Illness in Iran. Culture, Medicine and Psychiatry 1:25–58.
Good, B. J. and M.-J. D. Good
1981 The Meaning of Symptoms: A Cultural Hermeneutic Model for Clinical Practice. In L. Eisenberg and A. Kleinman (eds.), The Relevance of Social Science for Medicine. Pp. 165–196. Dordrecht: D. Reidel Publishing Company.
Hahn, R. A. and A. Kleinman
1981 Belief as Pathogen, Belief as Medicine: "Voodoo Death" and the "Placebo Phenomenon" in Anthropological Perspective. Paper presented at Society for Applied Anthropology meeting, April, 1981, Edinburgh, Scotland.
Harris, C. M.
1980 Lecture Notes on Medicine in General Practice. Oxford: Blackwell Scientific Publications.
Hawkins, C. F.
1975 The Alimentary System. In W. N. Mann (ed.), Conybeare's Textbook of Medicine. P. 326. London: Churchill Livingstone.
Haynes, R. B. et al.
1978 Increased Absenteeism From Work After Detection and Labeling of Hypertensive Patients. New Eng. J. of Med. 229:741–744.
Helman, C. G.
1978 'Feed a Cold, Starve a Fever' – Folk Models of Infection in an English Suburban Community, and Their Relation to Medical Treatment. Culture, Medicine and Psychiatry 2:107–137.
1980 An Anthropological View of the Modern Hospital. MIMS Magazine 1, July. Pp. 37–41.
1981 Disease Versus Illness In General Practice. J. Royal Coll. Gen. Pract. 31:548–552.
1981 Observations from General Practice. Social Science and Medicine 15B:415–419.
Henker, F. O.
1979 Diagnosis and Treatment of Nonorganic Pelvic Pain. Southern Med. J. 72:1132–1134.
Herman, M. V., P. F. Cohn and R. Gorlin
1973 Angina-Like Chest Pain Without Identifiable Cause. Ann. Int. Med. 79:445–447.
Hunt, J. H.
1964 The Renaissance of General Practice. In J. Farndale (ed.), Trends in the National Health Service. Pp. 162–191. London: Pergamon Press.
Hurst, W. J. et al.
1974 The Heart. 3rd Edition. Pp. 1552–1555. New York: McGraw-Hill.
Jeffcoate, N.
1975 Principles of Gynaecology. 4th Edition. Pp. 499–500. London & Boston: Butterworths.

Julian, D. G. (ed.)
  1977 Angina Pectoris. Edinburgh: Churchill Livingstone.
Kimani, V. N.
  1981 The Unsystematic Alternative: Towards Plural Health Care Among the Kikuyu of
         Central Kenya. Social Science and Medicine 15B:333–340.
Kleinman, A.
  1978 Concepts and a Model for the Comparison of Medical Systems as Cultural Systems.
         Social Science and Medicine 12:85–93.
Kleinman, A., L. Eisenberg, and B. Good
  1978 Culture, Illness and Care: Clinical Lessons from Anthropologic and Cross Cultural
         Research. Ann. Int. Med. 88:251–258.
Kleinman, A.
  1980 Patients and Healers in the Context of Culture. Berkeley: University of California
         Press.
  1982 Personal Communication.
Lévi-Strauss, C.
  1967 Structural Anthropology. Pp. 161–180. New York: Anchor Books.
Levitt, R.
  1976 The Reorganized National Health Service. London: Croom Helm.
Lewis, G.
  1975 Knowledge of Illness in a Sepik Society. Pp. 146–151. London: The Athlone Press.
Lex, B. W.
  1977 Voodoo Death: New Thoughts on an Old Explanation. In D. Landy (ed.), Culture,
         Disease and Healing: Studies in Medical Anthropology. New York: Macmillan Pub-
         lishing Company.
Lum, L. C.
  1981 Hyperventilation and Anxiety State. J. Royal Soc. of Med. 74:1–4.
Matthews, W. B. et al.
  1978 Spasmodic Torticollis: A Combined Clinical Study. J. of Neurol. Neurosurg. &
         Psychiatry 41:485–492.
McHugh, P. R.
  1979 Psychiatric Illness in Medical Practice. In P. B. Beeson, W. McDermott, and J. B.
         Wyngaarden (eds.), Textbook of Medicine, 15th Edition. Philadelphia: W. B.
         Saunders.
Mechanic, D.
  1972 Social Psychologic Factors Affecting the Presentation of Bodily Complaints. New
         Eng. J. of Med. 286:1132–1139.
Morrell, D. C.
  1971 Expressions of Morbidity in General Practice. Brit. Med. J. 2:454.
Ockene, I. S. et al.
  1980 Unexplained Chest Pain in Patients with Normal Coronary Arteriograms: A Follow-
         Up Study of Functional Status. New Eng. J. of Med. 303:1249–1252.
Oram, S.
  1971 Clinical Heart Disease. P. 441. London: William Heinemann Medical Books.
Press, I.
  1978 Urban Folk Medicine: A Functional Overview. American Anthropologist 80:71–
         84.
Short, D.
  1981 Diagnosis of Slight and Subacute Coronary Attacks in the Community. Br. Heart
         J. 45:299–310.
Smith, H. C. T. and E. J. Eastham
  1973 Outbreak of Abdominal Pain. Lancet 2:956–958.

Stacey, M. (ed.)
  1976 The Sociology of the National Health Service. London: Croom Helm.
Stimson, G. and B. Webb
  1975 Going to See the Doctor: The Consultation Process in General Practice. London:
         Routledge and Kegan Paul.
Sussman, L. K.
  1981 Unity in Diversity in a Polyethnic Society: The Maintenance of Medical Pluralism
         on Mauritius. Social Science and Medicine 15B:247–260.
Titmuss, R. M.
  1964 The Hospital and Its Patients. In J. Farndale (ed.), Trends in the National Health
         Service. London: Pergamon Press.
Toffler, A.
  1970 Future Shock. London: Pan Books.
Waites, T. F.
  1978 Hyperventilation – Chronic and Acute. Arch. Intern. Med. 138:1700–1701.
Waller, S. L. and J. J. Misiewicz
  1969 Prognosis in the Irritable Bowel Syndrome. Lancet 2:753–756.
Waxler, N. E.
  1981 The Social Labeling Perspective on Illness and Medical Practice. In L. Eisenberg and
         A. Kleinman (eds.), The Relevance of Social Science for Medicine. Dordrecht:
         D. Reidel Publishing Company.
White, A. E.
  1978 The Vital Role of the Cottage-Community Hospital. J. Royal Coll. Gen. Pract. 28:
         485–491.

James Cooper, M.A. (Clinical Psychology)*; Doctoral Candidate, Department of Psychiatry, University of California at Davis School of Medicine, Davis, CA.

Atwood D. Gaines, Ph.D. (Anthropology), M.P.H. (Behavioral Sciences); Assistant Professor, Departments of Anthropology and Psychiatry, Case Western Reserve University and Medical School, Cleveland, OH; Adjunct Assistant Professor, Department of Psychiatry, Duke University Medical Center, Durham, NC.

Byron J. Good, Ph.D. (Anthropology); Assistant Professor of Medical Anthropology, Department of Social Medicine and Health Policy and Lecturer, Department of Anthropology, Harvard University and Medical School, Cambridge, MA.

Mary-Jo DelVecchio Good, Ph.D. (Sociology); Assistant Professor of Medical Sociology, Department of Social Medicine and Health Policy and Lecturer in Sociology, Harvard University and Medical School, Cambridge, MA.

Robert A. Hahn, Ph.D. (Anthropology); Acting Assistant Professor, Department of Psychiatry and Behavioral Sciences, School of Medicine, University of Washington, Seattle, WA.

Cecil G. Helman, M.D.; General Practice and Research Assistant, Department of Anthropology, University College, London, England.

Henry Herrera, M.D.; Associate Professor, Department of Psychiatry, University of Rochester School of Medicine, Rochester, NY.

Thomas M. Johnson, Ph.D. (Anthropology); Assistant Professor, Department of Anthropology, Southern Methodist University and Clinical Assistant Professor, Department of Psychiatry, University of Texas Health Science Center, Dallas, TX.

Pearl Katz, Ph.D. (Anthropology); Assistant Professor, Department of Psychiatry, University of Maryland School of Medicine and Research Candidate, Baltimore-D.C. Institute for Psychoanalysis, Baltimore, MD and Washington, D.C.

Margaret Lock, Ph. D., (Anthropology); Associate Professor, Department of Humanities and Social Studies in Medicine, McGill University Medical School, Montréal, Quebec, Canada.

Thomas W. Maretzki, Ph.D. (Anthropology); Professor, Departments of Anthropology and Allied Medical Sciences, University of Hawaii and School of Medicine, Honolulu, HI.

William Rittenberg, Ph.D. (Anthropology); Assistant Professor of Pediatrics and

* Field of academic degree.

333

Human Development, College of Human Medicine, Michigan State University, East Lansing, MI.
Ronald C. Simons, M.D., M.A. (Anthropology); Professor, Department of Psychiatry, College of Human Medicine and Adjunct Professor, Department of Anthropology, Michigan State University, East Lansing, MI.

AUTHOR INDEX

335

SUBJECT INDEX

341